MENTAL HEALTH,

RACISM, and SEXISM

MENTAL HEALTH,
RACISM, and SEXISM

Edited by   Charles V. Willie
                Patricia Perri Rieker
                Bernard M. Kramer
                Bertram S. Brown

UNIVERSITY OF PITTSBURGH PRESS

Pittsburgh and London

Published by the University of Pittsburgh Press,
Pittsburgh, Pa. 15260

Copyright © 1995, University of Pittsburgh Press
All rights reserved
Manufactured in the United States of America
Printed on acid-free paper

Library of Congress Cataloging-in-Publication Data

Mental health, racism, and sexism / edited by Charles V. Willie . . .
[et al.].
    p. cm.
    Includes bibliographical references and index.
    ISBN 0-8229-3869-3. — ISBN 0-8229-5549-0 (pbk.)
    1. Minorities—Mental health services—United States.   2. Women—
Mental health services—United States.   3. Discrimination in mental
health services—United States.   4. Sexism in mental health
services—United States.   I. Willie, Charles Vert, 1927–   .
RC451.5.A2M48   1995
362.2'08'693—dc20
                                               94-41407
                                               CIP

A CIP catalogue record for this book is available from the British Library

Eurospan, London

The editors and the contributing authors
gratefully acknowledge the continuing
support of the Maurice Falk Medical Fund
which has, since its establishment in 1960,
played a significant role in the nation's struggle
against prejudice and discrimination; they also
acknowledge the helpful advice, encouragement,
and unending patience offered by its president,
Philip B. Hallen.

This book is dedicated to the memory of
JUSTICE THURGOOD MARSHALL
of the U.S. Supreme Court,
who wrote the foreword for
Racism and Mental Health, 1973

and to
ROSALYNN CARTER,
First Lady and Honorary Chairperson of the
President's Commission on Mental Health,
1977–1978

CONTENTS

FOREWORD

Before his death, Mr. Justice Marshall had agreed to write a foreword for Mental Health, Racism, and Sexism. In recognition of the timeless wisdom contained in the foreword for Racism and Mental Health (1973), we are reprinting it in this volume. (Eds.)

M ENTAL health and the law—what if anything do they have in common? Both are concerned with the aspirations and problems of the human condition, and both deal with human rights and human responsibilities.

The age-old problem is to balance individual freedom and social responsibility. Racism is demeaning to individuals and the nadir of social irresponsibility. Racism condones oppression and tramples on fundamental rights.

Thus I welcome the first exploration in depth of the complex relationships between racism and mental health. Discrimination based on race, creed, color, sex, and national origin interferes with opportunities for individual expression by some and blinds others to their normal obligations. There is no health in a society afflicted by racism and discrimination.

The authors of this volume tell us that racism is oftentimes deliberate and sometimes unintentional. Nevertheless, the consequences are the same. The call for institutional change to overcome racism is a central theme in this book.

There are many ways of bringing about changes in the institutions of a society. The enactment of laws by way of democratic procedures is one way of effecting the necessary changes. But this is only part of the process of achieving a just and healthy society. People must support the law if it is to be effective. Such support is forthcoming only when the people have participated directly or indirectly in the lawmaking process. Through their participation, they achieve a feeling of belonging. This feeling in itself is something of value.

This book calls our attention to an aspect of social action that is often overlooked. It indicates how the struggle to achieve one's human rights is strengthening as well as debilitating. The story of despair is written in the pages of history and on the faces of the oppressed. This is a well-known story that need never have been written, according to the Constitution of this nation. Yet, it was. Some of the oppressions of the past have been overcome today simply because some of the oppressed had sufficient faith in the Constitution to confront the anomalies in society and to insist that they conform with the basic principles upon which this nation was established.

In the process of confronting injustice, the oppressed members of society have often grown strong, even stronger sometimes than those who maltreat them. Consequently, the self-concept of the children in many oppressed families has become exceedingly high, as pointed out by some of the authors in this book. It is my guess that this is an important finding for mental health as well as for the Civil Rights Movement.

That we can achieve two goals with one action is an idea worthy of considering. In overcoming racism and its debilitating effects, we may, at the same time, be achieving a better and more healthy society. This book is a contribution toward achieving these goals.

PREFACE

"R ACISM is tearing this country asunder." So begins the preface to *Racism and Mental Health* (Willie, Kramer, and Brown, eds. 1973). As we write this preface today in the summer of 1993, that sentence still captures the present state of the national mood. To be sure, much has changed for the better since the era when race and sex discrimination and segregation were legal. The promises of the civil rights and the women's rights movements, however, face unremitting opposition from radicalized conservatism and prejudice at the centers of national power (public as well as private). The task of achieving justice becomes harder and harder.

In 1990 Charles Willie, Bernard Kramer, and Bertram Brown joined with Patricia Rieker to organize the publication of a sequel to *Racism and Mental Health*. We wanted to bring together a new group of specialists to write for a new generation of mental health workers in what we supposed would be a new set of conditions in the 1990s. We wanted not an encyclopedic, contemporary compendium but rather a range of fresh perspectives. At our initial meeting we decided, for example, that the new book must recognize the enormous influence of the contemporary women's movement. Ergo, the title *Mental Health, Racism, and Sexism*.

Mental health leads the title because that term highlights the obligation of the mental health community to do its part in understanding the role of social and psychological well-being. Likewise, we say *mental health* rather than *mental illness* because it conveys our concern for the positive and preventive dimensions inherent in common problems of living. We wanted, as well, thereby to promote social and psychological models of the connections between racism, sexism, and mental health.

We chose the word *racism* rather than *race* because we wanted to investigate the impact of prejudice and discrimination upon people's well-being rather than to discuss racial differences. It is impossible to ignore the universal use of *racism* as the key word for an ingrained system of subordination, oppression, and victimization. Similar reasoning informs our decision to use the word *sexism* in the title. Although it was not a dictionary word before 1968 (*Webster's New Collegiate Dictionary* 1993, p. 1073), sex discrimination has always existed and still does. What is new in this era is the conscious, organized recognition of its myriad consequences and the determination to change its enduring pattern. That determination however, continues to face resistance in much the same way as the struggle against racism continues to encounter opposition.

We anticipate that the federal government will be required to face the issues of racism and sexism as it confronts health and welfare reform. We hope this volume will contribute to that task.

Many standard issues and conflicts make their appearance in this collection of essays—such as diagnosis, treatment, etiology, research, training, and the like. Less common but equally pressing contemporary issues put a special stamp on the character of this book, including interracial adoptions, teenage motherhood, chronic mentally ill women, gender bias in diagnosis and therapy, homeless families, prison as a substitute for hospitals, and violence on the college campus. These issues are informed by our analysis of gender and race.

Throughout this book, we strove to be action-oriented as well as theoretically sound. We focus on sexism as a form of oppression that injects itself into the matrix of mental health practice, training, and research. Recognizing that sexism shares with racism the qualities of being both pervasive and persistent, we have taken special pains to articulate the manifold ways through which the field of mental health suffers from acts of omission and commission.

Contributors to this volume are of multiracial, multiethnic, and gender-diverse backgrounds. The existential experiences of these scholars are reflected in their discussions and have made possible enriched analyses of pressing mental health and mental illness issues.

The editors would like to acknowledge David Breakstone, who provided excellent and extraordinary assistance as executive editor and editorial collaborator, and Kathy George, whose help as project secretary we very much appreciate.

A note on usage: We deliberately continue our earlier practice of capitalizing the words *Black* and *White* to recognize the status of each as a people. Moreover, we use *Black* and *African American* interchangeably as well as *White* and *Anglo*.

Summer 1993

> CHARLES V. WILLIE
> PATRICIA RIEKER
> BERNARD M. KRAMER
> BERTRAM S. BROWN

INTRODUCTION

I N the four introductory essays in Part I, the Conceptual Overview, six authors with diverse experience as teachers, researchers, and clinicians present a wide-ranging critical survey of selected major issues and topics within the associated disciplines of mental health to provide readers with a context within which to read, analyze, and interpret the individual chapters and interpretations to come. Castellano B. Turner and Bernard M. Kramer, in "Connections Between Racism and Mental Health," present a concise critical history of mental health as a research discipline and a clinical practice, with special attention given to the past thirty years. It was during this relatively brief period that enormous strides were made to legitimize public mental health care and provide it with adequate federal funds and supervision. Turner and Kramer document the structures and services that federal legislation and appropriations made available to a range of minority populations who never before had been able to afford mental health care.

The authors describe vividly the kinds of explicit and implicit racism existing even in a system intended to assist all minorities. A moving first-person account of the training of a Black clinical psychologist in a public hospital documents in cautionary detail the dismaying depth of institutional racism still present in a presumably nondiscriminatory program. The authors describe the initial benefits when the Community Health Centers Act of 1963 became law. They critique the subsequent painful realities when, over time, services are curtailed as funding and staffing are first cut back, and then eliminated.

Patricia Perri Rieker and M. Kay Jankowski, in "Sexism and Women's Psychological Status," comment upon the condition and status of women in American society. They evaluate the impact of societal sexism and sexist attitudes upon contemporary American women. As they observe early in their study: "we shall describe the social and emotional costs of sexism and show how as a routine aspect of daily life sexism intersects with racial and cultural differences to shape women's experience, identity, and psychological well-being."

Rieker and Jankowski point to the 1991 Supreme Court confirmation hearings for then Judge Clarence Thomas as one demonstration of how race and gender intersect. In their analysis, they observe that when women experience severe emotional stress, many factors usually are involved; moreover, because many women objectively lack personal power and resources, anxiety and depression often result. Depression, when internalized, can lead to silence—a literal and symbolic loss of voice and personal power. Becoming mute, losing her voice, embodies the final stage in an all-too-common American phenomenon of the devaluing, even effacing, of a woman's identity, competence, even credibility. In their discussion, Rieker and Jankowski explore the complex chain reaction in which women's strong voices can be silenced and their capabilities discounted or dismissed.

Elaine R. Brooks, Maria Zuñiga, and Nolan E. Penn, in "The Decline of Public Mental Health in the United States," present an in-depth analysis of the methods by which diagnoses of mental illness are manipulated by discriminatory treatment policies to deprive people of color, minority ethnic populations, and youth—especially young Black males—of needed therapy. Through narratives, historical analyses, clinical accounts, and data analyses, the authors describe the ways in which incarceration so often has replaced treatment. In large measure punishment has replaced remediation. The authors demonstrate through a variety of persuasive illustrations the need for responsible administrators and funding agencies to take prompt and appropriate remedial measures.

To begin reforming the multitude of abuses now operative in the American public mental health system may require rebuilding, not simply reforming, the existing structures. The present public mental health system is often insufficiently supervised and unevenly evaluated. Replacing it with a cost-effective, human being-effective system might reduce the wasteful cycle of relegating potentially productive individuals to impotent lives of stigmatized anger and despair.

John Townsend, in "Racial, Ethnic, and Mental Illness Stereotypes: Cognitive Process and Behavioral Effects," demonstrates with skill and insight the myriad ways in which the established procedures of the American public mental health system rely—deliberately or otherwise—upon the labeling and controlling of minority individuals. The present system often places these individuals in standard, stereotyped diagnostic categories—and then may prescribe ineffective or inappropriate treatment regimens. Such unscientific, impersonal "processing" of those in need of knowledgeable, effective care in many cases reflects the social prejudices of American society at large.

As Professor Townsend bluntly, if chillingly, observes in his conclusion: "if hospital staff expect female patients to suffer from emotional problems, and Black patients to be paranoid and potentially violent, their own treatment of the patients may help to fulfill their prophecy." His searching, meticulously specific critique of existing misuses of authority in many sectors of the U.S. public mental health system is shocking. It serves to expose how minority citizens—and especially the young—are more often victimized than assisted when they seek public-funded, professional help in dealing with critical personal and vocational problems.

In a trio of provocative chapters in Part II, Individuals and Families, an eminent Black physician, psychiatrist, and researcher, James P. Comer, and three expert sociologists in the fields of the emotional development of children of color and minority status, Professors Joyce A. Ladner, Ruby M. Gourdine, and Constance Willard Williams, explore the impacts of current popular American culture and mores upon young women and men in a range of powerless situations. These individuals often find themselves on the psychological, physical, and vocational defensive as a result of many types of institutional discrimination embedded in American culture.

Comer, in "Racism and African American Adolescent Development," carefully documents the long history of oppression and second-class citizenship that Black people in the United States have been forced to endure. The resultant deficits in education, training, vocational opportunities, and social mobility have severely limited the advancement of young Black men and women. It is the conscious, deliberate nature of this deprivation by the dominant White society that Comer illustrates with powerful, sometimes daunting specificity. To attempt to cope with the minority individual's contemporary second-class citizenship, status, and vocational prospect (or lack thereof) Comer sets forth a "modest proposal" that would involve setting aside "a significant percentage of the federal taxes paid by African Americans to be used to establish an endowment as an economic base and other structures in the community." This "set-aside" endowment could form the material basis of a renaissance of hope and tangible projects to turn opportunities into realities. This is obviously not another sweeping restitution scheme; Comer's plan would aim to accelerate the development—hitherto obstructed—of leadership roles for Black adults within their own communities as well as nurturing African American independence locally and, by extension, within the larger community of the United States.

Ladner and Gourdine, in "Transracial Adoptions," recount a fascinating and complex history of how attitudes toward transracial adoption among communities of color have shifted over time in the United States. Their research reveals how nearly uniform is the broad consensus of present policy positions as articulated, for example, by the National Association of Black Social Workers. What is striking is their finding of near unanimity of policy and conviction among national organizations concerned with the long-term welfare of children of color and other national minorities: they agree that adoption of these children by White individuals or families is harmful to the identities and self-concepts of children of color and other American minorities. Ladner and Gourdine present their findings and persuasively advocate a number of comprehensive, constructive transracial-adoption policy procedures.

Williams, in "Teenage Motherhood," examines comprehensively and thoughtfully the perplexing issues inherent in the problems—and opportunities—of teenagers with children. The topic of children who have children has received extensive but not always accurate coverage in the press. Invariably these popularizations of highly complicated individualized situations distort or obscure the intricacies of the social, economic, educational, and political issues bound tightly together in this growing social phenomenon. The virtues of Williams's research insights and sensitive interpretations shine most cogently as she sets forth feasible policies and plans to improve the lives and prospects of both teenage mothers and their children. Notable in Williams's study is her summary of recommendations regarding what could realistically be done now—regionally and nationally—to assure the financial solvency of these one-parent families and to assist young mothers in finding productive, independent livelihoods.

In Part III, Social Problems and the Community, a group of experienced physicians and sociologists chooses a number of the most pressing societal problems that have grown worse during the past decades. Major social dislocations have marked the tumultuous history of American society over the past thirty years. Racial conflict, class inequality, economic instability, and political disillusion have each substantially stretched, frayed, even torn, the fabric of American society and hurt those with limited financial resources. In the area of public community mental health, the most needy often get the least attention exactly because of their poverty and, in many cases, because of their very homelessness. Two of these essays concentrate upon the violence that so often is directed at the most vulnerable, and that has called into question repeatedly the stability of our own communities and neighborhoods. The other two deal with the financial and ideological conflicts that characterize many sectors of public mental health and American higher education.

Elaine (Hilberman) Carmen is the chief administrator of a public community mental health clinic in one of the most economically deprived, educationally marginalized sections of Boston, Massachusetts. In "Inner-City Community Mental Health," her eyewitness accounts of what it means to be a member of a racial, ethnic, and financial minority convey the anxiety-ridden lives of people who are just barely surviving. What Carmen points out so poignantly is that there are appallingly few therapeutic choices available to people without adequate educational and financial resources. Accordingly, the capacities of the community mental health center to help such individuals in the long term are severely limited. Too often, such an underfunded public facility is unable to provide the types of minimally adequate, ongoing assistance required by many of its most troubled and needy clients.

Carmen expresses special concern about the increasing numbers of abused children and battered women. She recommends the establishment of facilities and self-help groups that could begin to systematically address these growing problems. She also identifies and describes sexually transmitted diseases, especially AIDS, as principal threats to the very existence of many of her emotionally disturbed patients. In a trenchantly candid final section, Carmen makes a series of suggestions and recommendations that, among other types of assistance and care, would both offer greater physical protection from the spread of HIV and provide more effective counseling and educational programs to reach out to the populations most at risk—the mentally ill, the intravenous drug abusers, and the homeless.

Ellen L. Bassuk has fashioned a groundbreaking project in working extensively and intensively with the homeless, especially with homeless women. Some of the results and insights of her longtime association with the homeless are described in bold strokes in her gripping chapter, "Lives in Jeopardy: Women and Homelessness." What the reader rediscovers immediately is the near omnipresence of homeless individuals, especially women of all ages, in the United States. Their numbers are not confined to highly visible individual street people and panhandlers. The growing populations also include large numbers of people under 25; entire families, usually headed by a single mother; and significant numbers of elderly who have lost their homes and finances because of the decline of the American economy.

As Bassuk observes in the concluding section of her description and analysis: what must be done as nominal first steps in a remediation process is to increase public education and consciousness of the magnitude of the problem. She looks carefully at potentially effective ways to "increase public awareness about the relationship among poverty, homelessness, and 'the invidious effects of the socialization of women and the limited opportunities for women.' " The victims are not only women. Homelessness and the violence daily perpetrated upon the homeless severely injure and scar female and male, old and young alike. High on any newly revised agenda for community-based public mental health efforts must be an energetic attack on the problem and the ramifications of homelessness from coast to coast and from border to border.

Charles Vert Willie and Jayminn Sulir Sanford, in "Turbulence on the College Campus and the Frustration-Aggression Hypothesis," survey in depth and breadth the highly complex issues and emotions associated with turbulence on the college campus, and the possible source of this turbulence in the frustration-aggression hypothesis. The growing phenomena of conflict and overt violence on college campuses across the United States has received extensive media attention and popular "analysis." The issues appear to span the spectrum of available audiences and participants: racial, religious, gender, political, economic, or ideological. It sometimes seems to an observer that if an opportunity or excuse for conflict could be found, some combination of students somewhere might well seize the opportunity. The incidence and intensity of these volatile confrontations could continue to escalate through the 1990s.

In this richly anecdotal study, Willie and Sanford provide a capsule history of recent campus turbulence. They select a number of cogent case studies to use as paradigms for a successful understanding and resolution of campus turbulence. Then, by describing a provocative group dynamic stratagem that has had a successful record of conflict resolution in selected instances over the past thirty years, Willie and Sanford propose its revivification and active implementation again today when certain types of campus conflict arise. The use of nonviolent collective action by like-minded people is as old as biblical times and as "new" as the strategy and tactics of the Reverend Martin Luther King, Jr., and the Student Nonviolent Coordinating Committee in the 1960s. Willie and Sanford insist that the usefulness of a powerful, collaborative strategy is timeless and efficacious even in a markedly different social and polticial context.

Chester M. Pierce, in "Stress Analogs of Racism and Sexism: Terrorism, Torture, and Disaster," assesses from both long- and short-term perspectives the awful modern "triad of the apocalypse": terror, torture, and disaster. His consideration centers upon how commonplace those strategies have become in our modern, "civilized" world. He suggests that these strategies may be seen and interpreted as stress parallels of racism and sexism. Implicit in Pierce's appraisal and evaluation is the assertion that the skillful, timely application of the tactical and strategic tools of terror, torture, and external disaster can be highly effective in perpetuating and maintaining the anger and outrage that often fuels racism and sexism. The predicament in which victims and their champions find themselves, faced by the unexpected occurrence of these terrorizing stress simulations (or analogs), is simply "What to do?" "How to do it?" "When—if ever—to do it?" Pierce offers both theoretical analyses and hypothetical options for putting such aversive situations into constructive contexts and provides some practical suggestions regarding how real-life confrontations might be more effectively comprehended, analyzed—and, perhaps, even defused or resolved. This exploration is a thought-provoking double approach, both theoretical and reality based, to several of the most perplexing, anxiety-producing social dilemmas of our time.

In Part IV, Teaching, Learning, Research, and Training Issues, we present two notable analytic descriptions of significant research affecting women's mental health today and, by extension, making discernible impacts upon the status of women in American culture. We also share two significant capsule case histories of public mental health institutions that have made—and continue to make—positive, health-restoring contributions to the welfare and well-being of their patients.

The tasks of strengthening the field, the approach, and the techniques of the practice of public mental health grow ever more urgent and complex. This near crisis situation in the United States is due in no small measure to the dearth of human and material resources devoted to public mental health through the 1980s and into the 1990s. It remains imperative to pursue quality research as well as to keep clearly in mind the notable successes of public mental health enterprises over the years.

Jean A. Hamilton has long been engaged in extensive research to determine the degree to which certain classes of prescription drugs may be appropriately and safely given to women. In "Sex and Gender as Critical Variables in Psychotropic Drug Research," she presents an eye-opening case study of how sex and gender biases may well have negatively affected the synthesis and testing of antidepressant drugs. For decades, pharmaceutical companies, with the tacit approval of federal regulatory agencies and other supervisory bodies, have systematically excluded females from the testing of antidepressant medications. The net result is to cast disturbingly substantial doubt upon the efficacy and safety of nearly all antidepressant drugs prescribed for women.

The clinical studies reviewed and summarized in Hamilton's article provide powerful substantiation for her evaluation and judgment of the errors of omission and commission in the testing and use of antidepressant drugs as a pharmaceutical class. Since well over half of all antidepressants prescribed in the United States are taken by women, crucial questions of safety and efficacy are raised. The ethical issue of the intentional exclusion of women from field trials during the final phases of drug testing is also one of Hamilton's serious concerns. At stake are not only the safety and efficacy of drugs given to women but never tested on or by them, but also the trustworthiness and reliability of a scientific industry and the oversight processes so intimately involved in the public health and welfare. The implications and repercussions of Hamilton's research and the conclusions that she draws are of vital importance for all Americans, regardless of gender.

Harriet P. Lefley and Evalina W. Bestman, in "Training for Culturally Appropriate Mental Health Services," describe in topical and chronological fashion the conception, planning, and operation of a successful mental health facility in Florida—the New Horizons Community Mental Health Center. The authors are prime movers in this model program, which was funded by the National Institute of Mental Health to serve the inner city of Miami. African Americans and Caribbean and Central and South American peoples constitute the major clientele groups using this new catchment-area facility. Among the keys to the notable success of this community mental health center are (1) meticulous planning to serve the diverse clientele; (2) sensitivity to their clientele's particular needs; and (3) an informed awareness that many of the center's clients would be mentally ill—members of the large inner-city deinstitutionalized population who rarely received adequate services following their release from hosptials or mental health facilities. Not only is this essay a blueprint for the successful implementation of this NIMH-sponsored center, but it also describes the Mental Health Human Services Training Center that then became a resource hub for the dissemination of training skills and models of successful in-service, client-centered programs.

Nancy Felipe Russo, in "Women's Mental Health: Research Agenda for the Twenty-first Century," concentrates on enumerating, evaluating, and setting priorities for the major mental health issues currently confronting women and those that are still likely to be in the vanguard of women's mental health issues into the next century. Professor Russo surveys the seminal research projects in the field of women's mental health in process since the convening of the President's Commission on Mental Health in 1978. Her overview critically evaluates what was pragmatically and theoretically successful from the points of view of recipients and providers of mental health care for women. Russo's review takes into account the major personal and professional events in women's lives and then spotlights those mental health initiatives and programs that have produced measurable, positive results. She identifies major causes of mental disorders in women nationwide, including violence, poverty, and the voluntary and involuntary assumption of multiple private and vocational roles. She weighs the probable effects of health threats to women such as the rising rates of abuse and sexually transmitted diseases, especially AIDS. Russo concludes by setting forth a formidable, urgent agenda of mental health research projects, along with a rationale for the primacy of the most pressing.

The Center for Minority Group Mental Health Programs at the National Institute of Mental Health was a pioneering pilot project in 1970 to provide a focus for the training of mental health professionals who would be qualified to become both clinicians in and administrators of centers throughout the nation. The conception, initiation, and implementation of this ambitious model program form the background and materials for the chapter that assesses its history.

Bertram S. Brown and K. Patrick Okura chronicle in detail the major successes, problems, and insurmountable policy obstacles that the center encountered. Their history represents a microcosm of the promise and accomplishments of a highly ambitious, potentially effective public mental health master plan. It also provides contemporary health care planners and governmental funding agencies with a still valid blueprint for reestablishment of such valuable public health resource centers—for both clinical care and teaching of the skills of mental health care to new practitioners.

This volume of essays is intended to provoke productive discussion and debate regarding our nationally depressed state of public mental health care. The authors and editors encourage such revived public discussion of national mental health care priorities that have languished too long for lack of adequate funding and staffing. If public mental health care can again attain its rightful place on our national agenda of human service necessities, then the purposes of this collection of informative and persuasive essays will have served its multiple purposes.

PART I

Conceptual Overview

Castellano B. Turner and Bernard M. Kramer

Connections Between Racism and Mental Health

T HIS chapter will examine some ways in which racism and mental health connect with each other. First, we shall try to link the two historically. Then we shall provide a framework, identifying a number of conceptual and clinical connections between racism and mental health. Because the future of our field depends on the way we educate the next generation of mental health professionals, our discussion toward the end of this essay focuses on training issues pertaining to racism and mental health.

We estimate that more than a million people are mental health workers in the United States. We think it is essential to consider what these individuals will need to know and what they will be called upon to do. They will need to provide services to populations that may be thought of as special today but will very likely be the everyday clientele of tomorrow. In concrete terms this means that every mental health worker must be culturally aware enough to respond effectively to those they hope to serve. This cultural imperative must not be ignored.

In this chapter we also aim to give shape to a field of interest that emerged out of the ferment of the 1960s. It was then that the Civil Rights Movement succeeded in obtaining passage of the Civil Rights Acts of 1964 and 1965, major landmarks in the quest for racial justice. It was then, too, that the Mental Health Movement succeeded in bringing about passage of the Community Mental Health Centers Act of 1963. These acts serve as symbolic guides for the field of racism and mental health.

In the 1960s many of those interested in advancing racial justice were also attracted to the cause of better mental health services; likewise, many mental health activists were drawn to the civil rights cause. Scholars and practitioners in one area would often turn up in the other. In the early 1970s several publications marked the emergence of a specialty concerned with the interrelationship of race relations and the mental health disciplines (Kovel's *White Racism: A Psychohistory*, 1970; Thomas and Sillen's *Racism and Psychiatry*, 1972; Willie, Kramer, and Brown's *Racism and Mental Health*, 1973). These volumes suggested that members of mental health professions were not doing their parts to counteract racism.

One stream of thought held that racism was to be found in only a fringe element of the mental health field. In another view, racism was at the core of the entire field. Less harsh was the charge that African Americans with psychological problems received poor treatment because of negative stereotypes. Another point of view maintained that few mental health professionals were African Americans or Latino, and that racial sensitivity was in short supply. Nonetheless, an impressive number of mental health professionals were looking for ways to infuse their work with an antiracist sensibility, believing that racism was itself a mental illness striking at the nation's health.

Meanwhile, civil rights activists knew that victims of racial discrimination often experienced considerable psychological stress and suffered accompanying mental health problems. It was no accident, therefore, that advocates of racial justice in many communities mounted efforts to establish mental health facilities under new federal, state, and local initiatives. While economic opportunity and political empowerment were surely at the forefront of civil rights objectives, mental health services were, likewise, natural foci of progressive change at the interface between race relations and mental health.

In short, then, a marriage was in the making between mental health and antiracist activists. The engagement period has been long, but the wedding is still to come. And (to continue the metaphor) the marriage contract has not even been written yet. Still missing is an analysis of the types of connections and linkages that might bring the two together in a durable alliance. This chapter is intended as a step in that direction.

Racism and Evolving Mental Health Systems

Each generation lives in its own time and intellectual space. Taking this as a given, we begin with a bit of history to provide a context within which to reflect upon racism and mental health. The key feature of race relations in the United States is the existence of White racism—in all its forms and manifestations. It lies inescapably at the core of the past and present state of race relations. Social scientists have repeatedly demonstrated that racism persists in American society (Brigham and Weissbach

1972; Dovidio and Gaertner 1986). The word *prejudice* has come to mean negative attitudes toward a specific group without sufficient warrant, whereas the word *discrimination* refers to the acting out of prejudices to the detriment of a specific group and its members. The most comprehensive meaning of *racism*, however, encompasses both attitudes and behavior (McConahay 1986). Racism, however, must also include the concepts of power, stratification, and oppression. That is, inordinate power is held by one racial group; society is stratified according to race; and the dominant racial group uses its power to maintain this system and to oppress those who have been subordinated against their will.

The history of racism in the United States is a history of both conflicting and converging interests. The primordial conflict occurred in the forced removal of Africans from their homes, for use as slaves. In the ensuing centuries the United States experienced a civil war, centered on the abolition of slavery; a period of reconstruction that ended with Jim Crow segregation as a substitute for slavery; a Civil Rights Movement that resulted in the outlawing of segregation; and a subsequent complex, extended backlash. Today, the conflicting interests of African Americans and Whites remain side by side with their common interests. American society is now experiencing a transition period during which the civil rights consensus of the 1960s has shifted to growing polarization in the 1990s. Economic growth has yielded to worldwide recession, spurring increased immigration into the United States. Conflicting interests between African Americans and Whites are mirrored in conflicting interests among the several minority communities, where political unity is in its infancy. In the society at large, pragmatic optimism contends with intensifying anxiety about racial issues.

The history of racism has also intersected in several ways with the history of mental health care. For example, a prominent explanation of mental illness has been that of genetic predisposition in some racial stocks. During the several surges of immigration to the United States, a dominant claim was made that the new immigrants would bring in inferior stock. An alleged indication of such inferiority was the presumed "scientifically demonstrated" prevalence of mental inferiority and mental illness in that population (Chase 1977). During the 1940s and 1950s the focus shifted to a belief that African Americans suffer from mental illness as a "mark of oppression" (Kardiner and Ovesey 1951).

Critics of the "mark of oppression" thesis argued that social factors, not the stigma of color, held the key to explaining mental illness among African Americans. Since the 1960s, mental health scholars have been divided between, on the one hand, the desire to take a color-blind perspective regarding the nature and treatment of mental illness, and on the other, the wish to fully acknowledge minority culture and status as central to etiology and treatment.

Even within the context of positive developments in mental health policy, racism has introduced a distorted angle. The Community Mental Health Centers Act of 1963 set the stage for implementing two related ideas: (1) "downsizing" the state mental hospital systems, and (2) creating a community-oriented system of comprehensive local mental health centers. These ideas were theoretically interlocked and practically appealing to political authorities with their potential to reduce costs. The unforeseen actuality, however, was that massive deinstitutionalization was not accompanied by the required community-based facilities. Nor were the required funds made available for the personnel and services needed to support the deinstitutionalized in the community. Homelessness among the mentally ill reflects the deep problems of the current mental health system. Moreover, large numbers of people with psychological problems are prisoners in the criminal justice system. African Americans and Latinos are vastly overrepresented among the homeless and imprisoned. Some research has demonstrated that the latter's incarceration is partially traceable to racial bias in clinical evaluations (Lewis, Balla, and Shanok 1979). In the context of today's economic problems, the task of reconstituting a working mental health system appears to have been placed on the back burner of national priorities. Communities of color will undoubtedly be disproportionately affected by this neglect.

Connecting Framework Between Racism and Mental Health

How are racism and mental health connected? Racism and mental health connect with each other in at least seven major ways, and these connections are themselves interrelated:

- in the *definitions* of mental health and illness;
- in the theories of the *etiology* of mental illness;
- in the *evaluation* process (assessment and diagnosis);
- in the provision of *direct services;*
- in the organizing and structuring of mental health *institutions and programs;*
- in *research* carried out to understand the mental health problems of racial groups;
- in the *training* of mental health professionals to provide direct service and organize intervention programs.

Definitions and Etiology

Our framework identifies the most general connections between racism and mental illness. How does racism influence basic definitions of mental illness? Dominant racial groups may construct definitions of mental illness that justify their superiority or the subjugated groups' inferiority. If behavior that is more common in one racial group is described as abnormal, then members of that group will more often be considered abnormal. In the history of mental illness in the United States, race has been the basis for claims not only of excess incidence, but also of relatively limited incidence. The well-known example in the United States was the theory that African slaves were not subject to depressive disorders (Prudhomme and Musto 1973). Although genetics was the main basis for explaining the lower incidence of depression in African Americans, this construction also bolstered the notion that the living conditions of slaves (lacking as they were in the need to make decisions and therefore lacking in the burdens of conflict) were really beneficial rather than oppressive.

Racism is implicated, as well, in the formulation of theories of mental health and illness. Theories about the origins of mental illness range from those that are biological in nature (genetic predisposition, biochemical imbalance, and so on) to those that view mental illness primarily as a social construction. Between these two poles are positions that recognize both the biological foundation and the cultural meanings attached to manifestations of aberrant behavior. As part of our understanding of the etiology of mental illness, we generally allow for the influence of causal factors that are proximal as well as distal, personal as well as social and situational.

Racism may have several impacts on the effort to understand the origins of mental illness. To the extent that racist thought explains abnormality as deriving from fundamental differences between racial groups, one would expect that such thought would lead eventually to theories of mental illness as based on genetic inferiority of an entire population. In this general way of thinking about differences between people, superiority and inferiority play critical roles. Abnormal behavior or mental aberrations might well be considered as expressions of genetic inferiority.

It certainly is not the case that anyone subscribing to theories of mental illness that depend upon a genetic explanation is thereby subscribing to racist notions of inferiority and superiority. Such notions become relevant only when those doing the theorizing add the assumption that a particular racial group exhibits a greater genetic predisposition to mental illness than do other racial groups. Even those severe forms of mental illness for which there is evidence of a genetic component (such as schizophrenia and severe depression) occur in all racial groups. What variations do exist are readily interpretable as emerging from cultural differences and ecological stressors. (Cross-cultural differences in mental illness can be understood as variations in specific symptoms rather than as essential differences in underlying conditions.)

Our analysis of linkage must examine how racism may influence thought not only about the origins of mental illness but also about its maintenance. For example, a racist perspective will explain continuing mental health problems as rooted in shortcomings of the individual and the family rather than social-structural contexts. The victims of mental illness may be blamed, just as the victims of racism are blamed. Inasmuch as the development of mental health problems is linked to stress (particularly sustained stress), racism must be regarded as a major source of stress for African Americans and therefore as the genesis of many of their mental health problems.

We must also examine the impact of racism on the incidence of mental health problems among African Americans and other oppressed minorities. Although the weight of existing evidence does not support the notion of a genetic basis for racial and ethnic differences in rates of mental health problems, real racial and ethnic differences are facts of life. If ethnic minorities appear to have higher rates of mental illness than Whites, what explains the difference? Part of the explanation is that ethnic minorities are subjected to stressors directly related to minority status: discrimination in education and occupation; assaults upon self-esteem that arise out of low status within society; relative lack of access to health care; segregation in isolated communities that are prone to social disorganization.

Social class, however, is another major explanation for differentials in mental health problems among African Americans and other ethnic minorities in the United States. Rather than understanding differences in terms of ethnic or racial status, the most consistent and robust finding in this area is that an inverse relationship exists between social class and sources of life stressors as well as an inverse relationship between social class and rates of mental health problems. The lives of poor individuals, families, and communities are full of stressors. If stress is implicated in the development of mental health problems, then connections between racism and mental health are interpretable in terms of the higher rates of poverty among ethnic minority populations—including African Americans.

Moritsugu and Sue (1982), however, have demonstrated persuasively that minority status alone is a source of stress, apart from any explanation based on social class. That poverty is an important source of stress is incontrovertible. It is largely because African Americans and other ethnic minorities are overrepresented among the poor that they are subjected to higher rates of stress and mental health problems. That is, social class cannot be thought of as independent of the effects of racism; rather, relative poverty is indeed *the* primary effect of racism. Poverty is not, however, the only source of stress nor of mental health problems. African Americans in the United States continue to be oppressed in many areas of life—personally, socially, and politically, as well as economically.

Evaluation—Assessment and Diagnosis

Although the range of positions held about assessment and evaluation is wide—from those who regard them as central to an ethical science of behavior to those who feel that assessment and evaluation are inherently racist and should be abandoned altogether—we believe that assessment and evaluation are necessary, valuable processes. They are, however, full of intricate problems, some of which interact with issues of racism. The impact of racism on psychological assessment and diagnosis has been a particular concern in the African American community for many decades. The primary setting for the battles about the use and abuse of psychological evaluation has been the public schools, where racism and cross-cultural biases have often led to misleading intelligence test scores for African Americans. These biases have contributed to tracking, the lowering of expectations, and finally, limitations on educational and occupational aspirations and achievement.

The abuse of psychological assessment, however, is not limited to intelligence testing. In mental health settings the use of diagnostic criteria that fail to take into account major cultural and social class differences between African Americans and Whites lead to invalid conclusions concerning the type and degree of mental health problems. What diagnosticians regard as abnormal behavior cannot be separated entirely from their own cultural backgrounds—including their educational experiences and the professional orientations that provide frameworks for both definition and judgment of mental illness and health. Diagnosticians typically have power over African American clients, based on the former's dominant race and class status, along with a set of beliefs which rationalize that power.

Snowden and Todman (1982) have described a wide range of solutions to the problems of racial and cultural biases in testing. Although the inadequacies and errors of measuring instruments are many and well documented, the most important problems involve the testers themselves. Even an inadequate instrument can be useful in the hands of an examiner who acknowledges its limitations and makes an adjustment in interpretation. Likewise, Jones and Thorne (1987) have outlined a number of approaches to cross-cultural clinical assessment. The major thrust of their argument is that one needs to emphasize the uniqueness of persons and evaluate psychological status from the individual's particular perspective. That perspective is often informed by cultural background, but it is just as important to understand differences among members of given cultural groups.

Direct Service

Beyond assessment and diagnosis, there is the problem of equal access to intervention services for ethnic minority populations. The impact of racism on the provision of direct services to African American populations has been documented and discussed at length (Sue 1977; Sue et al. 1974; Myers et al. 1991). Rather than review that literature, let us consider the case of individual psychotherapy, which many consider to be the "best" of mental health services. The first question is whether racism acts as a barrier to psychotherapy. Are African Americans and other minority group members given fair opportunities to enter psychotherapy? Do practitioners too often judge minority group members as being inappropriate for psychotherapy? Even when minority group clients are accepted into psychotherapy, is the length of treatment service adequate? More broadly, are mental health service providers sensitive to the importance of cultural differences in their interventions? Are interventions designed in such a way that they prove relevant to the needs and values of ethnic minority clients?

Racial bias in the selection of clients is the primary connecting point between racism and mental health care services (Yamamoto et al. 1967). African Americans and other ethnic minority clients are not given a fair share of the resources of society. Health care is one such resource. On any index of the provision of services and quality of health services African Americans receive significantly less. Mental health resources are also distributed unequally. Jones and Korchin (1982) have documented the relatively greater need for mental health services among ethnic minority populations in the United States. In spite of their greater need, ethnic minority clients are provided with significantly less services of highest quality. It may be argued that individual psychotherapy is not the most effective service for many mental health problems. It is, however, generally so regarded by the profession and also is the most expensive. Ethnic minority group members are less often chosen to be clients in individual therapy, and the length of their treatment is significantly shorter. Instead of psychotherapy, ethnic minority clients are much more often hospitalized and are most often treated with pharmacotherapy.

Even the pattern of inpatient hospital treatment appears to be distorted to the disadvantage of minority clients. In a recent report from the National Institute of Mental Health (Manderscheid and Sonnenschein 1990) two related findings are clear: first, African American and Latino clients have significantly briefer stays in psychiatric inpatient facilities; second, the recidivism rate for ethnic minority clients is much higher. One explanation for this phenomenon argues that minorities are more often discharged prematurely, only to be returned more frequently. The evidence from other sources indicates that mental health professionals are less than enthusiastic about treating ethnic minority clients. Although it could be argued that greater recidivism among ethnic minorities reflects the greater stress they experience after leaving psychiatric hospitals, we are left to contend with the question concerning significantly earlier discharge.

Ethnic minorities in the United States are also more likely than others to receive diagnoses of serious and long-standing psychopathology (Sue 1977; Griffith and Jones 1979; Mayo 1974; Korchin 1980). Although this might suggest that they would be overrepresented among those in psychotherapy, minorities are not as likely as others to receive psychotherapeutic services. Minority patients are more likely to receive pharmacotherapy and inpatient treatment rather than long-term psychotherapy (Sue et al. 1974).

Several explanations for the paradox of greater need but less psychotherapy given may be considered. First, minority clients may reject psychotherapy or may drop out because their needs are not adequately addressed. Second, institutional policy may in some way restrict those who are most needy from receiving the best available treatment. Third, psychotherapists may reject minority clients more than they do others. Smith, Burlew, Mosley, and Whitney (1978) have tried to allocate the causality for this underservice, and conclude that all three explanations are implicated. We believe, however, that making changes in the attitudes of potential minority patient populations would be less productive than understanding and changing the mechanisms that lead therapists to reject, directly or indirectly, minority clients.

Previous research has demonstrated that psychotherapists (like all other members of American culture) hold and apply stereotypes about different categories of people (Turner, Turner, and Ciano-Boyce 1988). Bloombaum, Yamamoto, and James (1968) found that psychotherapists hold negative stereotypes of several ethnic groups—including African Americans. Using the Bogardus (1958) Social Distance Scale, they also determined that therapists organized their preferred distances in the same order as other Americans, with African Americans listed at the greatest distance. Stephan and Rosenfield (1982) have shown that the structure of stereotypes held by therapists is similar to that of non-therapists. Geller (1988) has reported the findings of an unpublished study of psychiatric residents and young psychiatrists, which experimentally examined the effects of race of client on clinical evaluations. Although a Black and a White patient were described in exactly the same terms, a hypothetical Black client was judged to be less suitable for psychotherapy than a hypothetical White client. More remarkable was the finding that this pattern persisted even when the Black patient was described as having an IQ of 120 and the White patient as having an IQ of 85 (Stevenson and Geller 1969).

In a study of a large random sample of National Register psychologists (Turner and Turner 1991), therapist ethnicity was related significantly to the percentage of minority clients seen in practice. Whereas 35 percent of the White respondents reported having no minority clients, all of the minority respondents reported having some minority clients. This finding held whether the question focused on percentage of Blacks or percentage of other minority groups; it held also when the percentage of clients who were Blacks and other minorities were combined to create a variable of "Total Percent Minority Clients." The findings repeatedly indicated that minority therapists were significantly more likely to report having minority clients than were White therapists.

We must conclude, therefore, that minorities appeared to be more likely to treat minority clients, but it suggests that one reason African Americans and other minorities are underrepresented among those receiving psychotherapy is that there are relatively few minority therapists. Our general hypothesis can be conceived of as a series of interactions. White therapists, based on socialization and experience, have certain attitudes—including negative attitudes and stereotypes about various categories of people. Minority clients enter the mental health system and need to be evaluated and treated, but they also have attitudes about people who are likely to be the service providers. When therapists and clients meet, therapists' negative attitudes and stereotypes lead them to both expect certain behavior from the client and behave in certain ways. The client reacts to these expectations and behaves in such a way as to fulfill them. The therapist notes that the client has behaved in a way consistent with his or her racial attitudes and stereotypes and continues to behave in ways consistent with those attitudes and stereotypes. Since little authentic encounter takes place, one of the two usually gives up and leaves the relationship. Snyder (1981) has very clearly demonstrated the self-perpetuating nature of social stereotypes, and Ward, Zanna, and Cooper (1974) have shown that subtle nonverbal cues can reveal negative attitudes and stereotypes in dyadic interactions. Furthermore, experimental research on dyadic interactions indicates that targets of negative stereotypes are influenced by them to behave in ways that "affirm" the stereotypes (Deaux 1984).

Evans (1985) has described the range of perspectives on the issue of whether African American clients are helped by traditional psychotherapeutic methods. The criticism of psychoanalytic methods, in particular, as irrelevant to the needs of most ethnic minority clients seems to her unfounded. The findings of her study suggest that the problem of the use of psychoanalytic therapy by minority clients is much more likely to be based on the disinclination of psychoanalytically oriented therapists to accept minority clients. The need to attend to severe life problems is certainly real. If that is the rationale for avoiding minority clients, however, it is misguided.

The corollary of the notion that African Americans and other minorities cannot make good use of in-depth or long-term therapy is the idea that behavioral approaches are the most practical. That is, since more often than not the minority client presents with behavioral problems that must be changed to carry on life satisfactorily, why not use the most direct and practical approach? Clearly, the behavioral approaches are more focused and take a shorter period to work. If, however, such decisions are based more on expense and practicality than on therapeutic utility, racism again controls the mental health service system.

Institutions and Programs: The Case of the Ghetto Ward

The structure, organization, and functioning of mental health services are also affected by racism. Our focus here is on "the system" rather than on the person. How does our racially stratified social system influence the provision of mental health services? How, for example, does systemic racism affect the provision of such services to African Americans?

If racism is pervasive in American society, then the effects must be present in all professions, including that of mental health. In a racially segregated community what is the possibility that mental health services will not be segregated? In a society whose members are taught that race is a legitimate basis for differentiating individuals on a hierarchical scale, why should any occupational group—including mental health care professionals—be immune?

Even the progressive inspiration of the Community Mental Health Centers Act left hidden many of the family secrets of racism. The Community Mental Health Centers Act of 1963 made specific reference to the concept of "catchment areas." What began as a way of conceptualizing epidemiological data soon found its way into the design of mental health programs. To ensure community connectedness rather than isolation, and to ensure continuity rather than fragmentation of care among the state psychiatric facilities and community mental health services, clients in a given catchment area were to be cared for in a common place for that particular area. In some cases this was accomplished by the construction of a completely new facility. In others, the approach was to renovate or combine facilities. Still other areas around the country placed their community mental health centers' programs in preexisting state mental hospitals. No matter what pattern was chosen, individuals from the same community or neighborhood entering the state mental health system were to be housed together.

In the late 1960s one of the authors—Castellano Turner—was involved in a community mental health program in Chicago. Here is a portion of his personal recollection of how the deep structures of racism affect clinical services:

As part of a comprehensive community mental health effort, a ward was set aside in a state hospital specifically to provide inpatient treatment for a community program based on the South Side of Chicago. Whenever individuals were identified as residing in the community served by this program, they were sent to the community's "catchment area ward." This plan was basically sound within the model of community mental health service planning. Race and racism became important because the catchment area community was overwhelmingly African American. Although there were several state hospitals—as well as several nearby private hospitals—within or near Chicago, the site selected for the ward was a state hospital 50 miles away from the community which it was meant to serve. The hospital was located in a rural, predominantly White community south of Chicago.

In this large institution, White patients predominated. Thus, the catchment area ward, with its largely African American population, stood out. When the ward program was opened only White professionals worked there, but about half of the psychiatric nurse assistants were African Americans. When I was hired to be a staff psychologist, I was the first African American professional on the ward. Gradually the White nonprofessional staff requested transfers to other wards. They were invariably replaced by African American staff members. By the end of the first full year of the program the psychiatric assistants were all African Americans, but the composition of the professional staff remained unchanged: I was still the only African American professional.

By the end of that first year the patients on the ward were about 90 to 95 percent African American, the nonprofessional staff was totally African American, and one out of seven professional staff members was African American. These staffing patterns and changes themselves reflected the occupational structure of United States society. More striking, however, was the nature of the relationship between this ward and the rest of the hospital. After a time I began to receive disturbing reports from ward staff about the attitudes and behavior of hospital personnel working outside the ward. The former complained that it was difficult to get routine services for the ward—pickups and deliveries, repairs, and laboratory services. Rumors circulated throughout the hospital about rampant violence and sexual activity on the ward. When asked about their reluctance to deliver services or work on the ward, some White hospital workers apparently claimed that they feared for their safety.

What is striking about this pattern is the extent to which it matches the relationship of urban ghettos with their surrounding metropolitan areas. In this ward we had a "ghetto ward," which was first identified as a place for African Americans, then stereotyped as a place to fear, and finally treated as a place to avoid. In the ghettoization process, self-fulfilling expectations lead to the spiral of isolation and deterioration. Victims of isolation, who are denied access to needed resources for satisfactory living and social arrangements, are blamed for their own victimization.

The existence of so many segregated communities in American cities is primary evidence that society is implicitly organized along racial lines. In practice, segregation means not only isolation. It also means inequality of access to vital resources—from garbage collection and street cleaning to quality shopping centers and medical services.

The construction of a ghetto ward is possible simply because ghettos exist in the world outside of hospitals. Racism exists. The stereotyping and isolation of groups based on race and ethnicity are processes present in everyday life. Mental health professions and mental health settings (such as hospitals and clinics) are nothing more than specific contexts for the playing out of these grotesque but all-too-normal societal processes.

What about the quality of services in the ghetto? Do the benefits of a catchment area program outweigh the costs involved in creating yet another racially segregated environment, which will once again reinforce the existing social arrangements? A cogent argument has been advanced over the last thirty years that minority communities would be better off as separate entities, left to control their own destinies. Without the domination of the oppressor, the quality of life and services in the ghetto would improve. This proposition assumes that the ghetto also has equal access to resources and is completely self-contained. However, "separate-but-equal" systems have never been equal, for at least two reasons. First, separatism leaves intact the social dominance of Whites; second, whenever interactions would occur—and occur they must—domination would lead to unequal distribution of resources. The community control justification for the maintenance of the ghetto is most appealing in light of the notion that self-esteem, group esteem, and empowerment of oppressed people are critical elements in the improvement of the lot of ethnic minority groups. Even when separation is understood as a transitional necessity, however, the costs of resigning ourselves to separatism—whether supported by oppressors or victims—are much too high and their accompanying dangers too great. It is difficult, nonetheless, to ignore the pride (as well as the despair) that ignites the impulse to go it alone.

Research

Racism may affect the research enterprise by means of oppression, neglect, exploitation, and rejection.

Oppression. The oppression of one racial group by another is fundamental to our definition of racism. The ubiquity of racism in our society guarantees that social science research will be influenced by racist perspectives and values. Scientific research, and specifically social science research, is not value free. Researchers bring biased attitudes, stereotypes, expectations, and motives to the scientific enterprise (Chase 1977). If we agree that Americans have all been tainted by racism, then the best we can do is (1) be alert to its manifestations in our work and (2) correct distortions. Antiracist perspectives do not now dominate social science research, because changing perspectives would require a radical shift in orientation and methodology. Research whose overt or covert aim is to establish the inferiority of some or the superiority of other racial groups is oppressive. Likewise, research founded on assumptions of the cultural deficiencies in certain racial or ethnic groups suffers from a biased perspective. For example, preconceived conclusions that compensatory education programs will not change the racial differences in school performance go beyond the evidence provided and justify the lack of effort at changing the status quo.

Neglect. Racist research is bad research. It includes research carried out with biased measures, which systematically either overestimate or underestimate psychological problems in African Americans. Such research does not take into account differences in meanings and response styles across racial and ethnic groups. It ignores the need to establish African American norms for some standardized tests. Such research, moreover, takes little notice of the importance in psychological research of the experimenter's race and ethnicity. In general, racist research neglects important methodological and interpretive constraints when its studies involve African American subjects. Much of the research carried out by mental health professionals, including clinical psychologists, has used White middle-class samples. That is not, in itself, a problem. The difficulty is that based on such research, theory is built, policies are established, and programs of intervention are designed.

Exploitation. One of the most infamous examples of racist exploitation of African Americans is the case of the "Tuskegee experiment" (Jones 1981), in which Black men infected with syphilis were allowed to go untreated so that the U.S. Public Health Service could monitor the progress of their illnesses. It is difficult to imagine a more exploitative abuse of human subjects simply because of their race. Clearly, government researchers took advantage of African Americans without informing them that they were not being treated and without giving them an opportunity to refuse to participate in this study. Other instances of exploitative research led African American social scientists to speak out and confront the issue (Clark 1973). Many of the recommendations that emerged from those confrontations involved increased participation of African American communities as collaborators in the research process. Even more impressive has been the recent policy change in federal funding agencies that requires an explicit justification for *not* including women and minorities as research participants.

Rejection. The research agendas of many African American and other ethnic minority scientists have included the special needs of their communities. This agenda was for decades largely ignored by mainstream social scientists, and the latter often resisted providing support for such research. As Sue, Ito, and Bradshaw (1982) point out, innovative research foci and approaches must be supported if research on mental health service needs is to be carried out effectively. Staying within the existing topics and methodologies of social science research has not been sufficient to satisfy the needs of racial and ethnic minority communities. The rejection of grant applications and proposed publications because of the absence of a majority comparison group is a particularly egregious example of rejection of racial and ethnic minority mental health research needs. Ironically, the vast literature of American psychological research is limited to studies of Whites only, without thought of including the comparison groups that are considered so necessary in studies of racial and ethnic minorities. African American and other ethnic minority researchers are desperately needed to carry out this research agenda. Mechanisms must be found for increasing rather than limiting ethnic minority participation in research.

Training Issues

Wyatt and Parham (1985) have assessed the extent to which training programs use culturally sensitive course materials, and they have suggested a variety of means to improve training for work with diverse ethnic minority populations. The potential utility and efficiency of a shift in training focus should not be underestimated. Ethnic minorities are a rapidly increasing proportion of the U.S. population. To be effective in the world of the twenty-first century, clinical practitioners must be able to interact with and serve individuals who are very different from themselves.

Students undergoing training in diversity-oriented programs invariably find themselves better prepared to deal with the realities of the varied populations they meet in clinical practicum assignments. They also find themselves sharing this knowledge and perspective with other graduate students and the professional staffs of the settings where they go for practicum training. An example is that of language barriers in various clinical settings. A student in our training program, faced with a language barrier between herself and the population she was to serve, understood both the advantages and pitfalls of using translators to establish the therapeutic alliance. Although the need for translation is usually regarded as no more than a necessary expedient, this student pointed out the opportunities presented in the translation relationship: family members and neighbors could be involved in treatment, and community-based translators with potential to enter the mental health care professions could be recruited. This experience suggests that training about differences in backgrounds is of considerable utility in clinical settings. It also suggests that the goals of such training are indeed achievable. What is needed is (1) to recognize the importance of the issue, and (2) the will to modify training processes and materials.

As educators and practitioners, one of the dilemmas we face is whether to train minorities to serve other minorities or to train all mental health service providers to be sensitive to the needs and characteristics of minorities. Currently, there is more need for service than is being met. Too few ethnic minority professionals are available to answer all unmet needs. Non-minority mental health professionals are not as likely as ethnic minority professionals to provide services to ethnic minority clients. Should we concentrate on increasing the number of ethnic minority professionals to try to serve all the needs that exist? This does not appear to be warranted or practical. Declining numbers of African Americans and other minorities are entering the mental health professions. Moreover, serious ethical, legal, social, and political problems are associated with the widespread expectation that ethnic minorities be required to commit their practices to seeing members of their own ethnic group.

How should the mental health professions respond to the service needs of minority communities? This question implies that a clear need exists, that the professions could provide some answers, and that some answers are better than others. For example, would it be reasonable to focus on increasing the number of psychologists who have been trained in the most traditional models of service delivery, with the hope that these additional professional resources would go toward working with the underserved? The field must respond with new models and approaches to training for the provision of service, because the needs of the minority community may well prove to be different from those of the White majority.

It is important not to underestimate the strategy of increasing the numbers of minority mental health professionals. The presence of a larger number of minorities as clinical practitioners would have several results. First, some minority clients would benefit most from having a therapist of their own race or ethnic background. Second, the increased presence of minority mental health professionals may have the effect of demonstrating more generally to minority communities that services are, in reality, available to them. The idea of mental health services may itself be foreign in some cultures and subcultures. The presence of individuals from one's own culture may make help-seeking more appealing and acceptable. Third, the increasing presence of minority mental health professionals may lead more majority providers to think of cultural factors as critically important considerations, especially because these issues will become increasingly mainstream alongside the rise of multiculturalism and in spite of politically inspired accusations of "political correctness."

Still, the problem of available numbers of minority professionals will be with us for some time. The answer to the problem must, then, include changes in training of the non-minority mental health professionals. Most mental health service providers will have to become knowledgeable about and sensitive to other cultures and ethnic groups. Future mental health professionals of all persuasions will feel the need for increased ethnic knowledge so as to fulfill their helping potential.

This implies that mental health professionals as a group will have to receive appropriate training. Indeed, some establishments within each of the professions have responded with modifications in their training programs. The University of Massachusetts at Boston has recently established a Clinical Psychology Program that emphasizes cross-cultural and minority-related issues along with its multidisciplinary and developmental approaches. Students are recruited and admitted because of their interest in addressing the needs of underserved urban populations. In designing a training program to prepare clinical psychologists to serve such populations, several important components are needed. Our model includes the following components:

Goals. We aim to produce professional clinical psychologists who value diversity and multiculturalism. The individual completing this program should be sensitive to differences among people without stereotyping members of any group. Students should leave the program with knowledge of diverse groups as well as the skills necessary to provide valid assessment and design culturally appropriate interventions.

Students. The goals of individuals who pursue graduate education are not identical. Our students' goals, however, must correspond with those of the program. In this program students must be interested in working with underserved populations. Students should be open to learning about diverse cultures as well as learning the skills appropriate to the needs of groups very different from themselves. In a program that commits itself to training for cultural diversity, students themselves must represent as much diversity as can be managed. A program of this kind cannot hope to have credibility without admitting ethnic minority students in substantial numbers.

Faculty. If the students who are to be trained for helping underserved populations must begin with such an interest, so must the faculty share that interest and find concrete ways of preparing students for this work. Many reasons exist for having a diverse faculty. In the context of this discussion, however, here are the two major reasons: First, the presence of diversity within a faculty reflects an awareness that the world beyond the academy is diverse. Second, a diverse faculty provides students with a much richer range of experiences and perspectives.

Curriculum. Traditional training in clinical psychology and psychiatry has typically ignored considerations of cultural and racial differences. Our program, founded as it is on the principle that these factors are crucial, includes material relevant to racial and cultural differences—along with gender, age, class, and other types of diversity—throughout the curriculum. Since ours is a training program in clinical psychology, it must meet accreditation standards of the American Psychological Association. Therefore, the curriculum requires courses in general psychology, statistics, life-span development, psychopathology, psychological assessment, and intervention strategies as well as a required course in culture and mental health. Where possible, all of the required courses also contain material relevant to issues of cultural diversity.

Practicum and Internship. Since the program is committed to training professionals to serve various underserved populations, the clinical practicum requirement stipulates that at least one of two years be spent in a facility that serves an underserved ethnic minority or poor population.

Research. There are three avenues for encouraging graduate students to engage in research involving diverse racial and cultural groups: First, if the faculty are themselves carrying out research on the status and needs of diverse groups, students are much more likely to pursue such research themselves. Second, if the curriculum includes courses that emphasize the importance of cultural and racial differences, questions will emerge for students to pursue in their own research efforts. Third, if students have been exposed in their practicum experiences to diverse populations, they will be less likely to err by assuming that their own racial or ethnic group forms the normative standard of behavior.

Conclusion

Here, in summary, is a set of perspectives on and recommendations for understanding the complex intersection of racism and mental health.

These include the importance of historical analysis; of the simultaneous use of macro and micro perspectives; of continual research on epidemiology and provider personnel; of the impact of the cultural context; and of culture-sensitive clinical training.

First, the *perspective of history* is essential to understanding phenomena that have any sociocultural roots. Much that seems mysterious to us— about events in the world as well as the meaning of public policy—is clarified by the perspective of history. Surprisingly, many Americans are taken aback by the thought that the history of slavery in this country ought to be part of any explanation of current racial differences and strife. This is not to say that we should remain wedded to the past as providing the answers to our future. We can plan the future, however, only if there is understanding of how the present came about. This applies to the study of both racism and mental health. The link of racism to mental health is one we would like to break. Only the unfolding story of society will tell whether our wishes can be fulfilled.

The second perspective, related to the importance of history, is the need to use the critical lenses of the *micro and the macro perspectives*. As Jones and Thorne (1987) suggest, reality is experienced at the level of the individual. When we are too far removed from the way individuals experience their world, we are likely to construct theories and policies that apply to no one. On the other hand, large-scale social and ecological events affect us as individuals in important ways. Acknowledging the ubiquitous nature of racism, for example, does not free us from the responsibility of understanding its personal destructiveness and doing what we can to lessen its impact.

Third, among the ways that we can merge our sense of the larger picture with the necessity of keeping ourselves grounded in the reality of the human perspective is to regularly engage in monitoring and counting. *Epidemiology* is a fundamental tool with which we can observe variations and watch changes taking place that should alert us to the need to modify our explanations and intervention strategies. Observing that African Americans continue to receive more diagnoses of schizophrenia than do Whites, for example, requires our attention and attempts at explanation. Likewise, if we believe that there is value in having African Americans available to serve African Americans, personnel trends in the helping professions also require serious attention.

Fourth, we believe in the *centrality of culture* as a force in the lives of individuals and groups. Perhaps the most general way in which racism has affected mental health services for African Americans is the wholesale application of Eurocentric theory and constructions both to treat African Americans who need mental health services and to explain their behavior.

Fifth, as much as anything we have described here, we believe in the importance of *training in mental health*. Here we assert a special meaning: training not only in mental health, but also in non-racist practice and research. We have identified several dilemmas in training: The first dilemma concerns who should be trained to meet the mental health service needs of ethnic minority clients? Although we recognize that service is often most useful when the provider shares the background of the client, we do *not* recommend strict matching of mental health providers with clients. In the foreseeable future there will certainly not be a sufficient supply of African American mental health providers to serve all those in need. African American mental health providers, moreover, should not be expected to limit their work to other African Americans. On the other hand, if an assertion that race makes no difference leads us to avoid striving for diversity in the helping professions, racism will then have prevailed. Our response: increase the numbers of ethnic minorities in the professions and train nonminority professionals to serve a wider range of different populations.

The second dilemma concerns the content of the curriculum: How much are we to emphasize racial, cultural, and other group differences in our training? One danger is that our well-intentioned emphasis on being sensitive to diverse groups will lead us to reinforce stereotypes. Groups and cultures are not static; just as individuals constantly change, so does social ecology. Ethnic behaviors and beliefs shift, both between generations and across individual life spans (Luborsky and Rubenstein 1987). Because those who aspire to help others cannot hope to know the significant cultural elements of all groups they will encounter nor everything important about even one group, the indispensable thing to teach is an attitude, a stance, an open-minded way of approaching the helping process with humility and a willingness to learn.

The third dilemma also concerns the content of the training curriculum: How can we balance the training we offer, so that mental health providers of the future will have generic skills as well as knowledge of group-specific approaches? The helping professions have always experimented with new approaches that hold hope for improved service. Again, what is most necessary is not to memorize the particular "bag of tricks" that happens to be current during one's training, but rather to acquire an attitude about the work one does. Our final degrees should not mean we can continue forever without changing our approaches to meet new problems and serve new populations.

Every culture shapes its members' mentalities. In this culture we are all racists to some extent. We can only hope that most of us devote some of our time to being "in recovery." But just as the recovery from addiction often begins with an acknowledgment of the addiction, recovery from racism requires a stance of reflectiveness about racism. Trainees must begin not with denial but with awareness that racist biases will unavoidably creep into their work. Being alert to this danger can move trainees to challenge and change their own thinking and approaches. These changes apply most palpably with respect to the biases inherent in various psychological tests and in diagnostic processes. They also apply equally to choice of clients and intervention strategies. To be helpful to each individual and group encountered, clinicians must continuously examine and adjust their perspectives and criticize their own biases.

The sixth perspective we advocate is a critical, complex perspective on mental health research dealing with ethnic minority populations. On the one hand, a focused research agenda is desperately needed to understand and respond appropriately to the mental health needs of ethnic minorities. On the other hand, research findings based on majority populations should not be applied uncritically to minority groups. Any researcher working in the field of racism and mental health must be exquisitely alert to the consequences of and responses to his or her research for the particular group under study.

Some commentators fear that emphasis on ethnic groups and cultural awareness threatens to fragment the country. Our answer is direct: a nonracist sensibility honors ethnicity but affirms humanity's oneness along with the worth of each group and individual. Researchers and practitioners, trainers and trainees, scholars and activists, consumers and providers, all can work together to impart to the field of mental health a common concern for racial justice. That would be a priceless contribution toward genuine national integrity.

REFERENCES

Bloombaum, M., Yamamoto, J., and James, Q. 1968. Cultural stereotypes among psychotherapists. *Journal of Consulting and Clinical Psychology* 32:99.

Bogardus, E. 1958. Racial distance changes in the United States during the past thirty years. *Sociology and Social Research* 43:127–35.

Brigham, J., and Weissbach, T., eds. 1972. *Racial attitudes in America: analysis and findings of social psychology*. New York: Harper and Row.

Chase, A. 1977. *The legacy of Malthus: the social costs of the new scientific racism*. New York: Knopf.

Clark, C. X., ed. 1973. The white researcher in black society. *Journal of Social Issues*, 29. Special issue.

Deaux, K. 1984. From individual differences to social categories: analysis of a decade's research on gender. *American Psychologist* 39:105–16.

Dovidio, J. F., and Gaertner, S. L., eds. 1986. *Prejudice, discrimination, and racism*. New York: Academic Press.

Evans, D. A. 1985. Psychotherapy and black patients: problems of training, trainees, and trainers. *Psychotherapy* 22(2):457–60.

Geller, J. D. 1988. Racial bias in the evaluation of patients for psychotherapy. In *Clinical guideliines in cross-cultural mental health*, ed. L. Comas-Diaz, and E. E. H. Griffith. New York: Wiley Interscience.

Griffith, M. S., and Jones, E. E. 1979. Race and psychotherapy: changing perspectives. *Current Psychiatric Therapies* 16:225–35.

Jones, E. E., and Korchin, S. J. 1982. Minority mental health: perspectives. In *Minority mental health*, ed. E. E. Jones and S. J. Korchin. New York: Praeger.

Jones, E. E., and Thorne, A. 1987. Rediscovery of the subject: intercultural approaches to clinical assessment. *Journal of Consulting and Clinical Psychology* 55:488–95.

Jones, J. 1981. *Bad blood: the Tuskegee syphilis experiment*. New York: Free Press.

Kardiner, A., and Ovesey, L. 1951. *The mark of oppression; a psychosocial study of the American Negro*. New York: Norton.

Korchin, S. J. 1980. Clinical psychology and minority problems. *American Psychologist* 35:262–69.

Kovel, J. 1970. *White racism: a psychohistory*. New York: Pantheon.

Lewis, D. O., Balla, D. A., and Shanok, S. S. 1979. Some evidence of race bias in the diagnosis and treatment of the juvenile offender. *American Journal of Orthopsychiatry* 49(1):53–61.

Luborsky, M., and Rubenstein, R. L. 1987. Ethnicity and lifetimes: self-concepts and situational contexts of ethnic identity in late life. In *Ethnic dimensions of aging*, ed. D. E. Gelfand and C. M. Barresi. New York: Springer.

McConahay, J. B. 1986. Modern racism, ambivalence, and the modern racism scale. In *Prejudice, discrimination, and racism*, ed. J. F. Dovidio and S. L. Gaertner. New York: Academic Press.

Manderscheid, R. W., and Sonnenschein, M. A., eds. 1990. *Mental Health, United States, 1990.* National Institute of Mental Health. DHHS Pub. (ADM)90-1708. Washington, D.C.: U.S. Government Printing Office.

Mayo, J. A. 1974. The significance of sociocultural variables in psychiatric treatment of Black outpatients. *Comprehensive Psychiatry* 15:471–82.

Moritsugu, J. N., and Sue, S. 1983. Minority status as a stressor. In *Preventive psychology: theory, research and practice*, ed. R. D. Felner, L. A. Jason, J. N. Muritsugu, and S. S. Farber. New York: Pergamon.

Myers, H. F., Wohlford, P., Guzman, L. P., and Echemendia, J., eds. 1991. *Ethnic minority perspectives on clinical training and services in psychology*. Washington, D.C.: American Psychological Association.

Prudhomme, C., and Musto, D. F. 1973. Historical perspectives on mental health and racism in the United States. In *Racism and mental health*, ed. C. V. Willie, B. M. Kramer, and B. S. Brown. Pittsburgh: University of Pittsburgh Press.

Smith, W. D., Burlew, A. K., Mosley, M. H., and Whitney, W. M. 1978. *Minority issues in mental health*. Reading, Mass.: Addison-Wesley.

Snowden, L., and Todman, P. 1982. The psychological assessment of Blacks: new and needed developments. In *Minority mental health*, ed. E. E. Jones and S. J. Korchin. New York: Praeger.

Snyder, M. 1981. On the self-perpetuating nature of social sterotypes. In *Cognitive processes in stereotyping and intergroup behavior*, ed. D. L. Hamilton. Hillsdale, N.J.: Erlbaum.

Stephan, W. G., and Rosenfield, D. 1982. Racial and ethnic sterotypes. In *In the eye of the beholder: contemporary issues in stereotyping*, ed. A. G. Miller. New York: Praeger.

Stevenson, K. R., and Geller, J. D. 1969. *The effects of race and borderline intelligence on the evaluation of patients for out-patient psychotherapy.* Unpublished manuscript.

Sue, S. 1977. Community mental health services to minority groups: some optimism, some pessimism. *American Psychologist* 32:616–24.

Sue, S., Ito, J., and Bradshaw, C. 1982. Ethnic minority research: trends and directions. In *Minority mental health,* ed. E. E. Jones and S. J. Korchin. New York: Praeger.

Sue, S. McKinney, H., Allen, D., and Hall, J. 1974. Delivery of community mental health services to Black and White clients. *Journal of Consulting and Clinical Psychology* 42:794–801.

Thomas, A., and Sillen, S. 1972. *Racism and psychiatry.* New York: Bruner/Mazel.

Turner, B. F., and Turner, C. B. 1991. Through a glass darkly: psychotherapists' gender stereotypes for women and men varying in age. In *Growing old in America,* ed. B. B. Hess and E. W. Markson. 4th ed. New Brunswick, N.J.: Transaction Books.

Turner, B. F., Turner, C. B., and Ciano-Boyce, C. 1988. The factor structure of psychotherapists' sterotypes of mental health for young, middle-aged, and old men and women. Paper presented at the annual scientific meeting of the Gerontological Society of America, San Francisco.

Turner, C. B., and Turner, B. F. 1992. Who treats minorities? Paper presented at the annual meeting of the Eastern Psychological Association, Boston.

Ward, C. O., Zanna, M. P., and Cooper, J. 1974. The nonverbal mediation of selffulfilling prophesies in interracial interactions. *Journal of Experimental Social Psychology* 10:109–20.

Willie, C. V., Kramer, B. M., and Brown, B. S., eds. 1973. *Racism and mental health.* Pittsburgh: University of Pittsburgh Press.

Wyatt, G. E., and Parham, W. D. 1985. The inclusion of culturally sensitive course materials in graduate school and training programs. *Psychotherapy* 22:461–68.

Yamamoto, J., James, Q. C., Bloombaum, M., and Hattem, J. 1967. Racial factors in patient selection. *American Journal of Psychiatry* 124(5):84–90.

Sexism and Women's
Psychological Status

I N this chapter we shall describe the social and emotional costs of sexism and show how as a routine aspect of daily life sexism intersects with racial and cultural differences to shape women's experience, identity, and psychological well-being. Sexism embodies the inequality that is both a cause and an effect of the prejudicial evaluation of a person based upon sex/gender. As a philosophical concept, it is a gender-neutral term even though in practice it is more often used to describe either the process or consequence of discrimination against women. Sexism has institutional, cultural, interpersonal, and emotional dimensions and can be manifest in every form of behavior from subtle gestures and language to covert exploitation and undemocratic structures that foster and perpetuate gender inequality. Burstow (1992, p. viii) stated it more succinctly: "what is especially insidious and psychologically destructive about sexism is its closeness" and the baffling and disguised ways it enters our homes, our families, and the workplace.

The word *sexism* became part of the American vocabulary in the early 1970s as the feminist movement gained momentum and women joined together in the struggle for equality and self-determination. Although there is an overarching unity to personal experiences of sexism, it is at once a vague and a dynamic term whose meaning and configuration shifts along with changes in women's status and life circumstances. For example, not too many decades ago women fought to gain the right to vote; having gained that fundamental right, the movement shifted its goals and members began to concentrate on the political process of electing women to public office. In 1992, along with the election of Democrat William J. Clinton as president, more women were elected to the U.S.

27

Congress than at any time in its history. In the following year President Clinton appointed an unprecedented number of women to cabinet-level positions, and Ruth Bader Ginsberg—a women's rights advocate— became the second woman to serve on the U.S. Supreme Court.

In spite of these gains, women still remain vastly underrepresented in federal and state legislative bodies when one considers the fact that females slightly outnumber males in the general population. This is unfortunate because women's participation in these policy-making processes not only makes a tangible difference in terms of issues raised but also in terms of the discourse surrounding those issues. The visibility of women in such policy-making roles has far-reaching symbolic value as well because women's roles have changed much more rapidly than has the socialization of females.

By the 1990s, the term *sexism* had all but disappeared from our popular vocabulary, research agenda, and especially in political discourse. Following an extensive literature search we found very few articles and no recent books with the term listed in the title. One explanation for the term's disfavor may have to do with the lack of complexity of earlier arguments and the sweeping claims about how patriarchy and other forms of oppression caused mental illness in women (Chesler 1972). Or perhaps the change is, as Susan Faludi (1991) has written, part of the antifeminist backlash against the progress (minimal by some standards) toward equality that women have made in the public and personal aspects of their lives. Whatever the explanation, the change in rhetoric from the 1970s to the 1990s was dramatic. *Sexism,* always a provocative term, was deconstructed and defused into specific, more neutral topics that allowed scholars from varied disciplines to examine more systematically the complex intricacies of women's lives and experiences.

In academic settings, the new knowledge and understanding of women's lives and psychological development were incorporated into academic programs such as women's studies, centers for cultural and literary analysis, or gender study institutes that promoted sex role reseach, among other relevant topics. However, with this significant development in academia, a parallel semantic shift occurred in which we believe a crucial aspect of the meaning of sexism was transformed as well. As legal barriers diminished and increasing numbers of women entered male-dominated occupations and professions across the status spectrum (that is, medicine, law, and manual skill trades, and so on), intellectual interest in women's inequality and powerlessness understandably became redirected to topics such as women's nature, women's history, and women's health. One explanation for the redirection is provided by Mednick (1989), for example, who contends that attempts to bring about change in the structure of gender inequality became so frustrating and difficult that it was more acceptable to focus on women's essential nature and psychological development. Communities of scholars and activists began to examine women's nature—and expand upon what were generally understood to be essential differences between women and men—rather than focus on political and social inequality (Tavris 1992; Hare-Mustin and Marecek 1990); Mednick 1989; Westkott 1989, 1990).

In 1970, Broverman and associates found that clinicians associated psychological maturity and health with stereotypical masculine characteristics, and psychological immaturity and pathology with traditional feminine characteristics. One feminist agenda ever since has been to expose the cultural context of pervasive sexism deeply rooted in these widespread beliefs. The critical work of Jean Baker Miller (1976), Nancy Chodorow (1978), Carol Gilligan (1979, 1982) and others challenged the presumed "universal" models of psychological functioning by exposing their inherent male bias and by giving new value and importance to traditionally female characteristics. In an interesting review of nine current books that reconsider women's psychological development, Grosskurth (1991) argues that the new narrative accounts by contemporary feminists of the process of growing up female are really accounts of how an idealized woman would emerge if only conditions in the family were different, that is if gender equality was the norm. Thus even feminist reformulations cannot entirely escape the residual effects of culturally transmitted gender myths.

To refute culturally embedded assumptions that women's inherent traits were deficiencies or weaknesses, feminist writers reinterpreted gender differences to argue that previously denigrated qualities were actually often valuable strengths. Two influential examples of this reformulation are Carol Gilligan's (1982) work on the centrality of relationships and concern for others in women's moral reasoning and Jean Baker Miller's and associates' (Jordan et al. 1991) theories about the importance of relational bonds for women's psychological development and evolving senses of womanhood. Whereas this alternative conception has had positive impacts on women's sense of self-worth and sisterhood, it also has had some negative consequences. Paradoxically, the new formulation of women's psychological development has had the unintended effect of creating an "ideology of implied female superiority" (Grosskurth 1991) that does little to counter existing beliefs about polarized stereotypes. Such formulations also focus attention on internal psychological processes in ways that can obscure the social and political sexism that is a byproduct of inequality.

We believe mental health theories and practices that ignore or deflect attention away from social realities and contexts cannot be trusted, or expected to be gender neutral. In a recent article, Marecek and Hare-Mustin (1991) have provided an interesting analysis of what a feminist clinical psychology would be like that takes account of power as well as gender. In writing about the link between sexism and mental health, we intend to reemphasize the social and political context of sexism—to show that exaggerated gender differences are a by-product of social inequality—and to examine the effects of inequality and powerlessness on women's social identity and emotional processes.

In this essay, we shall address how sexism is reproduced in language and made manifest through various types of behavior such as sexual harassment, interpersonal violence, sexual abuse, or poverty, and how these sexist realities, in turn, contribute to psychological distress or disorder. Women's lived experiences and their silences will be explored through analysis of gendered social roles. We will also discuss intersections of race and sex and how the Anita Hill case exemplifies and caricatures this dynamic.

Sexism and Essential Difference Philosophy

Gender inequality is based on the essentialist assumption "that the physical differences between females and males are so significant that they should determine virtually all social and economic roles of men and women" (Hare-Mustin and Marecek 1990). From this perspective, men and women are understood to be not ony different, but also opposites who embody mutually exclusive traits. Gender-restricted social roles, a pattern that characterizes the history of human relationships, rests on the philosophical and "scientific" belief that women are essentially different from men. Measured against male experience and maleness as the implicit standard, women as the "other sex" are different and thus assumed to be substandard or inferior (Tavris 1992). The invisibility and pervasiveness of this normative misperception and the "naturalness" of the social inequities that follow help to explain how sexism has come to be embedded in both the culture and in the psyches of men and women.

Female gender role socialization, which explains the process of how women learn sex-appropriate behavior and develop an identity as the "other sex," is one of the pathways through which sexism is perpetuated and transmitted across cultures and generations. Unfortunately, the socially learned attitudes and behaviors are often misperceived to be women's essential qualities instead of being understood as the products of social norms that implicitly and subtly devalue women. According to the social philosophy of essentialism, there is a universal female essence that

Anita Hill–Clarence Thomas Case Example

In October 1991, the U.S. Senate Judiciary Committee held confirmation hearings for the nomination of Clarence Thomas to the U.S. Supreme Court. Thomas—a lawyer, a judge, and the second African American man ever to be nominated for this important judicial position—was to fill the seat vacated by civil rights advocate Thurgood Marshall. Nominated by former president George Bush and a conservative himself, Thomas gained his greatest support from the Republican party. From the beginning, the Black community was split over whether to support Thomas's confirmation. During the controversy-marked hearings, Anita Hill—a conservative African American law professor—came forward to allege that she had been sexually harassed by Clarence Thomas when she worked for him, both at the Department of Education and at the Equal Employment Opportunity Commission (EEOC), a decade earlier. She formally testified against the nominee's confirmation before the Senate Judiciary Committee in what became known as the "Thomas-Hill hearings."

Hill accused Thomas of making lewd remarks and pressuring her to become sexually involved with him while she worked for him. Thomas vehemently denied the allegation, and in one of the most dramatic moments near the end of the hearings, he accused Hill and the Senate Judiciary Committee of engaging in a "high tech lynching." Thomas finally prevailed and was eventually confirmed by a committee comprised entirely of White male senators.

The hearings were broadcast nationally on television and generated extensive controversy across the United States and among diverse communities and constituencies. Causes of the controversy were broadly based: some Americans were apprehensive about Thomas's conservative legal philosophy; questions about what specifically constitutes sexual harassment were raised; there were debates over whose claims were to be believed, Hill's or Thomas's; and the hearing proceedings made apparent the paucity of women and minorities in the U.S. Congress (among other organizations). Hill continues to hold her appointment as professor of law at Oklahoma University. In June 1993, the University of Oklahoma Regents proposed a law professorship in her name. The Anita Faye Hill Professorship of Law establishes an endowed chair dedicated to long-range studies of workplace equality.

For insight into the complicated events that surrounded the confirmation hearings, a volume of essays written by African American scholars and writers, both men and women, was collected, with an introduction by the novelist Toni Morrison. We highly recommend the book, *Race-ing Justice, En-gendering Power: Essays on Anita Hill, Clarence Thomas, and the Construction of Social Reality,* for anyone who wants to understand the intersection of race and gender in this watershed event. (See especially the essay by Kimberle Crenshaw, "Whose story is it anyway? Feminist and antiracist appropriations of Anita Hill.")

determines women's behavior. For example, in popular psychology, this essence has been represented by some Jungian psychotherapists as a goddess who dwells in every woman (Bolen, 1984). As a result of such premises, individual differences among women of race, class, and ethnicity are minimized, and women are often mischaracterized as a homogenous group.

Essentialist philosophy, with its emphasis on internal traits or states, in effect ignores the gender power imbalance and functions to decontextualize and depoliticize gender inequities. From our perspective the qualities that are assumed uncritically to be women's inherent traits or characteristic of women's voices can be understood more accurately as acquired, developmental qualities associated with their subordinate status and powerlessness (Miller 1976; Tavris 1992; Marecek and Hare-Mustin 1991). Our concern is that essential difference premises and the polarized stereotypes that evolve from them are consciously misused to justify a restricted division of labor in which men as dominants are entitled to highly valued positions of power and authority and women as subordinates are relegated to undervalued roles of service to and care for others.

Both Tavris (1992) and Hare-Mustin and Marecek (1990) have argued that cultural assumptions about essential gender differences, which can be found in most psychodynamic theories and research, not only mask inequality and conflict between men and women but, in a complex dialectic, may even preserve the staus quo. For example, Jean Hamilton (this volume) demonstrates how even in science, such assumptions pervaded the rationales for sex-biased practices and paradigms in psychopharmacology research that have had ramifications for drug testing studies and treatment of mental illness in both women and men.

Tavris (1992) and Hare-Mustin and Marecek (1990) also discuss how this thinking has exaggerated the number, extent, and depth of differences between and among men and women and minimized the similarities between them. The tendency to exaggerate difference can be found in explanations of women's development whether they view the female nature as *deficient* (for example, Seligman's [1991] claim that women's excess depression rate results from attitudinal pessimism, an inherent personality trait) or *superior* (for example, as in J. V. Jordan and associates [1991], who glorify traditional feminine characteristics by suggesting that qualities such as caring, expressiveness, and concern for relationships will form the basis for human regeneration and public morality). While we have oversimplified these complex works to make the point, in a critique of Jordan et al.'s (1991) self-in-relation theory, Westkott (1990) contends that the theory is abstracted from the wider culture of patriarchy without proper recognition of its influence and, further, that the idealized qualities of care and relationship are themselves informed by patriarchal meanings and purposes. Moreover, as Hare-Mustin and Marecek have noted, the "energies of feminists are deflected from questions of their own choosing in order to counter exaggerated claims of difference, refute claims of female deficiency, and oppose policies and practices based on those claims" (1990, 13).

The Interplay of Racism and Sexism: The Hill-Thomas Example

We are asserting here that essentialist philosophy constructs a framework for representing women and men as a dichotomy where implicitly men are the standard for normalcy and women are the deficient other. And further, that beliefs about gender polarities are fundamental both to gender role socialization and to sexism. What sexist and racist attitudes and behavior have in common, then, is the subconscious belief that the "other" is essentially different and, therefore, inferior to oneself. Essentialist claims are sometimes reversed when those who represent the other redefine the devalued characteristics. For both female and racial or ethnic communities (or any other subcultural minority), the rhetorical reversal functions to reinforce group solidarity through the affirmation of an elevated identity based upon a reconstructed sense of self. The natural dynamic of wanting to maintain group cohesiveness or to behave in ideologically correct and strategic ways makes it difficult for Black women (or any other woman in a devalued cultural minority) to fully address abusive behavior of Black or other men, or to expose any internal conflict that might contribute to negative racial and cultural stereotypes. As Crenshaw (1992, 420) notes, "this 'code of silence' is experienced by African Americans as a self-imposed gesture of racial solidarity." The same dynamic functions to silence women in other cultural minorities as well (such as Asian, Latina or Hispanic, Italian, and so on).

The Anita Hill–Clarence Thomas hearings provide a vivid example of overlapping margins of a contemporary race and gender discourse—a discourse that underlies the chapters in this book. In analyzing the dilemmas faced by Anita Hill, for instance, Crenshaw (1992) contends that sexism has been subordinated to the struggle against racism, that Black women are marginalized in ways that limit the development of narratives to convey their experiences, and that the complexities of racism present Black women with many particularities that are unfamiliar to White women. As one example, the self-imposed code of silence has coercive elements that only become visible when someone breaks the code. (The same dynamic occurs in abusive or incestuous families when abused children are coerced into silence about their pain and suffering by a loyalty oath never to reveal secrets that will harm the family [Rieker and Carmen 1986]). Crenshaw believes that the coverage in the American Black press illustrates both the subordination of women and the coercive element as Anita Hill was portrayed as a traitor (just as abused women and children are) for coming forward with her story. "Less interested," says Crenshaw, "in whether the story was true, most commentators speculated on why Hill would jeopardize the upward mobility of a Black man and seek to embarrass the African American Community" (1992, 420).

As evidence for her assertion, Crenshaw summarizes a *New York Times* article (October 20, 1991) by Harvard sociologist Orlando Patterson to illustrate how "he deployed race to normatively embrace Thomas's behavior and to ostracize Anita Hill for having been offended by Thomas's language and behavior" (421). Patterson argued that Thomas's sexual taunting of Anita Hill was defensible as a "down-home style of courting," which Black women (whom he seems to have assumed are all alike) are accustomed to and apparently find flattering. Patterson concludes "that in this case perjury was a justifiable means toward winning a seat on the highest court of the land because white America could never understand that such sexual repartee was in fact common among black men and women" (Patterson cited in Crenshaw 1992, 422).

By labeling Hill's reaction to Thomas's "flirtations" as disingenuous, Crenshaw believes that Patterson implies either that Hill was not, in fact, emotionally injured by Thomas's barrage of sexual innuendo or that if she was, she was influenced to reinterpret her experience through the lens of middle-class White feminism. Thus she is denied her Black identity because in speaking out against the behavior of a Black man she broke the bond of racial solidarity. Indeed, Patterson suggests that the harassment may have actually served to affirm their common origins. "This pattern of 'bonding' is apparently so readily acceptable that any black woman who is offended or injured by it must be acting on a white feminist impulse rather than a culturally grounded black female sensibility" (ibid., 423). With her analysis Crenshaw intends to show that Anita Hill's main disadvantage was that she lacked a widely understood narrative— because she was subject to both racial and sexual stereotypes—to communicate the reality of her negative experience as a Black woman to the world. This example illustrates how racism can be used to negate sexism and sexism to negate racism and the confusion that follows.

In talking about sexual harassment, Crenshaw goes on to note that Patterson's argument rests initially on a failure to draw any distinction between sexual practices that occur privately and those that occur within the work environment, as well as a refusal to understand the power imbalance that shapes those sexual practices in the first place. Moreover,

Black and White women share the burden of overcoming assumptions that sexual harassment in the workplace is essentially a "private" issue. "Silence," she writes, "contributes to some degree of confusion where the boundaries between desired camaraderie and unwanted intimacy exists" (ibid., 427). However this confusion does not account for the occasions when men (Black or White) intentionally use and abuse power over women. From our perspective the confusion is created by the refusal to see how power itself defines such boundaries. It was this *misuse of power* that Crenshaw asserts was consistently misinterpreted or deliberately mischaracterized during the hearings. Sexual harassment is an expression of hostility and one of the many microaggressive acts described by Pierce (this volume), which women and other minorities endure, usually in silence, on a routine basis.

According to Crenshaw, the subordination of gender to race helps to explain why Thomas was, in effect, justified and Anita Hill vilified by some of the Black community. The experiences of Black men provide the representation of all racial domination; this is captured in the near universal understanding of the "lynching metaphor." Female narratives of racism have been marginalized in a way that limited the means available to Anita Hill to convey her experience as a Black woman. Thomas, in contrast, had a powerful and well-understood representation and constituency to call upon when he referred to the congressional hearing as a "high-tech lynching." Thus, "her racial identity became irrelevant in explaining or understanding her position, while Thomas's play on the lynching metaphor racially empowered him" (Crenshaw 1992, 416).

Racial solidarity is demanded of all Blacks; however, the representations of racial inequality are actually of inequality between men. Thus, the racial alliance between Black men and women necessarily means subordination of women's struggle for sexual equality. However, Crenshaw also believes that the dominant or generally understood representation of sexual harassment is of White women. It is in this sense that she maintains that Black women are oppressed in numerous subtle and overt ways.

There are race-specific points to consider in analyzing sexual harassment and other forms of sexual abuse of Black women. (Just as ethnicity and the cultural fabric would be relevant in considering the abuse of other minority women.) Historically, Black women have been portrayed as lustful, sexually insatiable, and of questionable integrity and veracity (Giddings 1992). Black women, according to Crenshaw, have always been characterized as "fallen" women. White female sexual abuse victims have had to suffer the consequences of the polarized madonna/whore stereotype, whereas Black women have nearly always been denied the madonna image. Thus the sexual exploitation of Black women is often not acknowledged as victimization, whether perpetrated by Black or White men. Black women are supposed to like violent sex and are stereotypically portrayed as being tougher than White women. Patterson (1991) explains that because the common response of Black women to sexual harassment is humor and wit, they are not threatened or disturbed by it and may even enjoy those types of behavior. But given the dynamics of sexual stereotypes and women's subordinate status, such reactions (humor and wit) are probably the only calculatedly safe responses available to Black women. As Crenshaw poignantly asks, "After all, to what authority can women who have been consistently represented as sexually available appeal?" (1992, 429). When viewed from this perspective, Anita Hill's ten years of silence about her harassment not only become more comprehensible, but also highlight the social and emotional costs of women's restricted roles and silences (which are issues we shall elaborate in a subsequent section).

Restrictive Gender Roles, Social Status, and Psychological Distress

Nancy Tomes (1992) provides a historical analysis of the social patterns of women's emotional distress and mental illnesses that explores more deeply the "psychic costs of restrictive gender roles." After addressing the complexity of the link between gender and mental illness, she discusses the differences in mental disorders between women and men and reviews societal perceptions about women and their "nervous" symptoms. Based upon archival records from the nineteenth century—a century in which women are reported to have suffered more physical and mental disabilities than previous centuries—Tomes proposes the following thesis: women's discontent with gender role restrictions was expressed through "symptoms," which they and members of the newly emerging profession of medicine interpreted as illness or disorder. Illness, she asserts, functioned metaphorically as a "desperate communication of the powerless" and as an implicit yet direct escape from the emotional and sexual demands so prevalent in women's lives.

Women, then, were more likely to label their distress (that is, discontent) as symptoms of illness, whereas men who expressed their distress as alcoholism or through violence were perceived as fundamentally "bad." "Thus the historical record supports the argument that sex-role socialization may have predisposed men and women to gender specific reasons for and modes of expressing psychological distress" (Tomes 1992, 151–52). Carmen, Rieker, and Mills (1984) found a similar pattern of gender differences in the expression of distress in their study of the psychological consequences of physical and sexual abuse. The psychological trauma was the same, but women became self-destructive and disordered whereas men became violent toward others. Tomes concludes that even though the specifics of gender role socialization have changed throughout history, as have other social realities for women, the devaluation and powerlessness of women have remained unchanged. Her analysis and others (for example, Mirowsky and Ross 1989) suggest that a fundamental link exists across time between the experience of powerlessness and women's emotional distress. Thus it is not just gender or race per se but the demonstrable, objective lack of power and resources and the consequences that follow from that condition which produce distress.

Tomes (1992) also challenges prevalent misconceptions regarding the gender differences in rates and types of mental illness and psychological distress. In contrast to the representation of reality in literary texts where insanity was portrayed as a female malady (see Gilbert and Gubar 1979; Showalter 1985), empirical data from the nineteenth century to 1980 indicate that women have not outnumbered men in psychiatric hospital admissions and do not suffer from severe mental illness in greater numbers than do men. Available data indicate that women do report more emotional distress, anxiety, and depression than do men. According to Tomes (1992) these are also the disorders most poorly defined and most sensitive to cultural and social influences. Women are more likely to seek outpatient and office-based services of all kinds and more likely than men to receive drug treatment. Women outnumber men 2 to 1 in the incidence of some types of depression (see Hamilton, this volume). Men outnumber women in rates of alcoholism, drug abuse, and personality disorders that involve anti-social and violent behavior.

My own analysis (Rieker 1993) of current figures from the National Institute of Mental Health (NIMH) supports Tomes's assertions. For example, in 1986, the NIMH Division of Biometry and Applied Sciences surveyed a sample of persons admitted to, discharged from, and receiving continuing treatment in the inpatient, outpatient, and partial care programs. National estimates of the population under care at the beginning of the survey period on April 1, 1986, show that approximately 1.7 million persons were under care and 3.9 million persons were admitted during that year. The majority of patients were concentrated in outpatient programs (Manderscheid and Sonnenschein 1990).

The distribution of new inpatient admissions by sex, race, and type of facility for 1986 shows that males represented a larger percentage of admissions than did females (57 percent to 43 percent). This pattern was true for persons of color and Hispanic patients as well. Except for private psychiatric hospitals, where more females are admitted, males also accounted for significantly higher percentages (and particularly for Black males) of inpatient admissions across all types of facilities. This pattern was the same for prevalence rates, that is, patients already receiving inpatient care. Total admissions for people of color were higher in state and county mental hospitals and VA medical centers than in private psychiatric hospitals. For all inpatient programs combined, the inpatient admission rate for males was higher than for females (790 versus 551 per 100,000 civilian population), and the admission rate for other races was almost twice the rate for Whites (1,074 versus 594 per 100,000 civilian population) (Rieker 1993, based on Rosenstein et al. 1990, as cited in Manderscheid and Sonnenschein 1990).

In terms of admissions to outpatient psychiatric services, males and females were almost equally represented (52 percent to 48 percent). However, in contrast to the inpatient admissions, 85 percent were White and 15 percent other races. Only 8 percent of the people of color population were treated in private psychiatric hospitals. Clearly gender, race, and income affect where and how patients receive treatment for psychological problems. The most frequently occurring diagnoses among inpatient admissions were affective disorders (31 percent), schizophrenia (23 percent), and alcohol-related disorders (15 percent). Patients with affective disorders (mood disturbances, such as depression, mania, and so on) were more likely to be treated at private psychiatric and general hospitals (48 percent and 37 percent) than at other inpatient facilities. Schizophrenia was more common among admissions to state and county mental hospitals, multi-service mental health organizations, and VA medical centers. Alcohol-related disorders were particularly high among admissions to VA medical centers (32 percent versus only 8–16 percent in other organizational settings). VA hospitals are most likely to treat men (Rosenstein et al. 1990).

Even though men have higher rates of admissions to non-private treatment settings, Russo (this volume) shows that women report more psychological distress on surveys in the community. Community surveys conducted by the highly respected and reliable NIMH Epidemiological Catchment Area (ECA) Program have found women to have higher rates of depressive disorders (major depressive disorders), anxiety disorders (simple phobia, agoraphobia, panic disorder, obsessive-compulsive disorder), schizophrenia, and somatization disorders. In contrast, men have higher rates of alcohol abuse or dependence, antisocial personality, and drug abuse or dependence. Unfortunately, as Russo points out, these significant studies did not report their findings separately by gender within ethnic or minority groups.

These data raise many questions about how to explain the gender differences in rates of mental disorder and psychological distress. For example, why are women more likely to express their distress through depression and men through alcohol, drugs, and violence? As Russo indicates, variation in rates of mental disorder by marital status suggests a need to think not only about social roles that men and women fill but also about the experience within those roles. For example, married women have higher admission rates to mental health facilities than married men; in contrast, never married and separated or divorced men had higher admission rates than comparable women. This gender difference in relationship between marital status and admission rates has been found for both Blacks and Whites (Russo, this volume). In fact, depressive disorders represent the leading diagnosis for women regardless of race. According to Russo, it is likely that the overall gender difference in rates of mental illness is accounted for by the gender difference in rates of depression. Consequently, therapists need to delve into the specific experiences that women have in their social roles to identify the particular aspects (powerlessness or devaluation, for example) that may lead to depression.

The difference in rates of disorder between married and unmarried women depends on the quality of the marriage, with quality determined by the sharing of domestic responsibility and child care and decision making, in addition to other values. Wives in unhappy marriages experience more depressive symptoms than happily married or never married women (Weissman 1987, as cited in Russo, this volume). Using ECA data, Weissman reported that wives in unhappy marriages were three times more likely than husbands to be depressed. The depression rates for both sexes were lower in happy marriages, but the gap was larger; wives in happy marriages were nearly five times more likely to experience depression than husbands in such marriages.

Some authors have suggested that women's higher rates of depression, particularly for unhappily married wives, reflect the burdens of childbearing and child rearing (Gator, Dean, and Morris 1989), rather than the specific restrictions of the marital role (Russo and Green 1992). Although a greater number of children has been found to negatively affect women's self-esteem, even when marital status, education, income, and employment are controlled, the relationship between children and women's mental health remains unresolved (Russo, this volume). These findings underscore the importance of building a reliable epidemiological portrait of mental disorder that will clearly identify the interactive relationships among gender, race, ethnic group, and marital and parental roles (Russo, this volume; Mirowsky and Ross 1989). In the meantime, to have an adequate understanding of women patients, therapists have to obtain information about the subtle alienation and stresses that women experience, but may not always recognize, as they enact their roles as wives and parents.

To summarize, these figures illustrate that more men than women are admitted for inpatient treatment, and that men are more likely to be treated in non-private psychiatric settings. This pattern holds for Whites and minority populations. Men outnumber women in rates of alcoholism, drug abuse, and personality disorders that involve antisocial and violent behaviors. Women have higher rates of anxiety and depression than do men and seek more outpatient and private, office-based counseling services. Married women have higher admission rates to mental health facilities than do married men, whereas the reverse is true for never married or divorced women.

The Connection Between Sexism, Poverty, and Psychological Distress

Poverty and violence continue to be two central components of the social context of women's mental health. According to Bassuk (1993a, 339), the dramatic increase of homeless women (from 3 percent in 1950 to 20 percent in 1993) reflects the vast increase of American families headed by women and the economic hardships associated with single parent households. Female-headed families rose from 5.5 million in 1970 to 9.9 million in 1984, representing 26 percent of all families with minor children (Sidel 1986, cited in Bassuk 1993b). Over the past two decades and more, women have accounted for the increasing numbers of people living below the poverty line. This phenomenon has been referred to as the feminization of poverty and has been argued to be, in part, a direct result of institutional sexism. More single mothers receive no child support; there is an increase in out-of-wedlock births; women are overrepresented in low-paying, low-status occupations; and there is a lack of adequate affordable child care, making it impossible for large numbers of mothers to work at all. Bassuk (this volume) provides a vivid portrait of the link between poverty, violence, sexual exploitation, and mental illness in homeless families, which not surprisingly consist mainly of women and children. Bassuk and Weinreb (1993) also describe the adverse intergenerational outcomes that follow homeless pregnant women. And Carmen (this volume) elaborates on that portrait to show how the same factors intersect with race in chronic mentally ill women. In fact, Carmen's clinical case examples demonstrate how an understanding of the powerlessness and alienation produced by these social realities can become an effective therapeutic strategy for assisting these women in their struggle to function in the face of persistent vulnerability.

Poverty continues to be a problem for all women, but especially for minority women (Belle 1982, 1988). These women tend to be living in more extreme poverty and for longer periods of time than comparison White populations. Persistent rather than temporary poverty is common among single mothers and even more among women of color. Minority women also may face other chronic stresses associated with poverty including being "ghettoized in 'dilapidated territorial enclaves that epitomize acute social and economic marginalization'" (Belle 1990, 385). Women at all levels of society are marginalized, and lack of material resources makes it doubly difficult for them to overcome the social and psychological barriers that help to keep some women poor.

It is well known by now that poverty is correlated with psychological distress and mental illness. Available data also indicate there is a consistent relationship between financial strain and depression in women. A longitudinal study by Kaplan, Roberts, Camacho, and Coyne (1987) found that insufficient finances were associated with an elevated risk of depressive symptoms over a nine-year period. A study by Hall, Williams, and Greenberg (1985) of depressive symptoms in low-income mothers of young children found significant symptomatology in almost half the women. In that study, low income, unemployment, and single parent status were positively correlated with the magnitude and extent of depressive symptoms.

The term *poverty* incorporates and signifies much more than just insufficient income or financial problems. It is associated also with other chronic stressful conditions, including parenting and child-care problems, unemployment, inadequate and dangerous living conditions, homelessness, and dependence on public assistance. Ultimately, these women feel they have little control over their lives or their future. Poverty also can undermine the quality of an individual's social support network which compounds the stressors already discussed. Social relations are often strained when there are financial problems, and social networks themselves can sometimes be more stressful than supportive. Riley and Eckenrode (1986) found that large social networks of poor women and women with little education tended to be sources of stress rather than support as demands for care exceeded women's ability to respond. Chronic, stressful conditions and a diminished support system are the typical, recurrent characteristics of poor women with depression. Both Bassuk and Carmen (this volume) provide a graphic demonstration of this complex dynamic in homeless and chronic mentally ill women. According to Belle (1988), income is related to depression indirectly as it produces other stressors and erodes support networks, which in turn affects women's distress levels.

Caretaking and Psychological Processes

Gender role socialization is an ever-changing process that varies across time, culture, race, and class. However, the unchanging cross-cultural commonality for women is socialization to a subordinate status and responsibility for the care of others. This fundamental gender role restriction manifests itself in the form of expectations about the way that women should behave in most social roles. Although the nurturant or caretaking element of female socialization may be a more relevant aspect of certain roles (such as parent or spouse) more than others, it has come to be seen as an involuntary, predictable part of a woman's behavior in both the home and the workplace.

Caretaking involves strong demands, both externally imposed and internalized by women, as a mandate to be aware of and meet the needs of others. For example, Marge DeVault's (1991) analysis of the skills, strategies, and organizational abilities that women employ as part of the daily task of caring for and feeding the family suggests that these activities are a central ritual in the production and maintenance of family life. Producing meals requires coordination, management, preparation, and interpersonal skills. Moreover, the ability to perceive and manage the diverse needs of others—even when they themselves are unaware of such needs—leaves women in a constant state of planning and apprehension. According to DeVault, the repetitiveness of the work can be deceiving, so much so that those who do the work barely appreciate how much they do. The skills that women use involve complex planning and coordination, but the mental work often is invisible to women themselves and to family members. Women, Devault concludes, develop a compelling sense that care for others is their permanent duty; thus commitment to the work of caretaking has become a "natural" part of women's sense of self.

Not surprisingly, studies show that women are named significantly more often than men as confidantes, companions, and counselors by both women and men (Fisher 1982, cited in McGrath et al. 1990). Women provide almost all of the care for children and elderly relatives (Brody and Schoonover 1986, cited in McGrath et al.). The stress of caring for an aging parent is likely to increase the risk of depression (Jarvik and Small 1988). Dychtwald and Flower (1989) found that approximately 80 percent of older Americans receive care from their families. The typical American woman will spend more years caring for parents than for children. The average age of these "women in the middle" is 57 years, the decade when women anticipate some freedom from caretaking responsibilities.

A complex relationship, then, exists between caretaking and women's mental health. Research indicates that involvement in roles that maintain social connections with others also has positive benefits for women's mental health. Much satisfaction and mutual benefit grow out of intimate relationships with others, and such activities constitute a large part of women's lives. However, women's relationships and the associated care-taking requirements also can be great sources of strain; too many ties and too few are both identified as risk factors for psychological distress (McGrath et al. 1990). The psychological and physical demands of care-taking often leave women with their own needs unrecognized, unmet, and even unfelt (DeVault 1991). Moreover, women traditionally have been at higher risk than men for feeling the stress of others, especially those for whom they feel responsible (McGrath et al. 1990). As Russo (this volume) points out, women are different from men in the way they respond to crises in their interpersonal network and this may reflect the cost of subordination as well as a cost of caring.

Silence of the Self and Psychological Distress

One of the most complex and vexing questions is: Why do women who are in situations or relationships where they are harassed, abused, or humiliated remain silent about their pain and distress and why do they not leave the job or relationship? In the case of Anita Hill, many people wanted to know why she waited ten years to reveal the abusive event and why she remained in contact with the person she accused of harassing her. Hill's silence—and the silence of victimized women gener-ally—can best be understood as one of the psychosocial consequences of powerlessness and gender inequality. Crenshaw (1992) claims that the doubting of Anita Hill by Black women and men (with many exceptions) across a political and class spectrum provides a telling testament of the extent to which gender conflicts are suppressed by the desire for racial solidarity. Among the most painful of the lessons to be drawn from the Thomas versus Hill confrontation is that feminism must be recast in order to reach women who do not see gender as relevant to an understanding of their own disempowerment.

Silence is one of the most central elements of the social context for understanding the connection between psychological distress (or psycho-logical disorders) and sexism. We use the term *silence* to refer to the actual loss of voice, and metaphorically to the silencing or loss of the self. As Dana C. Jack puts it, "Voice is an indicator of self" (1991, 3). In her book, Jack (1991) acknowledges women's exclusion from social and economic power, and she writes about the process of the silence of the self and its relation to depression. She believes that women become silenced through a combination of inequities within their social context, conflicting demands of adulthood, and cultural imperatives that require women to sacrifice the fulfillment of their own needs for the benefit of others. Loss of self is a process of self-betrayal that can eventually result in depression.

Central to the process of silencing of the self is a gender imperative to internally subordinate or "sacrifice" oneself for the growth and prosperity of others. Harriet Lerner (1974) contends that the practice of sacrifice of the self can be understood only in the context of the pervasive devaluation of women. All women are socialized to believe that they will achieve the most important goals of intimacy and self-growth by giving to and bolstering the egos of others. Women give the "gift" of themselves to those they love; the gift is the giving up of self so that the other may gain in self (Lerner 1984, 1987). Unfortunately, this process of "de-selfing" often results in exactly the opposite of what women were striving for; instead of connection, it results in loss of self (or self-betrayal) and interpersonal distance.

It is the internalization of a devalued and sacrificing self that forms the basis for women's low self-worth, their self-alienation, vulnerability to victimization, and silence. "To be willing to risk arguments and explore difference, one has to believe in the legitimacy of one's point of view" (Jack 1991, 33). One consequence of this internalized cultural imperative is that women believe that their needs are not as important or do not have as much value as those of others. This belief is acquired from a culture that does not value women's needs as highly as men's. "Women both silence themselves and are silenced by the social context within which they live" (Jack 1987, 180).

Jack identifies three kinds of fears that may lead a woman to silence herself. (1) a threat of annihilation of herself and/or her children; (2) a feeling that she is unlovable; and (3) thinking that her feelings and perceptions are wrong or that her credibility will be questioned. As Jack says, to silence one's self can be a way to stay "safe" (1991, 182). Silencing the self is an act of protecting one's self when some potential threat is perceived or when the woman fears she will not be heard or understood. For example, it might occur in situations where a woman has been, or is fearful of being, devalued or attacked. She sacrifices her expression and defense of herself—her feelings, opinions, and beliefs—because she is afraid of not being understood or of being retaliated against. Such hidden, defensive responses may occur in marital and other relationships, in the workplace, and even in therapy. She may feel hopeless and frustrated because she fears she will not be listened to or validated for the person that she is.

Open conflict and anger are not as available for women as they are for men, in large part because of their relative inequality and the socialization that follows (Lerner 1985). In her pathbreaking book *Toward a New Psychology of Women* (1976) Jean Baker Miller has explained the qualities that dominants (men) and subordinates (women) acquire by virtue of their unequal status. Dominants have more freedom to communicate anger directly than do subordinates, whose survival depends on pleasing those in positions of power. Expressing anger is an act of asserting power. Women often respond to a male partner's, a boss's, or men's anger with fear (Jack 1991, 42). If a woman feels "unsafe," figuratively or literally, often she may shut down the capacity for expression in order to protect herself. Jack has preliminary data from 140 depressed women living at three different battered women's shelters that support this understanding of silence as a fear reaction. Her data indicate a relationship between depression and women's being silenced by an abusive partner as measured by her "Silence of the Self Scale."

Both the ability to express oneself and to be understood and validated are critical to mental health. Jack and others believe that it is through the mechanism and function of voice that women are able to get beyond the barrier of silence. She understands voice as an indicator of self and dialogue as a metaphor for movement out of despair (Jack 1991, 190). Self-expression requires women to believe in their point of view, to be taken seriously, and to feel affirmed. Having voice that is validated and understood is critical to insuring personal and social identity.

Is there a way for the debilitating, dehumanizing experience of silence of the self to be reversed or eliminated? Silence accounts not only for women's loss of voice but also for inadequate narratives for communicating their experience. The behavioral manifestations of loss of self are sometimes misjudged by women and others as passiveness, masochism, deception, or lack of agency. When Anita Hill regained the use of her voice, she spoke out metaphorically for all women against sexual exploitation. Her actions provided a context for understanding the contemporary meaning of sexism and racism. Women all across the United States connected her actions with the power of speaking out. Hill demonstrated that she could prevail, that she could survive the ostracism, dissention, and conflict with her racial community, though not without the emotional consequences that follow from public complaints of sexual harrassment or sexism (Hamilton et al. 1987). Two powerful statements of self-determination by African American women appeared in the *New York Times* on November 17, 1991. One was an article in the *New York Times Magazine Section* by Rosemary L. Bray, "Taking Sides Against Ourselves," the other was an ad signed by 1,603 women titled "African American Women in Defense of Ourselves." Both statements in essence testified to the conflicting loyalties to race and gender that Black women experience, and they both affirmed that Black women will speak for themselves about social injustice regardless of the color of the oppressor.

Little did Anita Hill or anyone else know that her courageous step would set in motion the election of more women (and the first African American woman elected to the U.S. Senate, Carol Mosley Braun from Illinois) to state and federal legislatures than at any time in the history of the United States. Women's understanding of Hill's experience helped to unify them, and their common understanding was expressed through the votes they cast in 1992. The hearing also generated more complaints of sexual harassment than ever before. Such positive developments do not mean that the struggle for equality is by any measure over. But it does mean that women have acquired a new metaphor and perhaps a narrative for conveying the experience of sexism.

However, the lessons of Anita Hill's experience and the ground gained for women's equality and mental health by old and new feminist agendas will be lost if therapists do not continue to find ways to address the social and political context of sexism in their practices, theories, and training. Women's elevated rates of depression are due in part to gender role imperatives to sacrifice and to suffer inequities in silence. The psychological impact of social arrangements that restrict women's freedom to choose the nature of their careers, the extent of their ambitions, the shape of their personal lives, and expressions of their experiences must be explored in every therapeutic context.

There are several ways that therapists can take account of the ways women's lives are blunted by sexist social arrangements and the psychological distress that follows. I think that what my colleague, Elaine Carmen, M.D., and I wrote in our 1984 book, *The Gender Gap in Psychotherapy: Social Realities and Psychological Processes* is still relevant. We asked clinicians to examine the gender values concealed in their theories and practices because it would improve mental health outcomes. We thought it was appropriate to make some of our most basic assumptions more explicit: (1) Intrapsychic explanations alone are insufficient for understanding psychological distress. Elements of the social context of patients' lives are critical to that understanding. (2) It is especially important to identify those taken-for-granted gender norms (for example, sex-role stereotypes, homophobia, and patriarchal ideologies) shared by patients and therapists that, if left unexamined, will negatively affect outcomes. (3) All modes of psychotherapy are limited in their ability to change the gender inequality that contributes to psychological distress; inevitably, change of that magnitude requires political action. (4) The myth of value-free psychotherapy is no less pervasive than the myth of value-free sociology—both positions derive from the more general myth of value-free science. (5) The continuous self-monitoring of personal and professional gender values as they influence clinical performance is hard work; mental health care and training programs must teach value-clarification methods in addition to new knowledge and skills. (6) Although there are differences between male and female therapists that need to be explored further, neither sex nor ideology guarantees one's skill as a clinician.

Finally, as we have said elsewhere, a competent therapist has the ability to stand outside the self, to observe the cognitive-value interaction, and to question her or his gender values and intellectual framework without the paralyzing fear of personal or professional annihilation.

REFERENCES

Bassuk, E. L.
> 1993a. Homeless women: economic and social issues—introduction. *Am J Orthopsychiat* 63(3):337–39.
> 1993b. Social and economic hardships of homeless and other poor women. *Am J Orthopsychiat* 63(3):340–47.
Bassuk, E. L., and Weinreb, L. 1993. Homeless pregnant women: two generations at risk. *Am J Orthopsychiat* 63(3):348–57.
Belle, D.
> 1982. *Lives in stress: women and depression.* Beverly Hills, Calif.: Sage Publications.
> 1988. *The women's mental health research agenda: poverty.* NIMH Occasional Paper Series. Rockville, Md.: NIMH.
> 1990. Poverty and women's mental health. *American Psychologist* 45:385–89.
Bolen, J. 1984. *Goddesses in everywoman: a new psychology of women.* San Francisco: Harper and Row.
Brody, E., and Schoonover, C. 1986. Patterns of parent-care when adult daughters work and when they do not. *The Gerontologist* 26:372–82.
Broverman, I. K., Broverman, D. M., Clarkson, F. E., Rosenkrantz, P. S., and Vogel, S. R. 1970. Sex-role stereotypes and clinical judgments of mental health. *J Con and Clin Psychol* 34(1):1–7.
Burston, B. 1992. *Radical feminist therapy.* Newbury Park, Calif.: Sage.
Carmen, E. (H.), Rieker, P. P., and Mills, T. 1984. Victims of violence and psychiatric disorders. *Am J Psychiat* 141(3):378–83.
Carmen, E. (H.), Russo, N. F., and Miller, J. B. 1984. Inequality and women's mental health: an overview. In *The gender gap in psychotherapy,* ed. P. P. Rieker and E. (H.) Carmen. New York: Plenum Press.
Chesler, P. 1972. *Women and madness.* New York: Doubleday.
Chodorow, N. 1978. *The reproduction of mothering: psychoanalysis and the sociology of gender.* Berkeley: University of California Press. Chaps. 4–5.
Crenshaw, K. 1992. Whose story is it anyway? feminist and antiracist appropriations of Anita Hill. In *Race-ing justice, en-gendering power: essays on Anita Hill, Clarence Thomas, and the construction of social reality,* ed. T. Morrison. New York: Pantheon Books.

DeVault, M.
  1990a. Novel readings: the social organization of interpretation. *Am J Sociology* 95(4):887–921.
  1990b. Talking and listening from women's standpoint: feminist strategies for interviewing and analysis. *Social Problems* 37(1):96–116.
  1991. *Feeding the family: the social organization of caring as gendered work.* Chicago: University of Chicago Press.
Dychtwald, K., and Flower, J. 1989. *Age wave: the challenges and opportunities of an aging America.* Los Angeles: Jeremy P. Tarcher.
Faludi, S. 1991. *Backlash: the undeclared war against American women.* New York: Crown Publishers.
Fisher, C. 1982. *To dwell among friends: personal networks in town and city.* Chicago: University of Chicago Press.
Gater, R. A., Dean, C., and Morris, J. 1989. The contribution of childbearing to the sex difference in first admission rates for affective psychosis. *Psychological Medicine* 19(3):719–24.
Giddings, P. 1992. The last taboo. In *Race-ing justice, en-gendering power: essays on Anita Hill, Clarence Thomas, and the construction of social reality,* ed. T. Morrison. New York: Pantheon Books.
Gilbert, S. M., and Gubar, S. 1979. *The madwoman in the attic.* New Haven: Yale University Press.
Gilligan, C.
  1979. Woman's place in man's life cycle. *Harvard Educational Review* 49(4):431–44.
  1982. *In a different voice: psychological theory and women's development.* Cambridge: Harvard University Press.
Goldner, V., Penn, P., Sheinberg, M., and Walker, G. 1990. Love and violence: gender paradoxes in volatile attachments. *Family Process* 29(4):343–64.
Grosskurth, P. 1991. The new psychology of women. In *New York Review of Books* 28(17):25–32. October 24.
Hall, L. A., Williams, C. A., and Greenberg, R. S. 1985. Supports, stressors and depressive symptoms in low-income mothers of young children. *Am J Public Health* 75:518–22.
Hamilton, J. A., Alagna, S. W., King, L. S., and Lloyd, C. 1987. The emotional consequences of gender-based abuse in the workplace: new counseling programs for sex discrimination. *Women and Therapy* 6(1–2):115–82.
Hare-Mustin, R. T., and Marecek, J., eds. 1990. *Making a difference: psychology and the construction of gender.* New Haven: Yale University Press. See esp. chap. 1 (On making a difference) and chap. 2 (Gender and the meaning of difference: postmodernism and psychology).
Jack, D. C.
  1987. Silencing the self: the power of social imperatives in female depression. In *Women and depression: a lifespan perspective,* ed. R. Formanek and A. Gurian. New York: Springer. Chap. 11.
  1991. *Silencing the self: women and depression.* Cambridge, Mass.: Harvard University Press.
Jarvik, L. S., and Small, G. 1988. *Parent care: a commonsense guide for adult children.* New York: Crown.
Jordan, J. V., Kaplan, A. G., Miller, J. B., Stiver, I. P., and Surrey, J. L. 1991. *Women's growth in connection: writings from the Stone Center.* New York: Guilford Press.
Kaplan, G., Roberts, R., Camacho, T., and Coyne, J. 1987. Psychosocial predictors of depression: prospective evidence from the human population laboratory studies. *Am J Epidemiology* 125:206–20.

Kaplan, M., Winget, C., and Free, N. 1990. Psychiatrists' beliefs about gender-appropriate behavior. *Am J Psychiat* 147(7):910–12.

Lerner, H. G.

1974. Early origins of envy and devaluation of women: implications for sex-role stereotypes. *Bulletin of the Menninger Clinic* 38:538–53.

1984. Female dependency in context: some theoretical and technical considerations. In *The gender gap in psychotherapy: social realities and psychological realities,* ed. P. P. Rieker and E. (H.) Carmen. New York: Plenum Press.

1985. *The dance of anger.* New York: HarperCollins.

1987. Female depression: self-sacrifice and self-betrayal in relationships. In *Women and depression: a lifespan perspective,* ed. R. Formanek and A. Gurian. New York: Springer. Chap. 13.

1993. *The dance of deception: pretending and truth telling in women's lives.* New York: HarperCollins.

McGrath, E., Keita, G. P., Strickland, B. R., and Russo, N. F., eds. 1990. *Women and depression: risk factors and treatment issues.* Washington, D.C.: American Psychological Association.

Manderscheid, R. W., and Sonnenschein, M. A., eds. 1990. *Mental Health, United States, 1990.* National Institute of Mental Health. DHHS Pub. (ADM)90-1708. Washington, D.C.: U.S. Government Printing Office.

Marecek, J., and Hare-Mustin, R. T. 1991. A short history of the future: feminism and clinical psychology. *Psychology of Women Quarterly* 15:521–36.

Mednick, M. T. 1989. On the politics of psychological constructs: Stop the bandwagon, I want to get off. *American Psychologist* 44(8):1118–23.

Miller, J. B.

1976. *Toward a new psychology of women.* Boston: Beacon Press.

1987. Women's psychological development: theory and application. In *Women's mental health occasional paper series—NIMH.* Washington, D.C.

Mirowsky, J., and Ross, C. 1989. *Social causes of psychological distress.* New York: Aldine de Gruyter.

Morrison, T., ed. 1992. *Race-ing justice, en-gendering power: essays on Anita Hill, Clarence Thomas, and the construction of social reality.* New York: Pantheon Books.

Patterson, O. 1991. Race, gender, and liberal fallacies. *New York Times,* October 20.

Rieker, P. P. 1993. Mental illness: framing the social problem. In *Sociology (introduction to social problems),* ed. C. Calhoun and G. Ritzer. New York: McGraw-Hill.

Rieker, P. P., and Carmen, E. (H.). 1986. The victim-to-patient process: the disconfirmation and transformation of abuse. *Am J Orthopsychiat* 56(3):360–70.

Rieker, P. P., and Carmen, E. (H.), eds. 1984. *The gender gap in psychotherapy: social realities and psychological processes.* New York: Plenum Press.

Riley, D., and Eckenrode, J. 1986. Social ties: subgroup differences in costs and benefits. *J Personality and Social Psychology* 51:770–78.

Rosenstein, M. J., Milazzo-Sayre, L. J., and Manderscheid, R. W. 1990. Characteristics of persons using specialty inpatient, outpatient, and partial care programs in 1986. In *Mental health, United States, 1990,* ed. R. W. Manderscheid and M. A. Sonnenschein, pp. 139–53. Washington, D.C.: U.S. Government Printing Office.

Russo, N. F. 1990. Overview: forging priorities for women's mental health. *American Psychologist* 45(3):368–73.

Russo, N. F., and Green, B. 1992. Work and family roles: selected issues. In *Handbook on the psychology of women,* ed. M. Paludi and F. L. Denmark. See also, in the same volume, Russo, N.F., and Green, B., Women and mental health: selected issues.

Seligman, M. E. P. 1991. *Learned optimism.* New York: Alfred A. Knopf.

Showalter, E. 1985. *The female malady: women, madness, and English culture, 1830–1980.* New York: Pantheon.

Sidel, R. 1986. *Women and children last: the plight of poor women in affluent America.* New York: Viking.

Tavris, C. 1992. *The mismeasure of women.* New York: Simon and Schuster.

Tomes, N. 1992. Historical perspectives on women and mental illness. In *Women, health, and medicine in America: a historical handbook,* ed. R. D. Apple, pp. 143–71. New Brunswick, N.J.: Rutgers University Press.

Weissman, M. M. 1987. Advances in psychiatric epidemiology: rates and risks for major depression. *Am J Public Health* 77:445–51.

Westkott, M.

1989. Female relationality and the idealized self. *Am J Psychoanalysis* 49(3):239–50.

1990. On the new psychology of women: a cautionary view. *Feminist Issues.* Fall.

3 Elaine R. Brooks, Maria Zuñiga, and Nolan E. Penn

The Decline of Public Mental Health in the United States

Racism is ultimately indivisible from the rest of
American life, a fact few of us wish to face.

—*Joel Kovel*

A REVIVAL of political conservatism in the United States during the 1970s and 1980s challenged several decades of direct federal involvement in domestic policy. New national domestic policies appeared with the conservative ideological trends evident in the 1970s. With the election of President Richard Nixon in 1968, a new ideology about governance was introduced (Conlan 1988; Nathan, Doolittle and Associates 1987) with a reemphasis of federalism. An uncertain reliance on states, local governments, private markets, and individuals was designated as the proper arenas for handling the nation's domestic affairs, eclipsing the dominant role that the federal government had played since the 1930s.

These ideas about federalism and the reduction of the role of the federal government in domestic affairs were expanded with the Reagan administration (Williamson 1990). Reagan issued an Executive Order in 1987 cementing the concept of federalism as the new national domestic policy, a document defining the relationship of the federal government to the states.[1] Overall, these new ideologies reflected a deep distrust of the involvement of the federal government in the lives of citizens and declared a mandate for a return to a set of traditional values of individualism and localism despite arguments that the federal government was better positioned to undertake many kinds of programs (such as health care), which were directly related to general welfare (Penn and Penn 1975).

In the wake of these ideological shifts, the provision of social welfare was dramatically transformed, including those public institutions providing housing, income maintenance, food, and medical care. Significant changes were introduced in the delivery of a variety of social services, as

51

responsibility for providing services was shifted onto new mechanisms that embodied the new concept of a limited role for the federal government. The Medicare and Medicaid programs at the federal level became the general models. These programs represented a new funding mechanism for brokering the expenditure of public money, not directly on public programs, but providing opportunities to use that money in private markets (Ruggie 1990, 1992). Ideally, in such a health-care system, all private physicians would treat clients eligible for Medicare or Medicaid. The needs for freedom of choice and private markets championed by the guilds would be preserved, and the health-care needs of the poor, disabled, and elderly would be met.

An immediate effect of this large pool of public money devoted to health care was an inflationary increase in the costs of health care overall (Freyman 1980). Cost containment became a central concern in the delivery of all medical care, whether that concern was motivated to preserve profits in private markets or motivated to reduce the costs to taxpayers. By the 1970s, the federal government began to resist the carte blanche approach to medical care and sought ways to contain spending (Freyman 1980). By the mid-1980s, through fundamental reforms in the system of reimbursement (Walsh 1988), the federal government was engaged directly in making treatment decisions through the development of the Diagnostic Related Groups (DRGs) system of reimbursement (Ruggie 1992). With these efforts at cost containment, many private physicians lost their interest in treating the poor, disabled, and the elderly. By the late 1980s, it was difficult to find a private psychiatrist who would accept a Medicaid patient, and within mental health, treatment intervention involving psychotherapy or counseling was more likely to be conducted by non-medical personnel such as social workers, psychologists, or marriage, family, and child counselors substituted for more expensive medical personnel. These substitutes were recognized in certain circumstances in third-party reimbursement.

This mechanism of service provision—created to transfer public money into private markets—was adopted widely for other services. In the area of housing for the poor, President Nixon directed a thorough review of the nation's housing policies, which resulted in the creation of the Section 8 program where the poor could take housing certificates into the private market to find subsidized housing instead of relying for shelter on expensive public housing projects (Carlson and Heinberg 1978). The Food Stamp program grew enormously under Nixon (Conlan 1988), allowing people to spend food stamps in the private sector. The Nixon administration worked to develop a Family Assistance Program that was designed to provide a direct income to poor people, eliminating the need for a collection of separate programs for providing basic need, but Congress refused to adopt this approach. Instead, through means-tested eligibility for specific federal programs, individual clients were given public funds to spend privately through food stamps, Section 8 certificates, and Medicare or Medicaid eligibility, thus bypassing the need for public programs designed and staffed by public agencies. Presumably these mechanisms for brokering the expenditure of public money in the private sector would lead to reduced administrative costs at the same time substantially reducing the direct role of government in people's lives.

Overall, these changes in political ideology and public policy had profound effects on the provision of general welfare in the country. By the end of the 1980s, the remnants of a set of national priorities, developed to alleviate poverty during the 1930s and revived and modified during the 1960s, were fragmented and scattered across a policy landscape cluttered with volunteerism, private charities, quasi-private contractors, corporate medicine, and residues of public agencies (Brooks 1992).

Two Decades of Change in the Provision of Public Mental Health

In the arena of mental health the new mechanisms created for providing for the social welfare needs of the poor contributed to a diminution of the traditional fiscal responsibility of states for providing public mental health services (Scull 1984; Ruggie 1990). States began to trim their public mental health commitment to residential care, particularly their inpatient programs, which were increasingly expensive to operate (Scull 1984). The creation of a system of eligibility for housing through Section 8 certificates, for income with Supplemental Security Income (SSI) and other disability payments, for food stamps and Medicare or Medicaid altered the economic demand for long-term public inpatient programs. This shift of public responsibility for maintaining mental health services actually began in the 1940s but accelerated through the 1960s and 1970s with the development of this system of means-tested federal programs for providing for basic needs that could be brokered in private markets.

New kinds of community-based treatment now seemed possible, treatment that would be both cost effective and efficacious. People could secure their basic needs individually, given their eligibility for federal programs. They could receive mental health services in their communities of origin and preempt the need for costly long-term inpatient residential facilities.

This policy of community-based care and general decentralization of services was further strengthened with the growing importance of biological psychiatry, which was promising safe and effective organic treatment

for mental illness (Gronfein 1985). The need for large and expensive inpatient programs supported with public funds seemed to diminish if
psychopharmacological intervention would reduce the symptoms of
major mental illness to the point that people no longer needed custodial
care for managing their illness.

These trends are most clearly symbolized in the reduced censuses of
state mental hospitals throughout the country (Ozarin, Redick, and Taube
1976), a process of deinstitutionalization of patients suffering major mental illness (Bachrach 1976). This policy was vigorously prosecuted during
the 1960s and 1970s as the community mental health movement expected
states to provide money for needed supportive services outside the hospitals in local communities.

By the 1980s, however, a new series of social problems emerged from
the unintended consequences of these new policies. Homelessness in the
1980s was caused partly by this policy of deinsitutionalization. Patients
unequipped for living autonomously were released from institutions
without adequate support services. Informal systems of care by family
and friends were strained to the breaking point (Johnson 1990; Task Force
on Homelessness and Severe Mental Illness 1992; Torrey 1988; Hopper
1988; Fischer 1989). The high prevalence of mental illness among the
growing numbers of homeless in the 1980s (Task Force on Homelessness
and Severe Mental Illness 1992) symbolized the major changes occurring
in the provision of services to the mentally ill throughout the health-care
system.

The loss of public inpatient psychiatric beds through the 1960s and
1970s was dramatic (figure 3.1). The number of patients began to decrease
in the late 1950s, declining steadily through the mid 1960s. This decline
then accelerated through the mid 1970s. What is evident today is that
there was not just a loss of public inpatient beds but an important shift of
service provision into the private sector (figure 3.2). Overall, given these
changes in funding social welfare, over the past twenty years there has
been a pronounced shift to private treatment (figure 3.2) and to outpatient
care (figure 3.3) with increasing fragmentation of services (Redick et al.
1990). With this "transinstitutionalization," (a term that more adequately
describes the changes in mental health service provision in the past two
decades), many of the most severely sick were left behind, no longer eligible for any care at all.[2]

The prevailing reason given for cutting inpatient psychiatric care beginning in the 1950s was the development of promising organic treatments for major mental illness (Gronfein 1985). A close examination of
this explanation does not show a direct relationship between the development of psychotropic medication and the release of patients. The data

FIGURE 3.1. Decline in number of patients residing in U.S. mental health facilities, 1950–1986 ("deinstitutionalization")

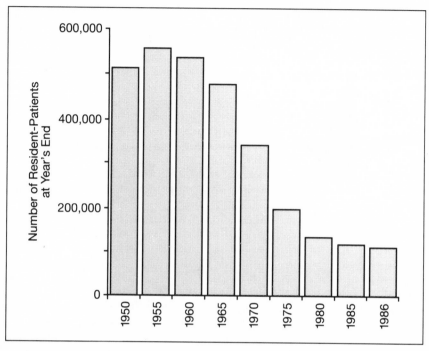

SOURCE: NIMH 1990b, table B.

show that the change in policy about inpatient public mental health treat-ment really began in the late 1940s. State legislatures around the coun-try—faced with the increasing costs associated with replacing or upgrad-ing an aging system of state hospitals, as well as the expansions needed to meet projected need—made critical budget decisions reducing funding for inpatient treatment (Scull 1984; Johnson 1990). Legislators were con-fronted by extraordinary new construction costs to build and refurbish the system of facilities needed, but also rising labor costs, the result of unionization and professionalization of hospital staff (Walsh 1988). More restrictive labor laws began to affect the use of patient labor for defraying costs (Black 1988). The operation of large inpatient facilities became an increasingly significant fiscal burden on state governments.

By 1955, public spending on mental hospitals was declining (Scull 1984). As with later reductions in all forms of public mental health care services throughout the 1980s, most changes in services have been the

FIGURE 3.2. Comparison of the change in proportion of inpatient beds available in different kinds of U.S. mental health facilities, 1970–1984

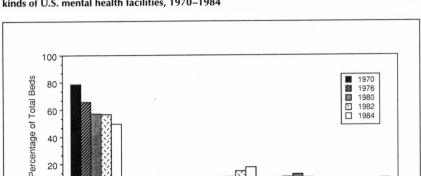

SOURCE: NIMH 1987, table 2.2.

outcome of budget, not medical, decisions, with medical or legal rationalizations applied post hoc or in parallel (Johnson 1990). The evidence for the pivotal role of the new availability of psychotropic medication in precipitating this policy of deinstitutionalization is weak. Chlorpromazine was introduced in 1954. Retrospective studies on the relationship of the use of this drug to discharge rates shows only weak associations (Gronfein 1985). (As figure 3.1 shows, the real acceleration in emptying beds did not occur until the 1970s.) Of greater importance to deinstitutionalization were the budget decisions made by state legislatures that were later linked to the expansion of federal health and welfare programs in the 1960s (Gronfein 1985; Scull 1984). Once these federal programs were in place, the changes in patterns of hospitalization accelerated from 1965 through 1980 (figure 3.1).

The most compelling evidence for the weak role of psychotropic medication in these policy decisions is Gronfein's (1985) comparison of discharge rates. The discharge rates from state hospitals increased steadily from 1946 onward, indicating that an increased discharge rate after the introduction of psychotropic medication (chlorpromazine) in 1954 was simply the continuation of a trend already underway. Occupancy rates in state hospitals were reduced as hospital stays became shorter (Ozarin et. al. 1976).

FIGURE 3.3. Increasing proportion of patients treated in outpatient settings in the United States, 1955–1985

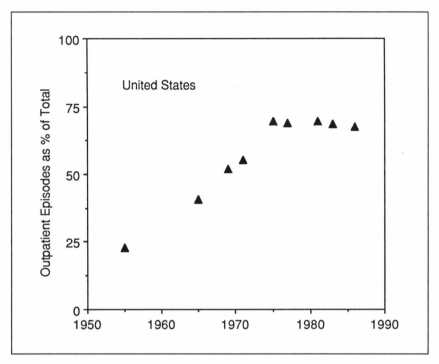

Source: NIMH 1990c, table 2.

State governments often seized any opportunity to back away from supporting public mental health services. That fiscal retrenchment has continued through the 1980s. In the interval from 1980 to 1986, per capita funding for mental health by the states decreased overall by 6.2 percent (figure 3.4). Although wide variation obviously exists among the states in their ongoing support of services, overall these changes are part of a trend of declining public support for mental health that stretches back to the 1940s.

Today, the budgets of public mental health services are favorite political targets for politicians at all governmental levels. The recipients of mental health services are politically weak. Consumer groups exist among mental health clients (Emerick 1991), but the stigma surrounding mental illness discourages high-functioning former psychiatric patients from maintaining an identification as patients long enough to be effective

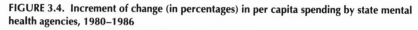

FIGURE 3.4. Increment of change (in percentages) in per capita spending by state mental health agencies, 1980–1986

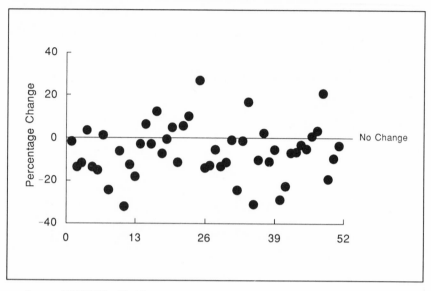

SOURCE: NIMH 1987, table 6.9.
NOTE: Each point represents the percentage change in spending by a particular state. If the point occurs above the line at zero, spending increased. If the point occurs below the line, spending decreased.

advocates. The social activism of professionals during the 1960s (Alvarez et al. 1976) was replaced with an exaggerated "careerism" as many professionals in the 1980s backed away from political advocacy on behalf of their clients.

Throughout the 1980s funding eroded for a wide variety of public treatment programs, both inpatient and outpatient. Special interest groups such as the National Alliance for the Mentally Ill (NAMI), composed of friends and family of the mentally ill, developed as important surrogates for consumers in the political arena (McLean 1990). Overall, however, no one has been fully effective in stalling or reversing the erosion of support to public mental health programs in the past twenty years.

The Privatization of Public Mental Health Care

Accompanying the decline of public mental health services was a transformation in treatment modalities in public settings away from expensive and prolonged individual approaches such as individual psychotherapy. The promise of a single drug for a single illness emerging from psychopharmacological research was financially attractive to public administrators as well as to insurance carriers and corporate boards (Sharfstein and Goldman 1989). In 1985, $1.45 billion was spent for outpatient purchases of psychotropic drugs in the United States, according to a survey of 2,250 pharmacies representing about 16 percent of all pharmacies in the United States (Zorc et al. 1991). Psychiatrists prescribed only 17 percent of all psychotropic medication. Most of it was prescribed by physicians in general practice. The biological treatment of mental illness and emotional distress is a growth industry throughout medicine.

Time-limited kinds of psychotherapy were evaluated and introduced in many treatment settings (Parloff 1982). Case management acquired a more important role in public treatment during the 1980s as increasing numbers of clients came to treatment with a much wider range of basic needs for food and shelter than previously. The need for a broker to help mentally ill people negotiate the difficult bureaucratic maze in a fragmented system of care became crucial (Anthony et al. 1988). With privatization and decentralization underway, a boom in the development of custodial arrangements in the private sector—such as board and care homes and nursing homes—was underwritten by the federal government through third-party payment (Scull 1984).

A diverse collection of outpatient settings sprang up, both public and private. Many services exist today as public-private blends. Local governments who were responsible for providing mental health services began to contract out their mental health care services to private providers who promised to run these programs more cost effectively. In fact, privatization became popular for a wide range of government functions during the 1980s (Starr 1987).

Public mental health locally became a hybrid public-private entity with a proliferation of new stakeholders who were the small, private professional businesses contracting with local governments to deliver mental health services to the poor. These new companies compete in local markets for local government contracts, and are seldom closely monitored, delivering a loosely coordinated set of services to the poor in local arenas. The whole public mental health system locally has become disconnected into a disparate collection of special economic interests where service coordination is rarely driven by client needs. Considerable anecdotal evidence exists that these arrangements are not working, but the thorough studies necessary to understand the impacts of funding and service fragmentation on client care are still in their infancy (Baldwin 1990; Cutler, Bigelow, and McFarland 1992).

Insurance in the private sector began to differentiate coverage for psychiatric problems from coverage for substance abuse (*Alcohol Health and*

Research World 1981; Hallan 1981; DeLuca 1981). Once treatment for substance abuse achieved its own standing, a new field of "addiction medicine" was born, which stimulated an increase in the number of private psychiatric hospitals as well as the expansion of psychiatric units in general hospitals through the 1980s (figure 3.2). The growth of separate treatment facilities for alcoholism accelerated in the mid 1980s (figure 3.5). Treatment philosophies for substance abuse diverged sharply away from traditional psychiatric approaches. The locus of treatment was a behavioral approach with abstinence the desired goal. Active participation in self-help programs was encouraged. Psychodynamic approaches based on patient insight into his or her problems were discouraged. The abstinence rules spilled over into a lot of traditional psychopharmacology, and the use of any kind of chemical was discouraged.

With the splintering of treatments for substance abuse and mental illness underway in both public and private systems, many dually or multi-

FIGURE 3.5. Comparison of the change in number of alcoholism treatment units in the United States, 1979–1984, for four different kinds of public and private facilities

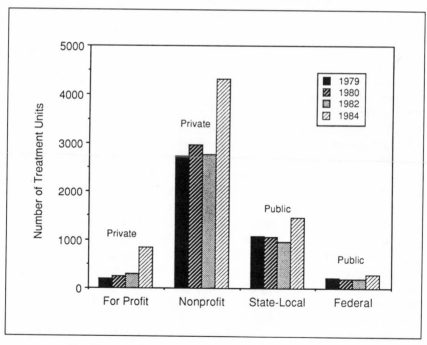

SOURCE: Reed and Sanchez 1986, table 11.

ply diagnosed individuals were left with no place for care (Cooper, Brown, and Anglin 1989). Eligibility for services, particularly for public services, came to be defined around single issues. Throughout the 1980s public service providers, challenged by shrinking budgets and rising demand, played a kind of shell game, eliminating clients from their own programs based on a client's eligibility for another kind of program. Thus, many mentally ill clients with substance abuse problems were turned away from drug and alcohol programs, and mental health clients involved with drugs and alcohol were discouraged in mental health care settings (Cooper et al. 1989). As a result, many patients with multiple problems never received any sustained services at all.

A significant number of these people represented a new generation of the mentally ill, young adult chronic patients (Bachrach 1982; Pepper and Ryglewicz 1984) who were appearing in large numbers by the late 1970s. These young people represented a new generation of patients who formerly would have been diverted into long-term care in inpatient treatment settings. These options no longer existed. Instead, these young people were streaming through the revolving doors of a poorly coordinated outpatient system punctuated with short-term hospital stays. Large numbers of them were deeply involved with alcohol and street drugs (Pepper and Ryglewicz 1984).

For those youth who had access to private insurance through their parents, their needs for psychiatric care stimulated the growth of new private ventures for treating teens (Weithorn 1988; Mason and Gibbs 1992; Hill and Fortenberry 1992). A variety of insurance plans—CHAMPUS (Civilian Health and Medical Programs for the Uniformed Services) for military dependents, commercial insurance, and Medicaid—underwrote the treatment of teens for substance abuse and emotional problems. Because of changes in the law related to the consent required to hospitalize juveniles, hospitalization of juveniles was simplified (Weithorn 1988). By 1988, 751,652 adolescents under the age of eighteen received mental health services, including inpatient residential treatment and outpatient care. This was 22.3 percent of all patients treated by the mental health care system in 1988 (Sunshine et al. 1991). Most of the adolescents receiving treatment were European American (Mason and Gibbs 1992). The reasons for this are complex but seem to be based on patterns of job discrimination, which deny good jobs with adequate benefits to proportionately more people of color, hence more European American families have access to insurance plans. At the same time there has been little development of drug and alcohol treatment programs for adolescents in the public sector. There are other issues related to the perception of deviance by law enforcement officers, who tend to divert juveniles of color involved with drugs into the juvenile justice system whereas European American youth are treated differently by police and the courts (Fagan et al. 1987).

The development of a new emphasis within private treatment on adolescent psychiatry was another significant trend in the privatization and disaggregation of mental health services throughout the country (Dorwart et al. 1989). This segmentation of medical care based on age was already memorialized in Medicare provisions for the elderly. For adolescents who did not have third-party coverage, their multiple problems received scant attention in what was left of the public system, and many of them have contributed to the growing youthfulness of the homeless population or are appearing in the juvenile justice system (Mason and Gibbs 1992).

By the early 1980s a variety of public and private insurers were picking up the overall costs of inpatient hospital treatment, mental illness, alcoholism, and other chemical dependencies (Hallan 1981). With this third-party coverage, new economic opportunities appeared in the private sector for psychiatric entrepreneurs. There was a proliferation of a variety of nonprofit and for profit inpatient facilities for the sole treatment of chemical dependencies as well as other specialized and reimbursable psychiatric services (Dorwart et al. 1989). The number of inpatient private investor and non-profit psychiatric facilities of all types grew remarkably through the 1970s and 1980s, and profits soared as private corporations came to dominate medical care (Stoesz 1986). The gross profits of four such companies are shown in figure 3.6.[3]

With these trends in services, there is an obvious impact upon people, which differs according to their access to private insurance or to private wealth. Because of this economic effect, people are sorted racially among the kinds of services available. The contrast is obvious in looking at the client mix in various sectors. White admissions constituted 85 percent of admissions to private inpatient programs in 1986, and White admissions were 98 percent of private outpatient treatment (Koslowe et al. 1991). Given the overall growing emphasis on outpatient treatment through the 1960s and 1970s (figure 3.3), only 2 percent of the outpatients treated privately were minorities. This is a clear example of the racial divisions in service delivery. Personal resources and commercial insurance paid for 71 percent of outpatient care. Medicare and Medicaid paid for 16 percent of private outpatient care (NIMH 1991). What has occurred in psychiatric treatment in the past two decades is an ongoing process of "transinstitutionalization." Inpatient treatment for mental illness has been sharply segmented into substance abuse disorders and then other mental illness, and treatment has been distributed according to third-party coverage over a variety of treatment systems that specialize in various aspects of

FIGURE 3.6. Growth in gross or operating revenues of four private for-profit corporations providing services for mental illness, 1976–1990 (in current dollars)

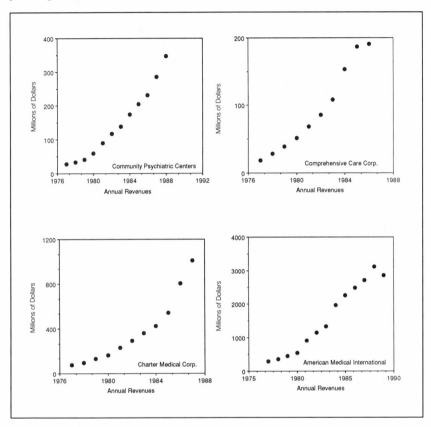

SOURCE: *Moody's industrial manual* 1975–1990.

these illnesses, with an increasing emphasis on the private sector as well as outpatient settings.

Making Do

A whole new set of institutions emerged to deal with those mentally ill who cannot afford to be treated in the private sector. These now include a potpourri of charities, demonstration projects, and occasional public services created to respond specifically to the problem of the homeless (Burt and Cohen 1989). For the middle class, the self-help movement became an important option and has grown dramatically over the past twenty years. Modeled on the original concept of Alcoholics Anonymous, which was started in the 1930s, a plethora of self-help groups devoted to a variety of single issues now exist. The self-help movement is resonant with a renewed emphasis on individualism in political ideology. Such groups as Alcoholics Anonymous (AA) or other 12 Step groups such as Narcotics Anonymous (NA) or Adult Children of Alcoholics (ACOA) are now viewed by professionals and treatment programs as integral parts of the treatment process. Much of the treatment philosophy in the medical field of substance abuse is derived from these approaches. Presently, it is estimated that membership in self-help groups ranges from 6 to 15 million persons (Powell 1987). Self-help became popular for a variety of reasons other than simply being inexpensive. These reasons included growing competition for professional services, questions about the quality of professional services, rising expenses in treatment with accompanying growth of regulations, and the unaccountability and inaccessibility of professionals as well as the tendency of professional treatment to focus on pathology rather than recovery (Gartner and Reissman 1984; Levin, Katz, and Holst 1976).

The new self-help movement remains predominantly a White, middle-class social movement. Experts in the self-help arena frankly admit that this movement does poorly in recruiting and maintaining people of color (Powell 1987). The experience of those in the helping professions supports the observation that underutilization by minorities is a critical issue (Gutierrez, Ortega, and Suarez 1990; Neighbors, Elliott, and Gant 1990). The reasons for this low utilization by minorities are varied. A major argument is that minorities are disinclined to air their problems with strangers (Powell 1987; Gutierrez et al. 1990). When the definition of self-help more closely approximates Gartner and Reissman's definition for the human services, then the lack of minority involvement is exaggerated. This definition includes such factors as face-to-face interactions, spontaneous origins, agreed-upon actions, personal participation, and recognition of powerlessness (Gartner and Reissman 1987).

The paradox is clear: for African Americans, Asians, Latinos, and Native Americans, self-help has been part and parcel of their cultural traditions for generations, but carried out differently. Using more general definitions of self-help, these cultural groups clearly have a range of self-help behaviors. According to Katz and Bender (1976), self-help groups are small groups structured for mutual aid in the accomplishment of a specific purpose. They are usually formed by people who have come together for mutual assistance in satisfying a common need, overcoming a common handicap or life-disrupting problem, or bringing about a desired personal or social change. The members of such groups perceive that their needs are not, or cannot, be met through existing social institutions (Remine, Rice, and Ross 1984). There are rich traditions of this kind of self-help in communities of color, but the focus is usually on external social or economic goals, accomplished through collective action, rather than on the self-examination and personal change that are prized in modern 12 Step programs. The small face-to-face encounters that characterize AA, ACOA, or Alanon meetings are the ones that clearly show minimal minority participation. Yet, there are unique groups spawned in minority communities to address their specific forms of need and powerlessness. For example, five years ago in Chicago, Frances Sandoval, a Latina mother whose son was killed by a gang member, formed Mothers Against Gangs (MAG), which now has seven hundred members in Chicago and Aurora, Illinois (Gutierrez et al. 1990). In the African American community there are local Sickle Cell Anemia support groups, the Urban League's Male Responsibility groups (which provide support and training in parenting for teen fathers), or Save Our Sons and Daughters, begun by and for Black mothers whose children were killed by other children (Neighbors et al. 1990).

Various factors contribute to the lack of minority involvement in established self-help groups, many of them reminiscent of the same arguments used to rationalize the underutilization of mental health services by people of color (Lum 1986; Becerra, Karno, and Escobar 1982). Underutilization occurs because these groups remain beyond the reach of people of color, because of economics, demands on time, lack of information, cultural and language barriers, racism, ethnophobia, culturally dystonic goals, as well as the history of these groups as part of a White middle-class social tradition.

The socialization and "training" to become part of a 12 Step program make it difficult for many people of color to develop competence and self-confidence in the program. Indoctrination occurs informally through direct participation and usually involves attending many meetings where the stories and testimonials of many individuals that form the core and the doctrine of the program are heard. It is the willingness to share these personal details with others publicly that forms the core of the "therapy" provided by a 12 Step program. For minorities who have learned important communication defenses for dealing with the majority race (one of which is minimal communication), involvement in such a group is difficult. This barrier becomes even more significant because people first presenting in self-help groups often feel extraordinarily vulnerable precisely because of their illness.

Other kinds of barriers persist. Alcoholics Anonymous is one of the oldest self-help groups of this type in the United States but meetings are rarely offered in other than the English language. For many Asian and Latino immigrants this presents a serious barrier. The goals and methods of self-help groups may be culturally inappropriate for many people. Some organizations have been willing to incorporate differing cultural values within their programs. The National Alliance for the Mentally Ill (NAMI) provides support to families of the mentally ill. In San Diego county, the Alliance recruited Spanish-speaking social workers to initiate a group for Hispanic families. Although the group started out following a model that engages only family members, soon the families brought with them their mentally ill kin, part of a cultural phenomenon that views the family as a collective unit that includes, rather than excludes, its mentally ill member. This has contributed to another level of education and empowerment for ill members and shows the critical need to acknowledge and incorporate the values of the diverse populations in such support groups support.[4]

Nowhere is this need for cultural sensitivity more critical than in the family dysfunctional movement, which addresses alcoholism, sexual and physical abuse, and family violence. Groups tend to be modeled on European American values around family and relationships. Therapeutic issues such as "enmeshment," for example, are central therapeutic concerns with considerable support given for member separation and individuation. Many traditional cultures (like Latino and Asian) are based on collective orientations espousing family cohesion over the life span rather than encouraging individualism. These groups often create painful conflicts for members who adhere to non-Western family mores. The interventions that are promoted are dissonant with cultural norms. If issues of self-revelation and speaking about private family themes violates cultural norms or threaten important defenses (Becerra et al. 1982), people do not participate. As with other mental health services there is a crucial need to incorporate diversity in a realistic way. Many of these criticisms were voiced about professional services by critics trying to achieve racial and cultural sensitivity in the 1960s and 1970s (Alvarez et al. 1976). They remain valid for the self-help movement.

The self-help movement grew in the 1970s and 1980s with the demand for inexpensive institutional arrangements for dealing with substance abuse and emotional problems, given the decline of public professional services through those decades. Overall, the self-help movement provides an important resource for the White middle class whose own household economies are also being challenged. So far, however, it has provided little direct support for African Americans, Latinos, Asian American, and Native Americans suffering the same illnesses. The modern self-help movement may be characterized as a functional equivalent to older kinship networks. In large metropolitan areas that have served as catchments for the redistribution of people throughout the country in the 1970s and 1980s, extensive kinship networks no longer remain (Perin 1988; Glick 1990). The European American middle class may be responding through the self-help movement to the needed support and connection formerly provided by families and neighbors of long standing, finding a formula for establishing a sense of community as the urbanization and anonymity of American life increases.

For African Americans, Latinos, and Asians, who have preserved more extensive kinship networks within localities, the support function of the extended family is the functional equivalent of self-help (Vega and Kolody 1984; Valle and Vega 1980). For those who do not have these consanguine resources, the choices for getting support remain severely limited. The effectiveness of informal social supports such as family and friends for supporting the severely mentally ill person in the community is problematic. The family, however constituted, tries to absorb decompensated behavior of the relative, which may often be connected to substance abuse, with little ability to address the worst symptoms. Particularly among the poor, families struggle to do this with few personal resources for meeting just the basic needs. They do this with housing that is inadequate to handle extra adult members. They are unable to provide close supervision because of work and other commitments. Yet families are the largest group trying to care for the chronically mentally ill particularly among the poor (NIMH 1991). When the symptoms cannot be contained any further within the family, people turn to the remaining professional services for which they are eligible. For people who are poor, what is left is this residue of public services. The private system of care generally excludes them.

Other opportunities for securing mental health services have included participation in the military. With the emergence of all-voluntary armed forces since the Vietnam war, African Americans and Latinos are overrepresented in their ranks. The percentage of African Americans in enlisted ranks rose from almost 13 percent in 1972 to nearly 22 percent in 1986 (Schexnider and Dorn 1989). Ironically, at the same time that there was better representation of people of color among the armed forces, medical services for veterans stagnated (see figure 3.2) as the generous medical care traditionally offered veterans became limited to clearly service-connected disabilities in the 1980s.

With the erosion of public resources for directly treating mental illness and with the demand for services continuing to rise, public agencies are constantly searching for ways to deliver services more inexpensively. The trends toward privatization of public services produced one such shift.

Within treatment programs themselves, vocational rehabilitation options have been proposed (Anthony, Cohen, and Cohen 1984). Genuine interest usually exists in improving the quality of life of patients with cost-effective treatment that can bring them back into the workforce.

The vocational rehabilitation option fits well with other government concerns. By the 1980s, the government was deeply involved in income-maintenance programs to the disabled with Supplemental Security Income (SSI) and Social Security Disability Income (SSDI). Disability expenditures for all adults aged 18 through 64 grew in constant dollars from about $60 billion in 1970 to $122 billion in 1982 (Berkowitz and Hill 1986). If significant numbers of patients could be returned to work, they would represent significant savings of tax dollars.

Few comprehensive vocational rehabilitation programs are yet under way for the mentally ill. It is really a new revival of an old concept of work for patients (Black 1988). A comparative analysis of existing programs leads to very few generalizations about the efficacy of rehabilitation compared to traditional medical approaches (Bond and Boyer 1988). People do recover from a major mental illness and assume a work role in society, but they may well do that on their own as effectively as they would without complex support systems. (Harding et al. 1987).

Little is known about the natural history of mental illness, hence little ability to predict the long-term needs of persons with major mental illness returning to the workforce (Strauss et al., 1985). But a great deal is known about the labor market. For the European American suffering a major mental illness, the opportunities for work, assuming adequate management of symptoms, remains problematic given the levels of discrimination against the mentally ill that exist in society.[5]

A reliance on a vocational outcome for a chronic mental patient, much less for one who might also be African American or Latino, does not meet the test of the reality of racism and discrimination in today's job market. In the 1960s, officials became concerned if the unemployment rate rose above 3 percent. Today, we routinely accept unemployment rates that are twice that figure (Harrington 1984). An effective vocational rehabilitation program for anyone is usually at the mercy of swings in the economy (Vachon 1989).

This approach is particularly problematic for the young adult chronic patient with an early onset of illness. Most have few educational or work acquired skills to bring to a job search. The young adult chronic patient as an unskilled worker competes in a labor market where the number of unskilled well-paying jobs continues to shrink as the economy continues to be transformed from an industrial to a service economy (Sassen 1990;

Reich 1991). If that young adult chronic patient is also a person of color, the chances for survival in the workplace are virtually nonexistent.

New varieties of institutions including self-help programs, charities, and public-private partnerships were created to deal with the changing trends in public mental health care. New approaches to treatment—including vocational rehabilitation and a separation of services for substance abuse—emerged in response to the changing patterns of funding for mental health services. But with these shifts has come an exaggeration of the impacts of these shifts on people of color, because these changes undermine more democratic approaches to treating mental illness, and they strengthen the tight correlation between class and race.

Different outcomes exist for the poor who are more often people of color. One outcome for people of color with a major mental illness in the 1980s has been life on the streets, part of the 1980s epiphenomenon of homelessness (Carter 1991; Rossi 1988). The second outcome, reserved for those with less debilitating pathology, has been the growth in "opportunities" in the criminal justice system. As funds were withdrawn from public mental health care during the 1980s, an enormous growth of budgets in the criminal justice system occurred. This is clearly seen in California (figure 3.7) where spending on criminal justice in constant dollars nearly doubled during the 1980s.

Scull (1984) originally described the 1960s and 1970s as "times of decarceration" as prisons and hospitals were emptied around the country. This trend was short-lived, however. Beginning in the early 1980s there was a national resurgence of interest in law and order. Incarceration rates in the nations jails and prisons rose precipitously (figure 3.8). A connection exists between the decline of public mental health care and the new trends in corrections. With the erosion of opportunities in the public sector for treatment of mental illness, the societal pressure to deal with the aberrant and disruptive behaviors that surround emotional distress and mental illness was redirected.

Perhaps there was a brief length of time in the late 1960s and early 1970s when there was an adequate supply of low-cost housing, when the resources of families were not yet strained to the limit, when adequate funds were being spent on community mental health care programs—that is, there was a time when the idea of community-based care could work. Redevelopment activities were only beginning in many cities in the early 1970s (Frieden and Sagalyn 1989). There was still a supply of lower-cost rental housing (Gilderbloom and Applebaum 1988). In 1970, the proportion of median income spent on rent was 21 percent in the United States. By 1983 it was 31 percent (Gilderbloom and Applebaum 1988). There was an infusion of federal dollars into community-based care

FIGURE 3.7. Increase in the yearly amount of money spent on criminal justice in the State of California, 1979–1989 (in constant dollars)

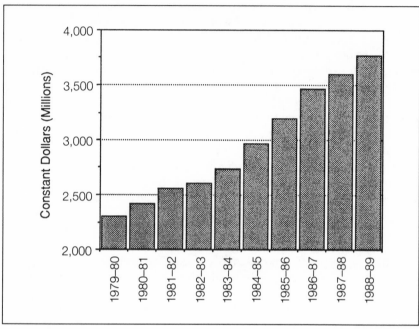

SOURCE: California Department of Justice 1990.

through the Community Mental Health Centers Act in the 1960s and more than four hundred comprehensive centers were in the process of development (Treadway and Brown 1972). But this relative abundance was short-lived, as other economic factors became important. In the early 1970s, federal money was withdrawn from the original commitment for 2,300 comprehensive mental health centers (Treadway and Brown, 1972) and the housing economy in the country underwent a radical transformation (Gilderbloom and Applebaun 1988). The loss of public mental health services and the eventual erosion of other public services providing housing, job training, income support, and other medical care are key factors explaining the transinstitutionalization of mental health care that is under way.

The ranks of the homeless are filled with extraordinarily high numbers of people of color (Carter 1991; First, Roth, and Arewa 1988; Rossi 1988), an indication of the economic vulnerability and marginality of

FIGURE 3.8. Incarceration rate for the United States, 1925–1985

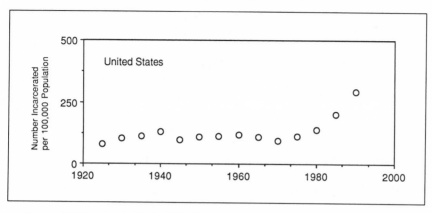

SOURCE: U.S. Department of Justice 1986, table 1.

NOTE: The incarceration rate is the number of people incarcerated in federal or state prisons per 100,000 population.

people of color in traditional American society as well as signaling the increasing racial and ethnic diversification around the nation. The problems accompanying chronic mental illness—as well as the problems arising from poor socioeconomic conditions, which range from substance abuse to adjustment disorders (including post–traumatic stress syndrome from living alongside the violence on the streets)—among the poor today are tended mostly by informal networks of family and friends.

The services that do exist for the poor are handling only the sickest. The use of strict legal considerations for involuntarily hospitalizing people during the 1980s was elevated as contributing to the problems of homelessness. This policy has been a scapegoat for an approach to find ways to limit the demand for a public system that is fundamentally unequipped to handle all the people who need services.

The civil rights concerns have also served policy makers as convenient post hoc explanations for the pattern of homelessness arising in the 1980s, much as policy makers have used the explanation of psychotropic medication to account for the deinstitutionalization phenomenon. Although there were important legal protections needed for patients, both of these arguments have been used to obscure what were fundamentally financial decisions by legislators; they are not sufficient explanations for the pattern of deinstitutionalization that has been observed. The popular focus on these two measures has diverted public attention away from the primary fiscal responsibility. The civil liberties arguments are usefully applied post hoc to hide what are fundamentally monetary decisions uncoupled from any objective legal or medical consideration.

A heightened visibility to law enforcement makes many people who are ineligible for any mental health treatment obvious targets for arrest, and the number of people now incarcerated in the nation's jails and prisons is increasing dramatically. This includes a high percentage of substance abusers as well as many suffering major forms of mental illness (Pallone 1991; Teplin 1990; Steadman et al. 1987). Overall, the individual patterns of dysfunction for European Americans are medicalized, whether caused by substance abuse or related to a mental illness. These problems are handled in a variety of private treatment settings because of the economic opportunities that exist for European Americans. Without these economic opportunities, besides increased risk for homelessness, many of the emotional problems of people of color have been criminalized in the past two decades because of inadequate economic resources that could lead to proper mental health care.

More and more behaviors associated with mental illness are labeled for African Americans and Latinos in terms of deviance associated with criminality. With the advent of the War on Drugs in the late 1980s, this formal national policy has legitimized the incarceration of thousands of young African American, Latino, and Native American men in the nation's prisons and jails whereas the drug-related problems of European Americans are diverted with third-party coverage into hospital and treatment settings. Thus, the justice system became another destination within the new configuration of institutions created in the wake of withdrawal of public support for public mental health care services, part of the transinstitutionalization created by these policies. The labeling of criminal behavior begins very early in communities of color, as the mainstream attention on gangs reveals (Mason and Gibbs 1992). The redefinition into criminality of the mental health needs of the poor is as dramatic in the 1980s as the emergence of homelessness, directly attributable to the decline of support for public mental healthcare.

Rules for Social Order: Criminalizing the "Other America"

The nation continues to diversify along gradients of race, immigration status, culture, religion, and language, and with this diversification, communication problems among groups multiply. Mediating conflicts among the many different kinds of people is a central public concern. The racial and ethnic tensions along these boundaries are exacerbated with the accompanying disparities in socioeconomic conditions among groups. Occasionally urban riots punctuate the changes underway.

The emerging process of racial and ethnic diversification is clearly seen in residential segregation patterns where people are sorted by skin color (Denton and Massey 1989; Massey and Eggers 1990; Massey and Denton 1993; Santiago and Wilder 1991). Settlement patterns of new immigrants into the country are strongly determined by the presence of people who are known to the immigrant, hence many new immigrants settle where they have friends or family, thus concentrating the direct impacts of immigration unevenly around the country (Vernez and Ronfeldt 1991; Massey and España 1987). These factors help create a generally patchy distribution of racial and ethnic groups at all geographic scales, whether examined nationally or locally.

Neighborhoods themselves may be more homogenous as groups segregate within larger metropolitan areas. Large, growing urban areas dominate domestic life today. As urbanization proceeds, there is a tendency in urban areas for differences among subcultures to be accentuated (Fisher 1982). Fisher studied social networks along a rural-to-urban continuum in the Sacramento–San Francisco area. He said, "the subcultural heterogeneity and vitality of urban centers leads to encounters between people who not only are personally strangers to one another but also are culturally strange, perhaps threatening, to one another" (1982, 234).

Two major institutions for managing deviance and maintaining social order are the nation's mental health system and criminal justice system (Scull 1984). Two quite different assumptions about personal responsibility support each system. The justice system presumes individual responsibility for one's actions and prescribes punitive measures for those who deliberately harm others. The mental health care system acknowledges the central powerlessness of the individual disabled by illness, uncouples personal responsibility for unacceptable behavior, and attempts to relieve the suffering of that person through treatment interventions, at the same time minimizing any further social disruption that the person might cause.

To a great exent, the elaborate system of state hospitals for the mentally ill serves primarily a custodial function, removing less desirable people from everyday life, only secondarily providing a place for treatment (Edwalds 1964). The reduction of capacity in this system during the 1950s, 1960s, and 1970s represented a significant loss of custodial facilities for removing aberrant people from society at a time when the overall population size of the country continued to increase. The American hospital system existed for well over one hundred years for handling the mentally ill who were obviously disruptive, as cities began to form and consolidate from an earlier colonial rural and small-town lifestyle in the mid-to-late nineteenth century (Jimenez 1987).

The community mental health care movement during the 1960s returned thousands of chronically mentally ill to communities and neighborhoods containing millions of people in rapidly growing metropolitan areas. The promise of real community-based treatment faded rapidly, partly because it was never fully funded, but also because modern social conditions in urban areas created conditions that were antithetical to the assumptions of this approach to care. Modern metropolitan regions were filled with people who were basically strangers to one another. Major changes in family structure occurring since the turn of the century (Glick 1990) added to the impossibility of this approach. The succeeding dimensions of urban anonymity increased because of the rapid urbanization of the country and the sheer growth in numbers of people.

The revival of a notion of community-based care in the 1960s was a return to a concept of inclusion of the mentally ill in the life of a mythical community that had long ago disappeared in the nation. In colonial times, neighbors and friends in smaller cohesive communities tolerated the mental illness of their kin and neighbors and included them in community life (Jimenez 1987). With the growth of modern urban centers containing millions of people, the mentally ill were no longer familiar as persons, no longer friends or relatives, but encountered as disruptive strangers who needed to be locked away (Jimenez 1988).

The increasing racial and ethnic diversification underway produced a new dimension of unfamiliarity. The major racial and ethnic groups in this country are strangers to one another despite a long history of coexistence (Williams 1989; Forbes 1990), and the consequences are a heightened wariness and scrutiny of strangers (Perin 1988). For instance, unless a White stranger walking through a White suburban neighborhood has other qualities (that is, is looking or behaving in bizarre ways, is talking to no-one, is singing loudly, is acting drunk, is naked, is wearing old dirty clothing and obviously has not bathed or shaved for weeks, or is, perhaps, carrying a weapon, or in any other way signaling behavior that may be disruptive or dangerous), the initial reaction is likely to be benign. However, the mere recognition of the skin color of a Black man or woman in a White neighborhood is likely to be interpreted by many of the White residents as a sign of potential problems. Likewise, a White person walking through a Black neighborhood will arouse suspicion. Skin color is loaded with other meaning for people depending on the context in which it is perceived. But the social consequences of that aroused suspicion are quite different for Blacks than they are for Whites. Because of the distribution of power in a society organized along racial lines, there is, by the majority group of European Americans, a societal presumption of innocence that is ordered racially with increasing degrees of culpability going from White to Yellow to Brown to Red, and then to Black, a measure for ordering people deeply embedded in European American history (Kovel 1970).

Although the concept of being a stranger will be socially constructed using different attributes than skin color for the Black stranger in the Black neighborhood, or the White stranger in the White neighborhood, the construction of the concept of the stranger in American society is powerfully determined initially by ideas of skin color. Based on a few simple perceptions of the physical characteristics of a person's skin color, sex, or age, these attributes are matched by a set of internalized notions of what constitutes a threat. The differential wariness that arises for White residents from the presence of a Black stranger in a White neighborhood (compared with a White stranger's presence in the same neighborhood) is a measure of the strength of our unthinking reliance on skin color for determining the social order. This difference in perception is then exaggerated by the social control exerted by a predominantly White criminal justice system. Although White people certainly are prosecuted and apprehended also, their construction of "strangeness and threat" by the criminal justice system is built on attributes other than skin color, whereas people of color bear an additional weight of suspicion by virtue of their skin color alone.

In a country of rising populations, informal "rules" such as these proliferate for identifying strangers and people who might be a threat. The social construction of mental illness is another way of handling the concepts of strangeness and of threat. The experience of mental illness is socially defined in important ways. Although the fear and emotional pain experienced by someone with mental illness is felt within, the degree of fear and the amount of pain is determined powerfully by the reactions of these around the individual. The irrational discriminations made about dysfunctional behaviors, which are labeled as mental illness or identified as something worse, are products of these interactions. If someone is a person of color as well, the predicaments of being considered both a stranger and a threat by the majority society (based on skin color alone) compound the interactions with others based on the stigma of mental illness.

Being mentally ill in this society is highly stigmatizing. The lifelong social consequences to an individual who has acquired the label "mentally ill" are often ignored by mental health professionals, who often reduce the individual to a set of symptoms or dysfunctional behaviors. The reimbursement for treating mental illness often requires focusing on this pathology (Baldwin 1990). The issue of stigma surrounding mental illness—whether it comes from mental health professionals or from friends, family, employers, or strangers—is far from trivial to the individual acquiring the label (Link et al. 1989). The label of mental illness is almost always acquired reluctantly. Studies of the identification process by which individuals come to see themselves in a sick role emphasize the resistance most people feel to acquiring this label, a resistance that cuts across racial and ethnic lines (Estroff et al. 1991; Whitt and Meile 1985; Link et al. 1989). Cockerham (1990) attempts to analyze this process for individuals who have lived the experience. One of the final stages in this process is accepting mental illness as a "normal state" for the individual. It becomes the "master status" (1990, 348) for that individual and is assumed only reluctantly as part of the general struggle an individual experiences with emotional dysfunction. Society shapes the very struggle itself.

Thoits (1985) describes this self-labeling process in a series of steps that the individual goes through. The process begins with a set of discrepant feelings, measured against a set of internal norms associated with those feelings. The individual then engages in various techniques for managing these discrepancies. Usually only after all other methods have failed to alter the feelings does a person seek psychotherapeutic help. At that point socioeconomic factors often enter to determine the outcome. Until then, an extensive array of culturally coherent, informal methods may be used to describe and to moderate the discrepant feelings.

Seeking formal psychotherapeutic help is usually the last step taken, usually voluntarily (Thoits 1985). More people seek out psychotherapy privately and voluntarily than are involuntarily treated in the mental health system. Estroff et al. (1991) demonstrate the lengths to which people who are hospitalized and who have spent significant lengths of time in the mental health system take to normalize their behavior by the way they talk about themselves. Their willingness to label themselves mentally ill usually depends on the context in which they are asked the question. Within a hospital setting, they may adopt the label, but outside, they undertake concentrated "identity work" to keep their self-definitions coherent with others who are normal. When a person gives up on this normalizing process, he or she accepts the deviant status and the label as a mental patient. In their sample of 169 individuals diagnosed with severe, persistent mental illness, Estroff et al. found that, "79 percent agreed with the statement, 'Like anyone else, I have some troubles, but I get along as well as most people do.' When presented (in the same scale) with the statement, 'In my opinion, I am mentally ill,' 77 percent responded that this was false" (1991, 363). The label of mentally ill carries enormous stigma and people vigorously defend against it.

Both roles of mental patient and of criminal are deviant social roles. Where people are able to control which label they acquire, they will opt for the least stigmatizing in the eyes of significant others. In many instances, criminality may be the preferred self-concept where acquiring one or the other status is negotiable. There are significant cultural differences in the perception and acceptance of mental illness (Kirmayer 1989; Angel and Thoits 1987) that will influence a person's adoption of such a label. Particularly, in communities that are routinely stigmatized racially by societal norms, a criminal label may simply reflect the dominant majority's unfair, hostile treatment of a subculture. The police and courts simply serve as agents of the majority. The label of mental illness, by contrast, implies that the individuals themselves are deficient in important ways and this threatens their status within their own social networks. Also, other cultures may view the mentally ill member more positively than the dominant group does, and these perceptual differences become significant in an individual's chances of recovery (Guarnaccia and Farias 1988; Jenkins 1988; Jenkins and Karno 1992).

Ample evidence exists that impoverished social and economic conditions can produce emotional and mental dysfunction (Mirowsky and Ross 1989; Dohrenwend et al. 1992). Minority status itself may lead to increased risk for mental health problems (Halpern 1993). Dohrenwend and colleagues demonstrate that rates of major depression in women, and substance abuse and antisocial personality among men, can be explained by a mechanism of "social causation" among lower classes of Israelis of North African background, suggesting that an "increment in adversity attaching to disadvantaged ethnic status produces an increment of psychopathology" (1992, 951). This study is particularly significant in defining the different roles of social causation and social selection in explaining the class differences among the mentally ill. People with schizophrenia tend to concentrate in the lower economic classes because they are unable to maintain their economic status as a result of their illnesses. As economic disadvantage keeps a larger fraction of a group in the lower classes, the number of cases of major psychoses that appear caused by biological mechanisms will be concentrated where the population is, in the lower classes. Their illnesses, however, are generally caused by intrinsic factors. Other problems such as depression and substance abuse (along with character disorders) seem to arise because of particularly difficult conditions associated with low socioeconomic status.

Mirowsky and Ross describe distress among people as a function of the control they exert over their own lives. Distress is more pronounced among minorities because "[i]t reflects the fact that any given level of achievement requires greater effort and provides fewer opportunities for members of minority groups. This is reflected in a lower sense of control, and consequent distress" (1989, 167). Mental health of the poor is challenged by their very living conditions, and the need for establishing programs to mitigate the worst outcomes of these conditions—including effective poverty programs and effective mental health services—is a central problem in the provision of all services.

Given the conditions of poverty and lack of opportunity in many communities of color, criminal activity as defined in the law (Padilla 1992) may be in fact functional, for individuals and families that are given few options. Unusual behavior of people of color is also more easily labeled as criminality by European Americans because of the socially constructed racial bias. These two factors appear to combine in a powerful way to create two quite different systems for managing deviance in this society—systems based on race.

Over the past twenty years, there has been a significant increase in the numbers of African Americans and Latinos in U.S. jails and prisons. This reality is accompanied by increasing problems of substance abuse, a renaissance in the variety of drugs available (Jarvik 1990), and the loss of opportunities for addressing discrepant behavior in the public mental health system because of loss of services. The reasons for the "browning" of the nation's corrections system are complex, but highly significant for people already denied full access to the opportunity structure in the country. The "choice" for an individual between a prison or a hospital is a complicated outcome of individual decisions coupled with societal perceptions. In cultures where mental illness is highly stigmatized, the individual may avoid seeking treatment for problems and behaviors that eventually attract the attention of the criminal justice system.

Treatment for substance abuse is one of those areas where social, cultural, and economic factors converge to discriminate against many people of color. Modern American organizations, both public and private, have instituted an array of employee-assistance programs that work to maintain the individual within the community and within the family. Given the problems of job discrimination in most of these organizations, European American employees are more likely to have access to the kinds of support services and interventions that keep them functioning in the community while receiving help. The differential availability of self-help programs to European Americans compared with others is another way for European Americans to avoid scrutiny by the criminal justice system. Proportionately more people of color with substance abuse problems are vulnerable to the legal consequences of substance abuse.

Rather than seeking out other kinds of services for earlier intervention before dysfunctional behavior becomes too disruptive, people often attempt to deal with their feelings by using a series of maladaptive behaviors that may lead them to jail. These are series of apparent "choices" that an individual makes in seeking help for mental and emotional problems, choices that are really fashioned by individual decisions converging with societal reactions to that individual and his or her behavior (Thoits 1985). For individuals in American society who are already affected by discrimination based on their race or ethnicity, adding the label of mental illness to the social baggage they already carry in their struggles for social and economic opportunity disproportionately affects their abilities to compete and survive. When this condition is coupled with culturally based stigma about mental illness, seeking treatment becomes highly unlikely. People turn to other informal strategies for managing their feelings—which may include substance abuse (Thoits 1985)—and find themselves in more difficulty because of it.

Antisocial behavior triggered by poverty, emotional distress, and substance abuse commands the attention of the legal system for people of color in ways that European Americans often escape (Reed 1991). Reed shows that the actual rates of illicit drug use for Blacks and Whites was about the same in 1985. In fact, Whites have a somewhat higher rate of drug use, but this level of drug use in the Black community creates a much different image in the media where drug use in Black neighborhoods is juxtaposed with images of crime and violence. The attention given by the justice system is also different.

Institutions that are created to deal with problems of substance abuse preserve the innocence of most European Americans, through institutional racism. A White adolescent drug addict is likely to be perceived as an individual in the minds of the White majority, a possible family member or friend or neighbor. Interventions made by the police, the schools, or mental health care services seem to protect this familiarity with medical interventions (Mason and Gibbs 1992). With the stereotypes of people of color that are harbored by most European Americans, the shadow of criminality is easily cast across the racial and ethnic boundary, redefining a whole class of people engaging in similar activity (Fagan, Slaughter and Hartstone 1987).

The numerical patterns of differences that are observed in the correction system require very little difference in applying labels of deviance to produce two quite different long-term outcomes, particularly if the labels once applied are difficult to alter. The numerical patterns are the result of incremental decisions integrated over many years (Schelling 1971, 1978). If a person is labeled criminal as an adolescent, it is very difficult to change that label. Thus, individuals so identified will nearly always be sorted into the criminal justice system, and if the rates of labeling are racially even slightly different, over many years one would see quite different distributions of people in one system or the other (Schelling 1971). The important sorting process begins during adolescence when society attempts to control the normal difficulties of adolescence (Weithorn 1988; Hill and Fortenberry 1992; Mason and Gibbs 1992). The process produces a tendency to medicalize the adolescent problems of European American children and to criminalize the adolescent problems of other groups (Mason and Gibbs 1992). With the growth of adolescent psychiatry in the past two decades, this difference can be exaggerated. A study of discharges of juveniles from California hospitals in 1987 (Mason and Gibbs 1992) showed racial differences in diagnosis, with White youths more likely to be treated for substance abuse than minority youths. Minority youths are seriously underrepresented in private hospital settings at the same time as they are the dominant group in juvenile detention centers (figure 3.9).

Five-year trends in juvenile court statistics (Allen-Hayen 1988) show a greater increase in delinquency cases among non-Whites (31.75) percent) than Whites (9.6 percent). This difference was greatest for drug offenses and may also reflect increased enforcement pressure on minority youth as compared to White youth. The War on Drugs has been a war on minority neighborhoods. Although formal drug cases declined for Whites (13 percent), they increased for minorities (111.4 percent) in that five-year period. At the same time, there was a healthy growth in private psychiatric treatment facilities for adolescents serving mostly White clients.

Similarly from 1984 to 1988, the number of delinquency cases detained between referral to court and disposition increased 7.3 percent. The greatest increase was for drug offenses (62.5 percent) as the War on Drugs got under way. This increase was caused mainly by the increase in the detention of non-Whites (268.5 percent). In contrast, detention in drug cases involving Whites dropped. During the 1980s, the number of adult felony drug arrests nearly doubled (figure 3.10) as the overall incarceration rate rose throughout the United States after having remained relatively stable for sixty years (figure 3.8). The 1980s reflected a politicized social demand for law and order that was disproportionately directed at the young and the urban poor.

These differences in labeling occurring in adolescence have profound implications for these individuals later in life. They lead to discernible patterns of permanent distribution of people into the justice system or mental health system, a sorting that changes with new policy or ideology (Gusfield 1967). For instance, society's attitude toward alcohol consump-

FIGURE 3.9. Hispanic, African American, and total juveniles in custody, 1985–1989

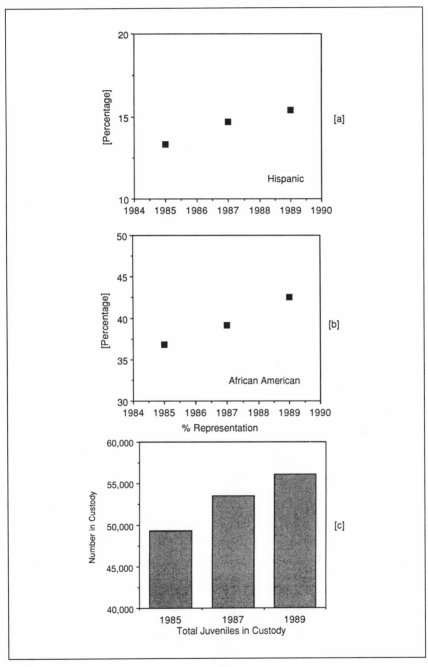

SOURCES: Allen-Hayen 1988, table 2; ibid. 1990, table 2.

FIGURE 3.10. Increase in number of felony drug arrests of adults in the United States, 1980–1987

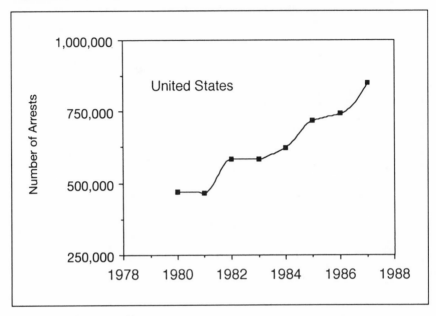

SOURCE: Cohen 1991, table 1.

tion during Prohibition created a new class of criminals involving alcohol use. Today problems with alcohol tend to be medicalized, with criminal penalties much different from during the days of Prohibition.

There is a strong tendency in our society to label major mental illness as a chronic condition and to assign the individual with a major mental illness to a permanent status as mentally ill (Jimenez 1988). Estroff et al. (1991) point out the semantic differences in saying "I am schizophrenic" as opposed to "I have schizophrenia." In the first description, the illness is a core identity. In the second, the illness is a kind of overlay, separate from the core of the person. These semantic patterns often differentiate major mental illness from other kinds of illness. Someone does not say, for example, "I am cancer." Labels for major mental illness become a permanent attribute of the individual: "I am White," "I am male," "I am 37 years old," "I am schizophrenic." Once so defined within the mental health system, a person assumes that status permanently.

Perceptions about criminality may not always contain the same kinds of messages implying personal deficits as do labels such as "schizophrenic," "manic-depressive" or "borderline personality disorder," but they possess similar permanence. Criminal labels may, in fact, signal only bad luck in getting caught, or they may acknowledge the only economic choices that are open in some communities. The perjorative aspects of criminality often have more importance for the group applying the labels in stereotypical, self-serving ways to other groups, emphasizing the status differences between them.

The overall greater availability of private mental health services to European Americans in comparison to others, because of economic discrimination, means that there is some chance of early intervention in the treatment of mental illness for European Americans. Emotional problems may not have to become severe persistent problems to receive attention. Early intervention and private treatment to mitigate dysfunctional behavior are constructed socioeconomically and may be the most important factors in shaping the outcomes of emotional dysfunction for European Americans and other Americans (thus, between the eventual assignment of status as a mentally ill person or as a criminal).

Although serious criticisms exist of the medicalization and reliance on psychiatric intervention to handle the normal problems of adolescence that evolved in the 1980s (Weithorn 1988; Hill and Fortenberry 1992), a European American youth is less likely ultimately to go to jail. The decisions made about handling adolescent difficulties are even more important for the new generation of young adult chronic patients who have grown up without the availability of inpatient treatment. Their early identification in the corrections system may preempt any future treatment for their underlying mental and emotional problems.

Incarceration rates around the country rose significantly during the 1980s (figure 3.8). The Omnibus Budget Reconciliation Act (OBRA) (PL 97–35) ended federal funding for community mental health centers in 1981. This was a significant retreat for the role of the federal government in providing mental health care services to inner-city and other poor neighborhoods. In California, felony arrest rates nearly doubled between the late 1970s and 1990, while expenditures on the criminal justice system more than doubled (figure 3.7). The national incarceration rate, which had remained relatively flat since the 1920s, tripled from 1980 to 1990 because of a national obsession with "law and order" (figure 3.8). The incarceration rate increased without a large increase in the number of law enforcement officers on the streets, but rather by increasing the money spent on prisons and jails. The enforcement activity of the police on the street was stepped up as more institutions were created to confine prisoners and more correctional officers were hired to tend them. Changes in staffing levels reflect these activities in the criminal justice system (seen

for California over a ten-year period from 1979–1980 to 1988–1990 in figure 3.11). The increase in law enforcement paralleled the population
growth. The number of parole officers was now reduced because people
were detained in prison. The number of public defenders increased as
more people were arrested. The number of corrections officers was raised
to guard prisoners after they were sentenced.

The number of people of color who were incarcerated rose through
the 1980s as the proportion in custody remained high. The number of
prisoners in U.S. jails continued to increase (figure 3.12). The number of
juveniles in custody increased (figure 3.9c). The average daily jail population of adults and juveniles nearly doubled from 1978 to 1988 (figure
3.12). Overall expenditures in constant dollars on mental health in the
United States stayed relatively flat, however (figure 3.13), and there was a
continual erosion of funding for state and county facilities. The per capita
expenditure on state and county psychiatric facilities in constant dollars
in the United States dropped from $10.13 in 1975 to $6.90 in 1986 (Witkin
et al. 1991).

The criminal justice system was reinterpreted and refocused as the
arbiter of social order in the 1980s, and heightened attention was given
the activities of the people in communities of color. This new focus on
criminal justice was consistent with the new conservative political trends

FIGURE 3.11. Percentage change in number of personnel employed in four sectors of the
criminal justice system in California, 1979–1989, compared to the actual change in
California's resident population

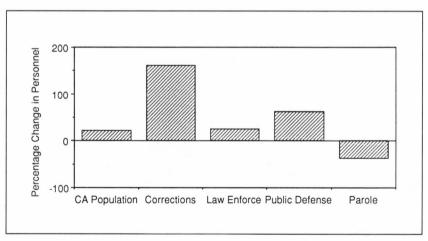

Source: California Department of Justice 1990, table 68.

FIGURE 3.12. Average daily jail population in the United States for five selected years, 1979–1990

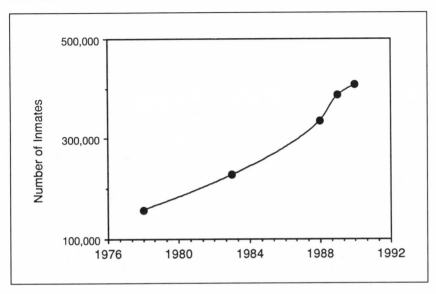

SOURCE: Stephan et al. 1991.

elevating individualism and individual responsibility as the important domestic policy for achieving the new American Dream. Individuals were responsible for their circumstances, and jails, not hospitals, were designated the appropriate institution for handling deviance (Gusfield 1967). The greatest impact of this new emphasis on corrections was felt by children of color as national attention to gangs through the 1980s demonstrates.

Demonizing the Children

The dramatic upsurge in violent youth gang activity in communities of color in the 1980s and 1990s was covered widely in the mainstream press. Across the nation juvenile gangs are obvious, not only in major cities but in suburbs and small towns. In cities like New York, Washington, Detroit, Los Angeles, and Boston, gang killings are reaching record levels and typically are drug-related (Ewing 1990). In 1987 in Los Angeles there were 387 gang killings; in 1988, 452; and in 1989, 500 (Ewing 1990). More and more children are dying in the crossfire, and homicide is now the leading cause of death for Black males and females (Ropp et al. 1992).

FIGURE 3.13. National expenditures on mental health care services in the United States (in constant dollars) for five selected years, 1969–1986

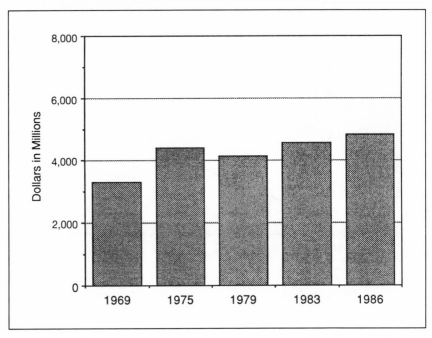

Source: NIMH 1990, table 1.2.

Most people killed in gang homicides are robbery victims and the innocent bystanders of drive-by shootings. The rest of the victims are gang members allegedly involved in either drug turf wars or drive-by shootings (Ewing 1990). Los Angeles has the highest prevalence of gangs in the United States. The counts range from a low of 300 gangs and 30,000 members (State Task Force on Youth Gang Violence 1986) to 600 active street gangs and over 70,000 members (Ewing 1990) to as many as 900 gangs with 100,000 members (Morales 1992). Although these seem like large numbers, 1,313 gangs were documented in Chicago with a prevalence of 65 gangs per 100,000 people in 1927 (Thrasher 1927) in contrast with 7 gangs per 100,000 in Los Angeles in 1987. In Los Angeles, two-thirds of the gangs are Hispanic, and the rest are composed of African Americans, Whites, and Asians. Ewing (1990) documented that in Los Angeles, the number of gang-related homicides has increased steadily: in 1988, 37 percent of homicides were related to gangs.

In the United States, gangs were identified as early as 1846. Violent behavior most often occurred when rival gangs intruded in each other's territories (Davis and Haller 1973). These were White gangs, as were the gangs in New York City evident during the pre–Civil War era (Asbury 1927). Between 1919 and 1927, there were 1,313 gangs in Chicago (Thrasher 1927). White ethnics such as the Polish, Italian, Anglo, Jewish, Slavic, Bohemian, Swedish, and Lithuanians were the major gang members (Thrasher 1927). As Morales notes, the drive-by shootings of present-day gang warfare reflect only changes in technology, with modern automobiles. In the turf wars of the early years, neighborhoods were terrorized for days at a time as gangs fought.

Recent societal reaction has been to increase the punitive actions toward these youths, the majority of whom are from racially or culturally diverse populations, and many of whom are immigrants or are members of immigrant families. There is rising antagonism toward immigrants, and an isolation and redefinition of their problems has emerged as characteristic only of communities of color. The current description neglects the rise of the youth cadres connected to hate groups such as the Ku Klux Klan or the White Aryan Resistance, and even the organized activities of fraternities on college campuses that have produced gang rapes and repeated crimes against property. These actions are often treated as "youthful exuberance" by White officials but as "criminal acts" if the same crimes are committed by minority youths in poor neighborhoods.

Various theories about gangs have developed over the years. Thrasher (1927) felt that gangs evolve mainly from immigrant communities. Cohen (1955) understood the delinquency of gang members as an angry rebellion against middle-class values. Similarly Moore (1978) felt that some of the gang activities focus as a protest to counter the "bureaucratic cruelties of minority status" (p. 50). Cloward and Ohlin (1960) theorized that gangs provide a deviant avenue to attain normal goals, when young people are blocked in their efforts to seek material gains or status through legitimate means.

Matza (1990) said that since adolescents are suspended between childhood and adulthood, they spend their time with their age peers, attempting to sort out their identity and to gain peer group acceptance. This theory does not explain the Chicano gang phenomena of adult and even middle-aged gang members (Morales 1992). Morales proposes that youths turn to gangs as surrogate families. His research has shown that gang members come from dysfunctional families, experience greater poverty, inadequate housing, substance abuse, chronic illness, and more family entanglement with correctional and law enforcement agencies. The gang provides what their families do not or cannot: affection, understanding, loyalty, recognition, and important emotional and physical protection (1992, 457). He notes that one of the largest Hispanic gangs call themselves "homeboys" or "homegirls," which are familial or domestic terms. Similarly, African American gang members call themselves "brothers" or "sisters." The use of the gang to replace what the family fails to provide, obviously, may be psychologically adaptive. However, when gang members maim or kill rival gang members for turf or gang motives, then the phenomenon changes to maladaptive.

According to Morales (1982), gangs are not merely a subcultural way of life. The gang is an epiphenomenon that appears in specific socio-economic conditions and tends to be absent when these conditions are absent. These conditions include low wages, unemployment, lack of rec-reational resources, urban slums, poor health, and other characteristics of urban decay. For minority groups, like Mexican Americans, gangs have existed for sixty years or more since the socioeconomic conditions that promote gang development remain unchanged for Latinos—as well as for African American and, more recently, for Asian populations.

Contemporary gangs reflect some fundamental differences from ear-lier groups (Vigil 1988). An exhaustive study of gangs in Milwaukee, Wis-consin (Hagedorn 1991), revealed that although gangs emerge because of common structural and economic constraints, current dramatic changes in the economy promote unique changes. The previous "maturing out of gangs" is not taking place among African American youth. The factory jobs that previously required mainly hard work are no longer available to provide incentives for gang members to graduate out of gang activity. Research demonstrated that by 1990, fewer than one in five African Amer-ican gang members had found full-time work. Rather than being reincor-porated into family and community life as adults, as Thrasher (1927) had postulated, these adults relied mainly on the illegal economy for survival. This results in an admixture of older members of drug posses modeling dangerous career paths for new generations of gang youths. Anderson (1990) in his studies found similar intergenerational effects, with older members promoting the values of "hustling," drugs, and sexual promis-cuity.

The increased violence first noted in the 1960s for Black gangs in Chi-cago has become the norm. Perkins (1987) identified the influence of drugs, corrupting prison experiences, and the ineffectiveness of commu-nity-based programs as contributing factors to these increases in violence. Although, historically, gangs fought to protect their turf, honor, and neighborhoods, two-thirds of those interviewed in a Milwaukee study felt the gang was mainly about making money, not helping their communi-ties (Hagedorn 1991). Similar conclusions were reached in a study of Puerto Rican gangs in Chicago (Padilla 1992).

The overall level of violence in poorer communities leads to differences in vital statistics based on race and ethnicity. The consequences of violence in minority communities shows up dramatically in mortality statistics from 1980 (table 3.1). Suicide rates, homicide rates (including those from "legal intervention"), and chronic liver disease and cirrhosis rates are shown for Hispanics, Blacks, and Whites further sorted by age for 1979–1981 in fifteen states across the nation. Homicide rates are nearly eight times higher for Blacks aged 15–24 years than for Whites, and nearly six times higher for Hispanics than for Whites.

Additionally, death by liver disease, or cirrhosis, where data are available shows the same kind of distribution in an older group. Blacks aged 25–44 years are nearly five times more likely to die of chronic liver disease than are Whites. In Hispanics, it is more than double the rate for Whites. Cirrhosis is strongly correlated with alcoholism. If these mortality rates reflect true incidence of alcoholism, the problems of violence and substance abuse in Hispanic and Black communities is alarmingly high by comparison with White communities. Paradoxically, White suicide rates are higher across all age categories compared with Blacks and Hispanics. Suicide in minority communities, of course, may be easily achieved by more indirect means. Morales (1992) explains gang homicide as inverted suicide, using the anger and frustration felt against oneself as a projection of the self's image onto the other's image. "That is why we see a young

TABLE 3.1. Mortality statistics from fifteen states by age and ethnicity

	Age		
	1–14 Years	15–24 Years	25–44 Years
Homicide			
Hispanic	1.80	5.87	5.55
White	1.00	1.00	1.00
Black	4.10	7.59	9.31
Suicide			
Hispanic	0.67	0.98	0.80
White	1.00	1.00	1.00
Black	0.33	0.61	0.68
Chronic Liver Disease and Cirrhosis			
Hispanic	N/A	N/A	2.42
White	N/A	N/A	1.00
Black	N/A	N/A	4.90

SOURCE: U.S. Department of Health and Human Services 1990, table 13.

NOTE: Numbers in this table are ratios of mortality rates for each group, compared to the rates for Whites only. Thus, the ratio for Whites is always 1.00.

gang member killing another gang member of the same age and ethnic-racial background. The intentional killing of an inner-city infant by a gang member may represent the ultimate rageful act of one symbolically killing himself to spare the life-long pain of being raised in the impover-ished inner-city, an environment created by years of neglect" (Morales 1991).

Alvin Pouissant, a prominant African American psychiatrist, found homicide the leading cause of death among young Black men, with gang activity contributing a substantial percentage to these statistics (Pouissant 1983). Both Morales and Pouissant see a tremendous unmet need to exam-ine and treat the psychological dynamics that contribute to homicide and gang homicide among minority males. Pouissant argues that just as sui-cide victims are psychologically impaired, we must also realize that those who commit homicide are similarly impaired. He notes that African Americans reflect emotional predispositions that facilitate their becoming homicide statistics for both environmental and political reasons (Pouis-sant 1983).

Yet despite this growing understanding of the conditions leading to gang behavior, the "normal" societal response to the psychological needs of minority youths is to lock them up rather than treat them. It is not simply coincidental that the psychological and emotional needs of gang members are addressed by the criminal justice system rather than by mental health experts. Institutional racism (Knowles and Prewitt 1969) is a critical factor that insures that the deviant behaviors of minority youths are assessed as criminal, when similar behaviors by Whites tend to be defined as mental health problems (Morales 1978; Mason and Gibbs 1992).

Public policy now evolves from a criminal justice basis to protect soci-ety against gang activities rather than addressing gang phenomena from a treatment perspective. Although there may be mental health care ser-vices in juvenile detention centers, it is often too late to mitigate the in-fluence that children are exposed to while detained, an influence that serves only to promote and strengthen gang ties and behaviors.

Prisoners or Patients: The Penrose Effect

In 1939, L. S. Penrose, a British physician who studied the biology of "mental defects," made an observation that by comparing the rates of incarceration for criminal offenses among eighteen European countries to the rates of incarceration for mental diseases in those same countries, one could see a significant negative correlation (Penrose 1939). These same data are analyzed here in a regression plot (in figure 3.14) using Penrose's

FIGURE 3.14. The Penrose effect plotted from the original data, showing the negative correlation between the rates of incarceration in asylums and prisons for eighteen european countries in the 1930s

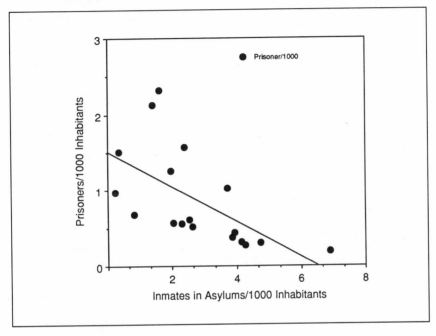

SOURCE: Penrose 1939.
NOTE: $y = 1.510 - 0.232x$; $R = 0.61$.

original data. As is obvious from this plot, there is a significant inverse relationship between incarceration for criminal offenses and incarceration for mental abnormalities. Pallone (1990) describes this Penrose effect in current data from the United States, as inpatient beds were dramatically reduced through deinstitutionalization with a dramatic increase in the corrections population through the 1980s.

Steadman et al. (1984) examined this effect in U.S. data from 1968–1978 for state hospitals and state prisons. They calculated a significant negative correlation, but in tracking individuals between these systems over that ten-year period, they were unable to find a significant rerouting of individuals who were former mental patients into the prison system with the loss of mental health services. The Penrose effect may be cumulative, a phenomenon that is less important in the short run and, thus, is a population phenomenon, not one that affects specific individuals who are already assigned to one system or another. It may be a long-term accumulation of the effects of overall policies for managing deviance that tend to concentrate "careers" as prisoners or patients in one system or the other, careers that are identified early in people's lives and that are difficult to alter. The effect may appear as overall shifts in aggregate numbers (Schelling 1971, 1978).

As Gusfield observed, "Deviance designations have histories, the public definition of behavior as deviant is itself changeable. It is open to political power, twists of public opinion and the development of social movements and moral crusades. What is attacked as criminal today may be seen as sick next year and fought over as possibly legitimate by the next generation" (1967, 187). Even more compelling data are presented in other Penrose data from South Africa (Penrose 1949). The rates of incarceration for criminality and insanity for Europeans (Whites) and for non-Europeans (presumably non-Whites) in South Africa in 1935 were nearly reciprocal (figure 3.15). Although the overall rates of incarceration were

FIGURE 3.15. The Penrose effect from Penrose data from South Africa in 1935, showing a transracial dimension with an inverse relationship between incarceration in asylums or prisons depending on whether one is European or Non-European (non-white)

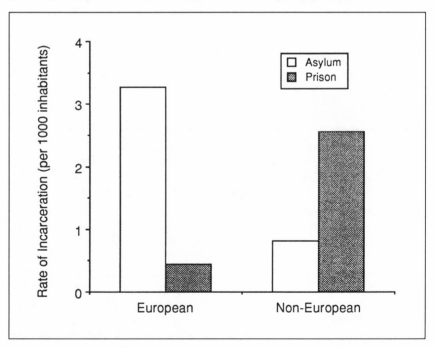

SOURCE: Penrose 1949.

about the same for both groups, far more non-Europeans were locked up for criminal offenses than Europeans, whereas Europeans were incarcerated for mental problems at much higher rates. Thus the Penrose effect demonstrates a pronounced transracial dimension.

Penrose, unfortunately, did not develop comparative data from other countries where similar heterogeneous populations may exist. At the time of Penrose's studies, there was a fair amount of racial homogeneity in Europe. His original data were not confounded by heterogeneous populations where racial differences existed in assigning deviance labels. It would be useful to look at European data today in light of the large immigration of non-White workers into Northern European settings.

The Penrose data from South Africa are important in examining the differential rates of incarceration for minorities in the United States today, the sorting of people into the justice system or the mental health system based not only on overall changes in public policy regarding mental health, but on differential effects of those changes based on skin color. The overrepresentation of African Americans and Latinos in the nation's criminal justice system is a well-known demographic feature (Moss et al. 1991; Hacker 1992). This disparity has become so great that a recent headline in the *New York Times* read, "42 percent of Young Black Men in Capital's Justice System" (DeParle 1992).

If "parity" existed between the general and the prison populations, the percentage representation of ethnic and subgroups should be the same throughout. This is clearly not the situation. The difference between these percentage representations is a measure of disparity. These differences are shown for five ethnoracial groups in the state and federal prison populations in five selected states across the nation in 1988 (figure 3.16). As is clear from this plot. African Americans and Latinos are generally overrepresented and Whites and Asians are underrepresented in prisons.[6] A histogram of the percentage differences in representation in 1988 for all of the fifty states and the District of Columbia (figure 3.17) in the non-White prison population compared to the general population has a mode of 30–35 percent with a broad distribution. Throughout the country, non-Whites are significantly overrepresented in the nation's prisons.

Regional distributions by race and ethnicity of federal and state prisoners in 1988 are shown in figure 3.18. Only in the West is the White prison population more than 50 percent of the total. Throughout the country, African Americans are incarcerated at significantly higher rates than other groups compared to their representation in the general population. Latinos compose an additional significant portion of prisoners in the East and the West where their representation in the general popula-

FIGURE 3.16. The over- and underrepresentation ("disparity") in prison populations compared to representation in the general population of five ethnic groups, shown for five states

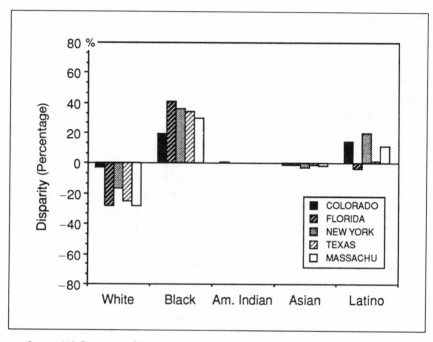

Source: U.S. Department of Justice 1991a.

tion is higher. Asian Americans tend to be underrepresented everywhere, but like Latinos their distribution within the country is quite uneven.

Crime, Poverty, Diversity Relationships

A quantitative expression of diversity can be used effectively to examine the relationship of diversity to a number of other variables.[7] Quantitative presentations of ethnic and racial data traditionally tend to locate separate groups—that is, African Americans, Native Americans, Latinos, or Asian Americans, or specific groups within these designations—and to analyze them separately. With increasing representation of Asians and Latinos in the U.S. population composed of quite different cultural groups, as well as increasing acknowledgment of the cultural complexity within African American and Native American communities (Forbes

FIGURE 3.17. Histogram of values for the "disparity" in representation of non-Whites in prison populations compared to general populations for data from the fifty states and the District of Columbia

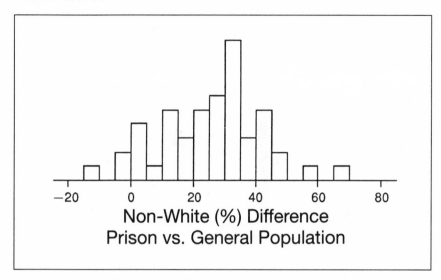

Non-White (%) Difference
Prison vs. General Population

Sources: U.S. Census Bureau 1992, table Z (preliminary data supplied on CD-ROM, "1990 Census of population and housing summary tape file 1A"); U.S. Department of Justice 1991a, table 5.5.

Note: "Disparity" = percentage non-Whites in prison minus percentage non-Whites in general population. The mode is at 30–35 percent overrepresented in prison populations.

1990; Vega 1992), the emergent concept of overall ethnic and racial diversity suggests a macrosocial feature with important analytic possibilities.

Each state in the United States has special features of history, law, economics, and governance, bound together by overriding national norms, customs, and rules. Each state also has different patterns of racial and ethnic diversity. These differences allow an exploration of the dynamics involved among variables. For instance, the variation among states for poverty rates, incarceration rates, treatment expenditures, and demographics allows one to explore quantitatively the cross-correlations between diversity and a number of other factors.[8] "Diversity" itself becomes a crucial analytic variable and becomes more important as the racial and ethnic complexity in the nation increases.[9] The following analyses support that contention.

Data on poverty rates for the states were obtained (Haveman, Danziger, and Plotnick 1991) and were compared for each state to the diversity index calculated for that state from 1990 census data. In this applica-

FIGURE 3.18. Ethnic distribution of prison population by region, comparing the percentage representation of six ethnic categories in state and federal prisons for four regions of the United States

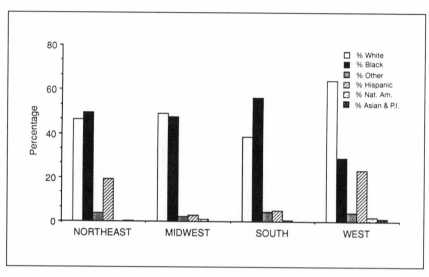

SOURCE: U.S. Department of Justice 1991a.

tion, a value of 0 means no diversity and a value of 1 is the most diverse (everyone is different). The index thus ranges between 0 and 1. Haveman et al. (1988) calculate a relative measure of poverty. Their index is the ratio of the mean family income of the upper quintile of the income distribution in each state divided by the mean family income calculated for the lowest quintile in the distribution.[10] The values range from 6.2 for New Hampshire to 15 for Louisiana. The larger the number, the larger the difference between rich and poor in a state. A linear regression of these data proved significant (figure 3.19). It indicates that there is a systematic linear relationship between increasing diversity and increasing income inequality among states. The states with the greatest diversity have the most income inequality.

The number of people incarcerated in each state in the United States for 1988 were obtained (Allen-Hayen 1988), and the values of the diversity index for each state were compared by linear regression (figure 3.20). Again, this relationship was statistically significant. As diversity increases in one state compared with another, the incarceration rate also increases.

This finding is verified in another type of calculation. The percentage difference between the representation of a group in the general popula-

FIGURE 3.19. Linear regression of the inequality index for each state versus the diversity index, showing increase in ethnic and racial diversity as income distribution becomes more unequal

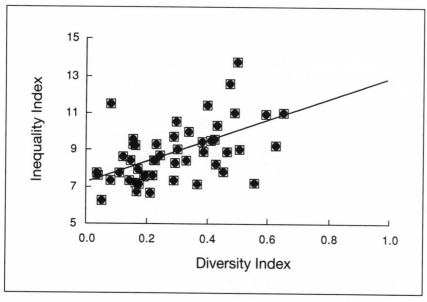

SOURCE: Haveman, Danziger, and Plotnick 1991; U.S. Bureau of the Census 1990a.
NOTE: The inequality index is the ratio of the mean income in the first quintile compared to the mean income in the fifth quintile of income distribution; the diversity index is a quantitative measure of racial and ethnic diversity based on the probability of selection from a population ($R^2 = 0.262; p = .001$; INEQINDX $= 7.262 + 5.638*$SIMPSON). See also note 7.

tion and the representation in a special population such as prisons is a measure of disparity (see figures 3.16 and 3.17). States vary widely in the proportion of the people maintained in their correctional systems. The percentage of the adult population of a state that is maintained in prison is a type of quantitative measure of the strength of punishment inflicted by the state. For 1988, this varied among states, who maintained from 0.5 to 3.8 percent of their adult population in prison. This was plotted against the percentage difference between prison and general populations for non-White prisoners (figure 3.21). The relationship is significant. This suggests that as a state locks up a larger fraction of its adult population, the overrepresentation of non-White people being locked up increases.

From these two relationships (figures 3.20 and 3.21), it is suggestive that as diversity within a state increases, community standards about punishment become more punitive and that the application of this in-

FIGURE 3.20. Linear regression of the diversity index for each state and the corrections rate, showing rise in rate of incarceration as ethnic and racial diversity increases

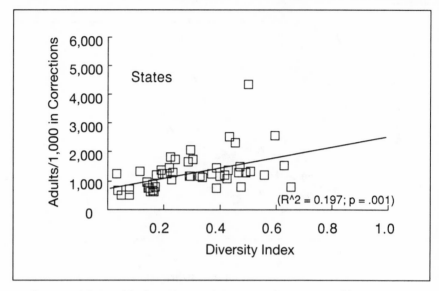

SOURCES: U.S. Bureau of the Census 1990a; U.S. Department of Justice 1991a, table 1.1.
NOTE: For calculation of diversity index, see note 7. The corrections rate is the number of adults held in prison per 100,000 population (Correction Rate = 733.938 + 1789.007*DIVE).

creased emphasis on punishment is more likely to be directed at non-Whites. These relationships were developed here using cross-sectional data (synchronic) in the kind of "natural" experiment available because of differing policies among states. One should also be able to see these relationships in time series data.

Between the 1980 and 1990 U.S. censuses, diversity as measured in the census increased in California (the overall value of the diversity index for the state increased from 0.349 to 0.432). Calculating values of the diversity index for each county in California for 1980, it is clear that diversity within the state is highly variable (range from <0.1 to 0.821). Thus, diversity is increasing spatially as well as over time. The felony arrest rate in California increased by half from 1980 to 1990, going from 980 arrests to 1,453 per 100,000 (California Department of Justice 1991b). Some of this change over time is related to the War on Drugs, but much of it may relate to the patterns of racial diversification underway in California. Within California, using 1980 poverty data obtained from the census for 1980, a

FIGURE 3.21. Linear regression of the percentage of adults in correction versus the difference in percentage representation in prison compared to the general population, 1990

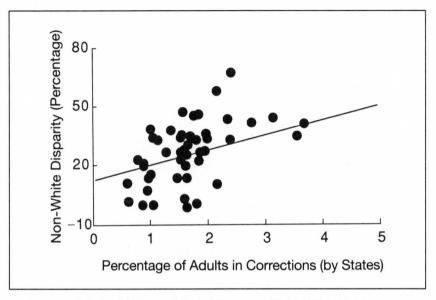

SOURCES: U.S. Bureau of the Census 1990a; U.S. Department of Justice 1991a, table 1.1.

NOTE: This figure shows that states with a larger disparity of ethnic groups in prison than in the general population are also more punitive overall, with a larger proportion of the people incarcerated ($R^2 = 0.167$; $p < .005$; NWHDISCR = 12.558 + 7.613*PCORRECT).

linear regression was calculated between poverty rate and arrest rates among counties. A significant relationship exists between poverty and arrest rates among California counties. The counties having less poverty also had relatively fewer arrests (figure 3.22).

There is, then, a complicated interaction involving poverty, ethnic diversity, and crime; the quantitative measures of these indicators allow an exploration of the possible relationships. There are important assumptions accompanying these analyses. So far the mathematical relationships between variables have been assumed to be linear, but there is no reason that they should be. The outcome measures in social statistics are influenced by many different kinds of factors, all of which may be interrelated. There is every reason to expect that more complicated mathematical expressions of these relationships should exist. This is validated in the following comparison.

The percentage difference in representation of non-Whites in the cor-

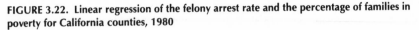

FIGURE 3.22. Linear regression of the felony arrest rate and the percentage of families in poverty for California counties, 1980

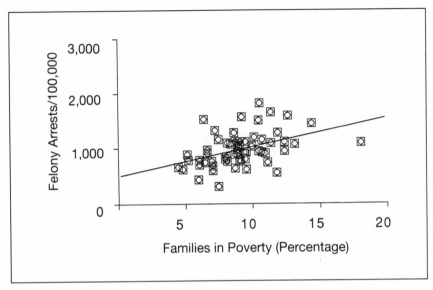

Sources: U.S. Bureau of the Census 1980b, table 180; California Department of Justice 1980.
Note: This figure shows that the poorer the California county, the higher the arrest rates for felonies. For California counties in 1980, there is a significant relationship (p = .001) between the felony arrest rate in each county and the percentage of families in poverty in that county. Poverty is taken from U.S. Census data as the percentage of families below the official poverty line (R^2 = 0.178; p = .001; FEARR80 = 503.730 + 52.124*PCFAPO80).

rections system for each state was compared with the diversity index calculated for each state (figure 3.23). A linear fit to these data points is given in figure 3.23A (R^2 = 0.20). This assumes that an increment of change in diversity produces a proportional increment of change in the representation of non-Whites in prison. However, a better fit to these data is given in the lower figure (figure 3.23B: R^2 = 0.411). A nonlinear regression was a better fit with the data and indicates that the relationship between diversity and incarceration of non-Whites is more complicated than simple linearity would suggest.

One interpretation is that, as diversity increases, the disparity in the prison population increases, but only up to a point. As the diversity of a state goes beyond a certain point, the disparity between corrections and the general population begins to moderate. A possible explanation is that there is some critical level of diversity at which the relationships among the different racial and ethnic groups become normalized, at which some

FIGURE 3.23. A comparison of the diversity index and the disparity between groups in prison and in the general U.S. population

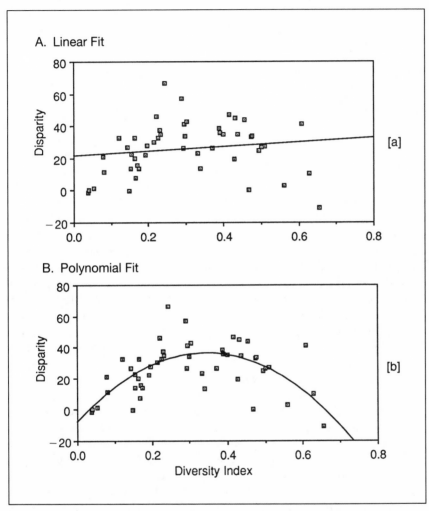

SOURCES: U.S. Census Bureau 1992 (see source for fig. 3.17); U.S. Department of Justice 1991b.
NOTE: The best fit to these data are compared. A polynomial or curvilinear fit is far better (R^2 = 0.411) than a linear fit (R^2 = 0.20). It shows that as ethnic and racial diversity increases, comparing the states, the disparity of ethnic and racial groups in prison compared to the general population increases, but only up to a point. Beyond a diversity index of about 0.4, this relationship moderates and, in fact, declines.

level of understanding or tolerance is institutionalized and further dis-crimination moderated. It may aslo reflect a monetary cap, whereby pub-lic opinion goes against incarcerating more people because increasing costs associated with corrections cannot be sustained. States cannot afford the costs associated with incarcerating any more people, thus the discrep-ancy moderates between non-White and White prisoners.

The Sorting Process

If the Penrose effect is still operating today, one should be able to see this relationship in the state-by-state data just as Penrose developed it for European countries in the late 1930s. One would expect that, as the corrections emphasis differs among states, the mental health emphasis also varies. Steadman et al. (1984) devised this mathematical correlation in the time series data they selected for the United States, but they could not establish the mechanism.

This relationship was explored in data for the states, taking advantage of the differences among states and the resources they direct toward men-tal health or corrections. This is the same kind of synchronic analysis originally done by Penrose for European countries. The assumption is that different policies about mental health treatment exist among political units represented by the states, thus allowing a range of influences that should generate an array of different outcomes in the correction system.

In this application, the number of inpatient and residential treatment beds per 100,000 state residents was compared to the number of adults incarcerated per 100,000 state residents for each state (figure 3.24). In these data the calculated relationship is ambiguous. As Pallone (1990) discusses, the rise in separate facilities for substance abuse obscures some of the relationship, as does the overall growth of private sector care. The actual number of inpatient or residential beds may not accurately reflect the availability of treatment, particularly with the new emphasis on out-patient treatment. A better measure of availability may be the per capita expenditure on mental health services for each state, which captures both inpatient and outpatient treatment. A plot of the per capita expenditures on mental health versus the adult incarceration rate in corrections is shown in figure 3.25. This, too, shows little correlation.

The Penrose effect must be highly sensitive to racial factors, as the early Penrose data from South Africa indicate and as the differences in populations within corrections in this country show. In the past two dec-ades, the proportion of people of different races and ethnicities has been increasing in relation to European Americans. The Penrose effect overall may be blurred by the differential treatment of the races. With large num-

FIGURE 3.24. Linear regression comparing the number of mental health inpatients and residential treatment beds to the number of adults in corrections

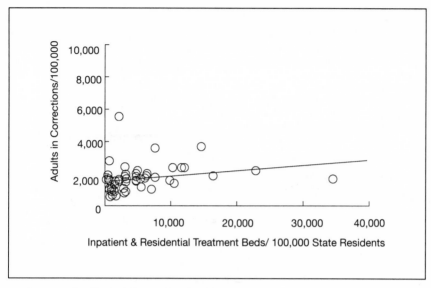

SOURCES: Allen-Hayen 1988; NIMH 1990b, table 1.11.
NOTE: $y = 1528.283 + 0.033*x$; $R^2 = .061$; $p = .08$.

bers of people of color diverted into corrections, dominating the populations there, it indicates that people of color are particularly sensitive to redefinitions of criminality, while European Americans are buffered against that change in labeling by economic access to private mental health treatment. The majority of the population of the United States is still European American, and they will dominate a medical market for handling deviance. If the separate systems of criminal justice and mental health are racially determined, the data for looking at the Penrose effect in heterogeneous populations must be disaggregated according to ethnicity and race and then analyzed separately for each group.

The increase in people needing mental health care and seldom receiving it in the nation's prisons and jails is now well documented (Teplin 1990; Metzner, Fryer, and Usery 1990; Lamb 1984; Lamb and Grant 1982; Steadman et al. 1987; Steadman, McCarty, and Morrissey 1986; Pallone 1990). The legal right to psychiatric care in prisons has been established based on constitutional grounds related to cruel and unusual punishment (Alexander 1989). The complex interrelationships among mental illness and criminality and violence have been explored in a variety of ways

FIGURE 3.25. U.S. mental health expenditures versus rate of imprisonment

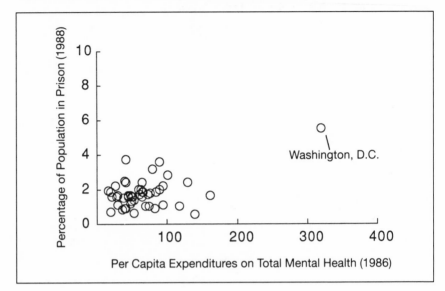

SOURCES: Sunshine, et al. 1990; U.S. Department of Justice 1991a, table 1.1.

(Davis 1991). Pallone's (1990) review of the epidemiological literature comparing mental disorders among prisoners and others shows that the rates of major mental illness in prisoners—particularly affective disorders, but also schizophrenia—are significantly higher than in the general population. Personality disorders are a prominent feature as well as organic mental disorders, along with substance abuse problems (up to 54 percent of prisoners have substance abuse problems according to Pallone).

The rates of drug use on arrest are high around the country (table 3.2). A study of drug use among jail inmates indicates high levels of drug use based on self-reports (figure 3.26) but with little difference among racial and ethnic groups. There was a higher involvement of Blacks and Hispanics in drug-related offenses. The leading group of offenses prosecuted in 1988 were for drug-related offenses (U.S. Department of Justice 1991b).

Although psychoactive substance use can be treated in a variety of treatment settings, most people are never treated; instead, they end up incarcerated (Jarvik 1990). Again, based on self-reports, the number of jail inmates reporting prior treatment for drug abuse according to race and number of treatment attempts is shown in figure 3.27. Proportionately

TABLE 3.2. Rates of drug use on arrest

City	Male Arrestees (% Positive for Any Drug)
San Diego	80
Portland	70
Phoenix	57
Dallas	57
New Orleans	75
Chicago	78
Detroit	69
Philadelphia	82
Washington, D.C.	68
New York	78
St. Louis	56
Birmingham	70

SOURCE: National Institute of Justice 1990.
NOTE: Drugs tested include cocaine, opiates, PCP, marijuana, amphetamines, Valium, Darvon, Methaqualone, barbiturates, and methadone.

more Whites have received some drug treatment, but the overall rates remain low for all groups—less than 30 percent.

In the past few years, in efforts to do something about the increasing numbers of mentally ill people who are unable to take care of themselves, compassionate police officers and courts have increasingly incarcerated homeless mentally ill individuals as a last resort, usually not having to look very far to find a legal reason to do so (Coates 1990). This has been happening at the same time that large numbers of people involved with drugs have been incarcerated. The dual effect attached a criminal label to large numbers of African American and Latino males who constitute the majority of these two populations.

An investigative report of this evolving relationship of the homeless with the courts in Los Angeles was written in 1991 by a *Los Angeles Times* reporter (Tobar 1991a, 1991b). Tobar presents statistics from the Los Angeles county jail system showing that the number of inmates served by mental health programs in the county jails rose from 5,103 in 1985–1986 to 8,479 in 1989–1990: 35 percent of these inmates had committed misdemeanors; 15 percent had felony drug charges, 15 percent had felony assault and battery; 17 percent had committed burglaries or grand theft; 5 percent had committed robberies; and 13 percent had committed murder and other felonies. Affective disorder was diagnosed in 16.2 percent of

FIGURE 3.26. Drug use among ethnic groups

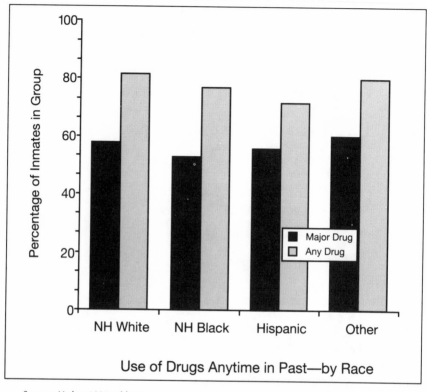

SOURCE: Harlow 1991, tables 2, 7.
NOTE: Drug use is based on self-reports by jail inmates. Major drug category includes heroin, cocaine, LSD, PCP, and methadone.

the cases; 14.9 percent had schizophrenia. An additional 35.5 percent had other psychotic disorders. Tobar wrote:

The worst problems date to the late 1980s when cuts in state funding forced the closure of eight county outpatient clinics. In fact, each time one of the outpatient mental health clinics closes, police and public defenders say they notice a corresponding increase in the number of mentally ill people arrested for crimes in the surrounding community.

The U.S. Department of Justice solicited an examination of the role of the police as a mental health resource (Teplin 1986), which concluded:

FIGURE 3.27. The history of drug treatment based on self-reports by people arrested in 1989 in the United States, comparing three ethnic groups

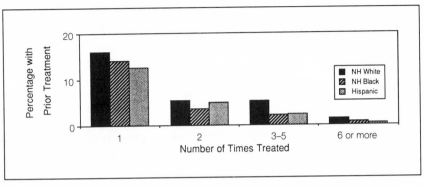

SOURCE: U.S. Department of Justice 1991b, table 4.13.

Given the many bureaucratic and legal impediments to initiating mental health referrals, police might consider arrest to be a less cumbersome and more reliable way of removing the person from the community. Due to the lack of exclusionary criteria, the criminal justice system may have become the institution that can't say no. Persons rejected as inappropriate for the mental health system are readily accepted by the criminal justice system. As a result, the jails and prisons may have become the long-term repository for mentally-ill individuals who have been institutionalized within a psychiatric facility. (1986, 16)

With the increased presence of African Americans and Latinos in the corrections system, the gatekeeping process is clearly biased. This bias is the outcome of many different factors including the racial and ethnic assymetry between the people working in criminal justice and those they arrest, prosecute, and incarcerate. There may be differences in the prevalence of mental illness and criminality among groups caused by socioeconomic differences. Obvious differences in availability of mental health services are affected by economic circumstances. Indirect socioeconomic effects on availability of care are based on the financial ability of households to provide informal care for a sick family member. In addition, local community norms that guide policing activity are often biased regarding race and ethnicity (William and Murphy 1990).

Further study of the dynamics of the interrelationships of racial and ethnic diversity, poverty, illness, crime, and the politics of treatment provision (which include cultural ideas about the maintenance of social order) must acknowledge the predominant tensions in a country of strangers whose most powerful measure of that strangeness is skin color. The Penrose effect includes a racial dimension that must be incorporated. The negative correlation between mental health treatment and society's emphasis on criminal justice is strongly determined by these demographic considerations.

Conclusions

The societal need for managing social deviance and maintaining social order becomes more important as the numbers and kinds of people increase. This process of growth and diversification amplifies problems among groups of people, and in recent years the issue of law and order has become a central public concern.

With the decline of public mental health over the past two decades, the mental health needs of the poor—who are more likely to be persons of color—are met primarily by traditional sources of support (that is, family and friends). The economic pressures placed on poor households make it difficult for families to manage the family member with a major mental illness, although this is the primary location of care for most of the poor today. Although new institutions such as the self-help movement met the demands for alternatives to care, this particular self-help strategy remains predominantly a middle-class European American social movement, omitting other groups through a variety of traditional mechanisms.

Besides contributing disproportionately to the growing homeless population, more and more of the mental health concerns of people of color have been labeled "criminal" during the 1970s and 1980s. This identification is made early in adolescence for increasing numbers of African American and Latino youths as evolving public policy created "opportunities" in a growing corrections system. The long-term consequences for these children are profound. Given access to third-party coverage because of economic opportunities, the adolescent difficulties for European American children have more frequently been dealt with medically, with less damaging long-term effects.

As natural growth and immigration continue to change the racial and ethnic diversity of the United States, new and more sophisticated strategies for maintaining social order will inevitably be shaped by the problems and opportunities created by this diversity. The logical outcome of the present emphasis on corrections may well be moderated because of simple budgetary pressure. The decline of public support for mental health services and a renaissance in the notion of community-based care turned into a nightmare of homelessness and imprisonment for the

"Other America" (Harrington 1962) in the 1980s. The costs to society of locking up ever larger numbers of people may eventually lead to a public demand for new ways of intervening to avoid these costs. Any intervention must address the central problem created because we are a nation of strangers whose traditional measure of strangeness is skin color.

NOTES

The thoughtful comments of Faustina Solís, M.S.W., and Henry Tarke, L.C.S.W., enhanced this project as it was underway and are gratefully acknowledged along with the comprehensive editorial review of Bernard Kramer, Ph.D., Charles Willie, Ph.D., and David Breakstone.

1. Executive Order 12612 entitled "Federalism," Section 2(h) states: "Policies of the national government should recognize the responsibility of—and should encourage opportunities for—individuals, families, neighborhoods, local governments, and private associations to achieve their personal, social and economic objectives through cooperative effort."

2. Weithorn (1988) attributes the first use of the word *transinstitutionalization* to a *New York Times* reporter in 1979; Lawrence Altman, "Release of Mental Ill Spurring Doubts," *New York Times*, November 20, 1979.

3. Data were obtained from *Moody's Industrial Manual* for the years shown in the figures. *Moody's* gives details of financial performance for American corporations, listed yearly. This presentation was suggested by David Stoesz, D.S.W., School of Social work at San Diego State University.

4. Presentation at NASW Conference, 1992, by Maria Zuñiga, Ph.D., and Piedad García, L.C.S.W.

5. This may improve once the American Disabilities Act is fully implemented and a body of case law develops around it.

6. The Native American numbers are so small that they don't show up in these presentations.

7. Quantitative expressions of diversity or heterogeneity have not been widely used in social science but have been proposed (Lieberson 1969; Blau 1977). Several mathematical expressions of diversity have had wide use in ecology (Magurran 1988). One of these, the Simpson Index, was evaluated for use on racial and ethnic data (Simpson 1949; Brooks unpublished manuscript).

8. The usual caveat is in order about interpreting this analysis. Correlations are only suggestive of possible relationships and, although it is tempting to see cause and effect, without additional supportive data these relationships are only suggestive. All statistical and graphical analyses were performed using software available for the Macintosh personal computer. Statistical packages used included "Fastat" and "Statworks." Graphical software included the graphics available on "Fastat" and "Cricket Graph."

9. Commentary and analysis in the wake of the urban riots in Los Angeles in the spring of 1992 indicate that the multiracial/multicultural complexity of Los Angeles must be accounted for in any explanation of the events that transpired.

10. The two-year difference between these two data sets was assumed to be insignificant because these measures change only very slowly over several years and, hence, could be compared.

REFERENCES

Alcohol Health and Research World. 1981. Fiscal and human resources. Summer, pp. 59–65.

Alexander, R., Jr. 1989. The right to treatment in mental and correctional institutions. *Social Work* 34:109–12.

Allen-Hayen, B.
  1988. Children in custody, public juvenile facilities, 1987. *Juvenile Justice Bulletin.* October.
  1990. Children in custody, 1989. *Juvenile Justice Bulletin.*

Alvarez, R., Batson, R. M., Carr, A. K., Parks, P., Peck, H. B., Servington, W., Tyler, F. B., and Zwerling, I. 1976. *Racism, elitism, professionalism: barriers to community mental health.* New York: Jason Aronson.

Anderson, E. 1990. *Street-wise: race, class, and change in an urban community.* Chicago: University of Chicago Press.

Angel, R., and Thoits, P. 1987. The impact of culture on the cognitive structure of illness. *Culture, Medicine, and Psychiatry* 11:465–94.

Anthony, W. A., Cohen, M., Farkas, M., and Cohen, B. F. 1984. Clinical care update: the chronically mentally ill. Case management—more than a response to a dysfunctional system. *Community Mental Health Journal* 24:219–28.

Anthony, W. A., Cohen, M. R., and Cohen, B. F. 1988. Psychiatric rehabilitation. In *The chronic mental patient: five years later,* ed. J. A. Talbott. New York: Grune and Stratton.

Asbury, H. 1927. *The gangs of New York: an informal history of the underworld.* New York: Alfred A. Knopf.

Bachrach, L.
  1976 *Deinstitutionalization: an analytical review and sociological perspective.* NIMH Series D. no. 4. DHEW Publication No. (ADM) 76-351, Superintendent of Documents. Washington, D.C.: U.S. Government Printing Office.
  1982. The young adult chronic patients: an analytical review of the literature. *Hospital and Community Psychiatry* 33:189–97.

Baldwin, D. M. 1990. Meeting production: the economics of contracting mental illness. *Social Science and Medicine* 30:961–68.

Becerra, R., Karno, M., and Escobar, J., eds. 1982. *Mental health and Hispanic Americans: clinical perspectives.* New York: Grune and Stratton.

Berkowitz, M., and Hill, M. A. 1986. Disability and the labor market: an overview. In *Disability and the labor market,* ed. M. Berkowitz and M. A. Hill, p. 219. Ithaca, N.Y.: ILR Press.

Black, B. 1988. *Work and mental illness.* Baltimore: Johns Hopkins University Press.

Blau, P. M. 1977. *Inequality and heterogeneity.* New York: The Free Press.

Bond, G. R., and Boyer, S. L. 1988. Rehabilitation programs and outcomes. In *Vocational rehabilitation of persons with prolonged psychiatric disorders,* ed. J. A. Ciardiello and M. D. Bell, pp. 231–63. Baltimore: Johns Hopkins University Press.

Brooks, E. R.
  1992. Domestic policy since the New Federalism: local response to the homeless and the environment in the San Diego, California, region. MSW thesis, School of Social Work, San Diego State University.
  1993. Measuring ethnic and racial diversity: analysis and application of a numerical method borrowed from ecology. MS.

Burt, M. R., and Cohen, B. E. 1989. Who is helping the homeless? local, state, and federal responses. *Publius* 19:111–28.

California, State of, Department of Justice. Division of Law Enforcement. Bureau of Criminal Statistics and Special Services.

1980. Criminal justice profile, 1980.

1990. *Crime and delinquency in California, 1980–1989.*

1991. *Criminal justice profile, 1990.*

Carlson, D. B., and Heinberg, J. D. 1978. *How housing allowances work: integrated findings from the experimental housing program.* Washington D.C.: The Urban Institute.

Carter, J. H. 1991. Chronic mental illness and homelessness in black populations: prologue and prospects. *Journal of the National Medical Association* 83:313–17.

Cloward, R., and Ohlin, Lloyd. 1960. *Delinquency and opportunity.* Glencoe, Ill.: Free Press.

Coates, R. C. 1990. *A street is not a home.* Buffalo: Prometheus Books.

Cockerham, W. C. 1990. Becoming mentally ill: a symbolic interactionist model. *Studies in Symbolic Interaction* 11:339–50.

Cohen, A. 1955. *Delinquent boys.* New York: Free Press.

Cohen, R. L. 1991. Prisoners in 1990. *Bureau of Justice Statistics Bulletin.*

Conlan, T. 1988. *New federalism.* Washington, D.C.: The Brookings Institution.

Cooper, L., Brown, V. B., Anglin, M. D. 1989. Multiple diagnosis: aspects and issues in substance abuse. White paper for the State of California Department of Alcohol and Drug Programs, Health and Welfare Agency Drug Abuse Information and Monitoring Project.

Cutler, D. L., Bigelow, D., and McFarland, B. 1992. The cost of fragmented mental health financing: is it worth it? *Community Mental Health Journal* 28:121–33.

Davis, A., and Haller, M., eds. 1973. *The people of Philadelphia.* Philadelphia: Temple University Press.

Davis, S. 1991. Are mentally ill people really more dangerous? *Social Work* 36:97–192.

DeLuca, John R. 1981. Health insurance coverage for alcoholism treatment: policy issues. *Alcohol Health and Research World.* Summer, pp. 2–3.

Denton, N. A., and Massey, D. S. 1989. Racial identity among Caribbean Hispanics: the effect of double minority status on residential segregation. *American Sociological Review* 54:790–808.

DeParle, J. 1992. 42 percent of young men in capital's justice system. *New York Times,* April 18, pp. 1, 6.

Dohrenwend, B. P., Levav, I., Shrout, P. E., Schwartz, S., Naveh, G., Link, B. G., Skodol, A. E., and Stueve, A. 1992. Socioeconomic status and psychiatric disorders: the causation-selection issue. *Science* 255:946–52.

Dorwart, R. A., Schlesinger, M., Horgan, C., and Davidson, H. 1989. The privatization of mental health care and directions for mental health services research. In *The future of mental health services research,* ed. C. A. Taube, D. Mechanic, and A. Hohmann, pp. 139–54. DHHS Publication No. (ADM) 89–1600. Superintendent of Documents. Washington, D.C.: U.S. Government Printing Office.

Edwalds, R. M. 1964. Functions of the state mental hospital as a social institution. *Mental Hygiene* 48:666–71.

Emerick, R. E. 1991. The politics of psychiatric self-help: political factions, interactional support, and group longevity in a social movement. *Social Science and Medicine* 10:1121–28.

Estroff, S. E., Lachicotte, W. S., Illingworth, L. C., and Johnston, A. 1991. Everybody's got a little mental illness: accounts of illness and self among people with severe, persistent mental illnesses. *Medical Anthropology Quarterly* 5:331–69.

Ewing, C. P. 1990. *Kids who kill.* Lexington, Mass.: D. C. Heath.

Fagan, J., Slaughter, E., and Hartstone, E. 1987. Blind justice? the impact of race on the juvenile justice process. *Crime and Delinquency* 33:224–58.

First, R. J., Roth, D, and Arewa, B. D. 1988. Homelessness: understanding the dimensions of the problem for minorities. *Social Work* 33:120–24.

Fischer, P. J. 1989. Estimating the prevalence of alcohol, drug, and mental health problems in the contemporary homeless population: a review of the literature. *Contemporary Drug Problems* 16:333–89.

Fisher, C. 1982. *To dwell among friends: personal networks in town and city.* Chicago: University of Chicago Press.

Forbes, J. D. 1990. The manipulation of race, caste, and identity: classifying Afroamericans, Native Americans, and red black people. *Journal of Ethnic Studies* 17:1–51.

Freidan, B. J., and Sagalyn, L. B. 1989. *Downtown Inc.: how America rebuilds cities.* Cambridge, Mass.: MIT Press.

Freyman, J. G. 1980. *The American health care system: its genesis and trajectory.* Huntington, N.Y.: Robert E. Krieger.

Gartner, A., and Reissman, F., eds. 1984. *The self-help revolution.* New York: Human Science Press.

Gilderbloom, J. I., and Appelbaum, R. P. 1988. *Rethinking rental housing.* Philadelphia: Temple University Press.

Glick, P. C. 1990. American families: as they are and were. *Sociology and Social Research* 74:139–45.

Gronfein, W. 1985. Psychotropic drugs and the origins of deinstitutionalization. *Social Problems* 32:437–54.

Guarnaccia, P. J., and Farias, P. 1988. The social meanings of nervios: a case study of a Central American woman. *Social Science and Medicine* 26:1223–31.

Gusfield, J. R. 1967. Moral passage: the symbolic process in public designations of deviance. *Social Problems* 15:175–88.

Gutierrez, L., Ortega, R., and Suarez, Z. 1990. Self-help and the Latino community. In *Working with self-help*, ed. T. J. Powell, pp. 218–36. Silver Spring, Md.: National Association of Social Workers.

Hacker, A. 1992. *Two nations: black and white, separate, hostile, unequal.* New York: Charles Scribner's Sons.

Hagedorn, J. 1991. Gangs, neighborhoods, and public policy. *Social Problems* 38:529–38.

Hallan, Jerome B. 1981. Health insurance coverage for alcoholism: a review of costs and utilization. *Alcohol Health and Research World.* Summer, pp. 16–21.

Halpern, D. 1993. Minorities and mental health. *Social Science and Medicine* 36:597–607.

Harding, C. M., Brooks, G. W., Ashikaga, T., Strauss, J. S., and Breier, A. 1987. The Vermont longitudinal study of persons with severe mental illness. II. Long-term outcome of subjects who retrospectively met DSM-III criteria for schizophrenia. *American Journal of Psychiatry* 144:727–35.

Harlow, C. W. 1991. Drugs and jail inmates, 1989. *Bureau of Justice Statistics Special Report.* August.

Harrington, M.
    1962. *The other America.* New York: MacMillan.
    1984. *The new American poverty.* New York: Penguin Books.

Haveman, J. D., Danziger, S., and Plotnick, R. D. 1991. State poverty rates for Whites, Blacks, and Hispanics in the late 1980s. *Focus* 13:1–7. University of Wisconsin-Madison: Institute for Research on Poverty.

Hill, R. F., and Fortenberry, J. D. 1992. Adolescence as a culture-bound syndrome. *Social Science and Medicine* 35:73–80.

Hopper, K. 1988. More than passing strange: homelessness and mental illness in New York City. *American Ethnologist* 15:155–67.

Jarvik, M. E. 1990. The drug dilemma: manipulating the demand. *Science* 250:387–92.

Jenkins, J. H. 1988. Conceptions of schizophrenia as a problem of nerves: a cross cultural comparison of Mexican Americans and Anglo Americans. *Social Science and Medicine* 26:1233–43.

Jenkins, J. H., and Karno, M. 1992. The meaning of expressed emotion: theoretical issues raised by cross-cultural research. *American Journal of Psychiatry* 149:9–21.

Jimenez, M. A.

  1987. *Changing faces of madness: early American attitudes and treatment of the insane.* Hanover, N.H.: University Press of New England.

  1988. Chronicity in mental disorders: evolution of a concept. *Social Casework.* December.

Johnson, A. B. 1990. *Out of bedlam: the truth about deinstitutionalization.* Basic Books.

Katz, A. H., and Bender, E. I., eds. 1976. *The strength in us: self-help groups in the modern world.* New York: New Viewpoints.

Kirmayer, L. J. 1989. Cultural variations in the response to psychiatric disorders and emotional distress. *Social Science and Medicine* 29:327–39.

Knowles, L., and Prewitt, K., eds. 1969. *Institutional racism in America.* Englewood Cliffs, N.J.: Prentice Hall.

Koslowe, P. A., Rosenstein, M. J., Milazzo-Sayre, L. J., and Manderscheid, R. W. 1991. *Characteristics of persons serviced by private psychiatric hospitals, United States, 1986.* NIMH Mental Health Statistical Note No. 201. September.

Kovel, J. 1970. *White racism: a psychohistory.* New York: Vintage Books.

Lamb, H. R. 1984. Alternatives to hospitals. In *The chronic mental patient: five years later,* ed. J. A. Talbott, pp. 215–32. New York: Grune and Stratton.

Lamb, H. R., and Grant, R. W. 1982. The mentally ill in an urban county jail. *Archives of General Psychiatry* 39:17–22.

Levin, L. S., Katz, A. H., and Holst, E. 1976. *Self care lay initiatives in health.* New York: Prodist.

Lieberson, S. 1969. Measuring population diversity. *American Sociological Review* 34:850–62.

Link, B. G., Cullen, F. T., Struening, E., Shrout, P. E., and Dohrenwend, B. P. 1989. A modified labeling theory approach to mental disorders: an empirical assessment. *American Sociological Review* 54:400–423.

Lum, D. 1986. *Social work practice and people of color: a process-stage approach.* Monterey, Calif.: Brooks/Cole.

McLean, A. 1990. Contradictions in the social production of clinical knowledge: the case of schizophrenia. *Social Science and Medicine* 30:969–85.

Magurran, Ann E. 1988. *Ecological diversity and its measurement.* Princeton: Princeton University Press.

Mason, M. A., and Gibbs, J. T. 1992. Patterns of adolescent psychiatric hospitalization: implications for social policy. *American Journal of Orthopsychiatry* 62:447–57.

Massey, D. S., and Denton, N. 1993. *American apartheid.* Cambridge: Harvard University Press.

Massey, D. S., and Eggers, M. L. 1990. The ecology of inequality: minorities and the concentration of poverty, 1970–1980. *American Journal of Sociology* 5:1158–88.

Massey, D. S., and García España, F. 1987. The social process of international migration. *Science* 237:733–38.

Matza, D. 1990. *Delinquency and drift.* New York: Wiley.

Metzner, J. L., Fryer, G. E., and Usery, D. 1990. Prison mental health services: results of a national survey of standards, resources, administrative structure, and litigation. *Journal of Forensic Sciences* 35:433–38.

Mirowsky, J., and Ross, C. E. 1989. *Social causes of psychological distress.* New York: Aldine de Gruyter.

Moody's industrial manual. Volumes for 1975 to 1990. New York: Moody's Investor Service.

Moore, J. 1978. *Homeboys.* Philadelphia: Temple University Press.

Morales, A.

1978 Institutional racism in mental health and criminal justice. *Social Casework.* July, p. 387.

1982 The Mexican American gang member: evaluation and treatment: In *Mental health and Hispanic Americans: clinical perspectives,* ed. R. Becerra, M. Karno, and J. Escobar. New York: Grune and Stratton.

1991 Latino gang violence: the suicide-homocide link. Paper presented at the Latino Males at Risk: Networking for Mental Health Service and Research Strategies Conference sponsored by San Diego State University, June 14.

1992 Urban gang violence: a psychosocial crisis. In *Social work: a profession of many faces,* ed. A. Morales and B. Shaefer, pp. 451–88. Boston: Allyn and Bacon.

Moss, E. Y., Austin, R., Jones, N., Krisberg, B. A., Locke, H. G., Radelet, M. L., and Welch, S. 1991. African Americans and the administration of justice. *Trotter Institute Review* 5:6–10.

Nathan, R., Doolittle, F. C., and associates. 1987. *Reagan and the states.* Princeton: Princeton University Press.

National Institute of Justice, U.S. Department of Justice. 1990. *Preventive file.* Winter.

National Institute of Mental Health (NIMH)

1987. *Mental health, United States, 1987.* Edited by R. W. Manderscheid and M. A. Sonnenschein. DHHS Publication No. (ADM) 90-1708. Washington, D.C.: Government Printing Office.

1990a. *Mental health, United States, 1990.* Edited by R. W. Manderscheid and M. A. Sonnenschein. DHHS Publication No. (ADM) 90-1708. Washington, D.C.: Government Printing Office.

1990b. *State and county mental hospitals, United States and each state, 1986.* By J. H. Sunshine, M. J. Within, J. E. Atay, A. S. Fell, and R. W. Manderscheid. DHHS Publication No. (ADM) 90-1706. Washington, D.C.: Government Printing Office.

1990c. *Patient care episodes in mental health organizations, United States: selected years between 1955 and 1986.* Mental Health Statistical Note No. 192. By R. W. Redick et al. Washington, D.C.: DHHS. August.

1991. *Caring for people with severe mental disorders: a national plan of research to improve services.* DHHS Publication No. (ADM) 91-1762. Washington, D.C.: U.S. Government Printing Office.

Neighbors, H., Elliott, K., and Gant, L. 1990. Self-help and black Americans: a strategy for empowerment. In *Working with self-help,* ed. T. Powell. Silver Spring, Md.: National Association of Social Work.

Ozarin, L. D., Redick, R. W., and Taube, C. A. 1976. A quarter century of psychiatric care, 1950–1974: a statistical review. *Hospital and Community Psychiatry* 27:515–19.

Padilla, F. M. 1992. *The Gang as an American enterprise.* New Brunswick: Rutgers University Press.

Pallone, N. J. 1991. *Mental disorder among prisoners: toward an epidemiological inventory.* New Brunswick: Transaction Publishers.

Parloff, M. B. 1982. Psychotherapy research evidence and reimbursement decisions: Bambi meets Godzilla. *American Journal of Psychiatry* 139:718–27.

Penn, N. E., and Penn, B. P. 1975. The role of the federal government in promoting general welfare. In *Mental Health: the public health challenge,* ed. E. J. Lieberman. Washington, D.C.: American Public Health Association.

Penrose, L. S.
    1939. Mental disease and crime: outline of a comparative study of European statistics. *British Journal of Medical Psychology* 18:1–15.
    1949. *The biology of mental defect.* London: Sidgwick and Jackson.
Pepper, B., and Ryglewicz, H. 1984. The young adult chronic patient: a new focus. In *The chronic mental patient: five years later*, ed. J. A. Talbott, 33–48. Grune and Stratton.
Perin, Constance. 1988. *Belonging in America.* Madison: University of Wisconsin Press.
Perkins, U. S. 1987. *Explosion of Chicago's Black street gangs.* Chicago: Third World Press.
Pouissant, A. 1983. Black-on-Black homocide: a psychological-political perspective. *Victimology* 8:161–69.
Powell, T. J. 1987. *Self help organizations and professional practice.* Silver Spring, Md.: National Association of Social Work.
Redick, R. W., Witkin, M. J., Atay, J. E., Fell, A. S., and Manderscheid, R. W. 1990. Patient care episodes in mental health organizations, United States: selected years between 1955 and 1986. U.S. Department of HHS-NIMH, Mental Health Statistical Note No. 192. August.
Reed, P. G., and Sanchez, D. S. 1986. Characteristics of alcoholism services in the United States, 1984. DHHS Public Health Service, ADAMHA.
Reed, W. L. 1991. Crime, drugs, and race. *Trotter Institute Review* 5:3–5.
Reich, R. B. 1991. *The work of nations.* New York: Vintage Books.
Remine, D., Rice, R. M., and Ross, J. 1984. *Self-help groups and human service agencies: how they work together.* New York: Family Service Association of America.
Ropp, L., Visintainer, P., Uman, J., and Treoloar, D. 1992. Death in the city: American childhood tragedy. *Journal of the American Medical Association* 267:2905–10.
Rossi, P. 1988. Minorities and homelessness. In *Divided opportunities: minorities, poverty, and social policy*, ed. G. D. Sandefur and M. Tienda, pp. 87–115. New York: Plenum Press.
Ruggie, M.
    1990. Retrenchment or realignment? U.S. mental health policy and DRGs. *Journal of Health Politics, Policy, and Law* 15:145–67.
    1992. The paradox of liberal intervention: health policy and the American welfare state. *American Journal of Sociology* 97:919–44.
Santiago, A. M., and Wilder, M. G. 1991. Residential segregation and links to minority poverty: the case of Latinos in the United States. *Social Problems* 38:492–515.
Sassen, S. 1990. Economic restructuring and the American city. *Annual Review of Sociology* 16:465–90.
Schelling, T. C.
    1971. Dynamic models of segregation. *Journal of Mathematical Sociology* 1:143–86.
    1978. *Micromotives and macrobehaviors.* New York: W. W. Norton.
Schexnider, A. H., and Dorn, E. 1989. Statistical trends. In *Who Defends America? race, sex, and class in the armed forces*, ed. E. Dorn, pp. 41–87. Washington, D.C.: Joint Center for Political Studies.
Scull, Andrew. 1984. *Decarceration: community treatment and the deviant, a radical view.* 2d ed. Cambridge: Polity Press.
Sharfstein, S. S., and Goldman, H. G. 1989. Financing the medical management of mental disorders. *American Journal of Psychiatry* 146:345–49.
Simpson, E. H. 1949. Measurement of diversity. *Nature* 163:688.
Starr, Paul. 1987. *The limits of privatization.* In *Prospects for privatization*, edited by Steve Hanke, pp. 124–37. Proceedings of the Academy of Political Science.

State Task Force on Youth Gang Violence. 1986. California Council on Criminal Justice, Final Report. January.

Steadman, H. J., Fabisiak, S., Dvoskin, J., and Holohean, D. J. 1987. A survey of mental disability among state prison inmates. *Hospital and Community Psychiatry* 38:1086–90.

Steadman, H. J., McCarty, D. W., and Morrissey, J. P. 1986. *Developing jail mental health services: practices and principles.* NIMH-DHHS Publication No. (ADM) 86-1458. Washington, D.C.: Government Printing Office.

Steadman, H. J., Monohan, J., Duffee, B., Hartstone, E., and Robbins, P. C. 1984. The impact of state hospital deinstitutionalization on United States prison populations, 1968–1978. *Journal of Criminal Law and Criminology* 75:474–90.

Stephan, J., Jankoski, L. W., and BJS Statisticians. 1991. Jail inmates, 1990. *Bureau of Justice Statistics Bulletin.* June.

Stoesz, D. 1986. Corporate health care and social welfare. *Health and Social Work* 11:165–72.

Strauss, J. S., Hafez, H., Lieberman, P., and Harding, C. M. 1985. The course of psychiatric disorder. III. Longitudinal principles. *American Journal of Psychiatry* 142:289–96.

Sunshine, J. H., Witkin, M. J., Atay, J. E., and Manderscheid, R. W. 1991. *Residential treatment centers and other organized mental health care for children and youth: United States, 1988.* NIMH Note No. 198. DHHS. July.

Sunshine, J. H., Witkin, M. J., Manderscheid, R. W., and Atay, J. E. 1990. *Expenditures and sources of funds for mental health organizations: United States and each state, 1986.* Mental Health Statistical Note No. 193. DHHS, Division of Biometry and Applied Science. August.

Task Force on Homelessness and Severe Mental Illness. 1992. *Outcasts on main street.* Interagency Council on the Homeless. DHHS (ADM) 92-1904.

Teplin, L. A.

   1986. *Keeping the peace: the parameters of police discretion in relation to the mentally disordered.* National Institute of Justice, U.S. Department of Justice. Research Report. April.

   1990. Detecting disorder: the treatment of mental illness among jail detainees. *Journal of Consulting and Clinical Psychology* 58:233–36.

Thoits, P. 1985. Self-labeling processes in mental illness: the role of emotional deviance. *American Journal of Sociology* 91:221–49.

Thrasher, F. M. 1927. *The gang: a study of 1,313 gangs in Chicago.* Chicago: University of Chicago Press.

Tobar, H.

   1991a A dumping place for the mentally ill. *Los Angeles Times,* August 25, pp. A1, A24, A25.

   1991b Mentally ill turn to crime in a painful call for help. *Los Angeles Times,* August 26, pp. A1, A18, A19.

Torrey, E. F. 1988. *Nowhere to go.* New York: Harper and Row.

Treadway, C. R., and Brown, B. S. 1972. Public policy and mental health. In *Progress in community mental health,* ed. H. H. Barten and L. Bellak, vol. 2, pp. 251–65. New York: Grune and Stratton.

U.S. Bureau of the Census.

   1980a. *1980 census of population. General population characteristics, United States summary.* PC80-1-D1-A. Table 62. Washington, D.C.: Department of Commerce.

   1980b. *1980 census of population. Social and economic characteristics—California.* Washington, D.C.: Department of Commerce.

   1990a. *1990 census of population and housing. Summary. Social, economic, and housing characteristics, United States.* CPH-5-1. Washington, D.C.: Department of Commerce.

1990b. *1990 census of population. General population characteristics, California.* CP-1-6. Washington, D.C.: Department of Commerce.

1992. *1990 Census of population and housing. Summary. Population and housing characteristics, United States.* CPH-1-1. Washington, D.C.: Department of Commerce.

U.S. Department of Health and Human Services. 1990. *Vital and health statistics: deaths of Hispanic origin, fifteen reporting states, 1979–1981.* DHHS Publication No. PHS 91-1855. December.

U.S. Department of Justice.
1986. State and federal prisoners, 1925–1985. *Bureau of Justice Statistics Bulletin.* October.
1991a. *Correctional populations in the United States, 1988.* Office of Justice Programs. Bureau of Justice Statistics. NCJ-12480.
1991b. *Correctional populations in the United States, 1989.* Office of Justice Programs. Bureau of Justice Statistics. NCJ-130445.

Vachon, R. A. 1989. Employing the disabled. *Issues in Science and Technology* 6:44–50.

Valle, R., and Vega, W. 1980. *Hispanic natural support systems.* Sacramento, Calif.: State Department of Mental Health.

Vega, W. A. 1992. Theoretical and pragmatic implications of cultural diversity for community research. *American Journal of Community Psychology* 20:375–91.

Vega, W., and Kolody, B. 1984. The meaning of social support and the mediation of stress across cultures. In *Stress and Hispanic mental health,* ed. W. Vega and M. Mirand. U.S. Department of Health and Human Services, NIMH, Rockville, Md.

Vernez, G., and Ronfeldt, D. 1991. The current situation in Mexican immigration. *Science* 251:1189–93.

Vigil, J. D. 1988. *Barrio gangs: street life and identity in Southern California.* Austin: University of Texas Press.

Walsh, A. M. 1988. Impact of DRG reimbursement: implications for intervention. *Social Work in Health Care* 13:15–23.

Weithorn, L. A. 1988. Mental hospitalization of troublesome youth: an analysis of skyrocketing admission rates. *Stanford Law Review* 40:773–838.

Whitt, H. P., and Meile, R. L. 1985. Alignment, magnification, and snowballing: processes in the definitions of "symptoms of mental illness." *Social Forces* 63:682–97.

William, H., and Murphy, P. V. 1990. *The evolving strategy of police: a minority view.* U.S. Department of Justice, Perspectives of Policing No. 13. January.

Williams, B. F. 1989. A class act: anthropology and the race to nation across ethnic terrain. *Annual Review of Anthropology* 18:401–44.

Williamson, Richard. 1990. *Reagan's federalism: his efforts to decentralize government.* Lanham: University Press of America.

Witkin, M. J., Atay, J. E., Fell, A. S., and Manderscheid, R. W. 1991. Specialty mental health system characteristics. In *Mental health, United States, 1990,* ed. R. W. Manderscheid and M. A. Sonnenschein. NIMH U.S. Department of Health and Human Behavior. Publication No. (ADM) 90-1708.

Zorc, J. J., Larson, D. B., Lyons, J. S., and Beardsley, R. S. 1991. Expenditures for psychotropic medications in the United States in 1985. *American Journal of Psychiatry* 148:644–47.

Zuñiga, M., and Garcia, P. 1992. A Spanish-speaking support group for Latino families of the chronically mentally ill. Paper presented at NASW conference, Los Angeles, California, April 1992.

Racial, Ethnic, and Mental Illness Stereotypes: Cognitive Process and Behavioral Effects

I N the past decade numerous researchers have reported that wide-spread acceptance and use of *The Diagnostic and Statistical Manual of Mental Disorders-III* (DSM-III) has increased reliability and validity of psychiatric diagnosis and minimized the influence of sexist and racist bias (Spitzer et al. 1980; Kass et al. 1983; Fabrega et al. 1990). Some researchers also report that clinicians' racial and sexual attitudes have moved toward more objective and less stereotyped views (Brems and Schlottmann 1988; Kaplan et al. 1990; Fabrega et al. 1990). In contrast, other studies suggest that racist and sexist biases persist in psychiatric diagnosis and treatment despite the widespread use of DSM-III, and that racist and sexist stereotypes play important roles in clinicians' perceptions and decisions (Loring and Powell 1988; Cleary et al. 1990; Redman et al. 1991; Fernando 1988; Waisberg and Page 1988; Lindsay and Paul 1989). The purpose of this chapter is to illuminate the dynamics and effects of stereotypes in the mental health field by comparing the stereotypes of mental illness with ethnic and racial stereotypes, and by examining recent empirical reports for evidence of the effects of racist and sexist stereotypes.

In his extensive study of prejudice, Ehrlich (1973) concluded that ethnic stereotypes are distinct, exclusive, consensual, persistent, and widespread. Because these stereotypes serve as guidelines and boundaries for social relations between groups, they do not change until the actual social relations change. Barth echoed a similar sentiment: "Revision only takes place where the category is grossly inadequate—not merely because it is untrue in any objective sense, but because it is consistently unrewarding to act upon, within the domain where the actor makes it relevant" (1969,

119

30). The evidence we will examine suggests that this is also true of stereo-types of mental illness. Stereotypes of gender, race, ethnicity, and mental illness persist until the actual relations between groups, including their relative power, begin to change.

Stereotypes

This chapter deals primarily with materials from the United States, but some research from other western nations will be included. For convenience, the terms, *attitude, conception,* and *image* will refer to any statement, depiction, or belief about gender, race, ethnicity, or mental illness in which no question of truth or falsity is at issue (Nunnally 1961; Brigham 1971). In contrast, the term *stereotype* will refer to those exaggerated beliefs and images that are popularly depicted in the mass media and folklore whose inaccuracy can be demonstrated (Brigham 1971; Scheff 1966; Nunnally 1961; Glassner 1979; Redman et al. 1991; Littlewood 1992; Fernando 1988; Loring and Powell 1988). The term *function* will be used not in the eufunctional sense but rather in that of a phenomenon having reinforcing effects, anticipated or inadvertent, upon other social processes or institutions (Hempel 1959; Davis 1959; Nagel 1961; Spiro 1961). These effects may have positive or negative implications for particular groups, or for society as a whole (Schrag 1978).

In his classic work *Public Opinion* (1930), Walter Lippmann introduced and explicated the concept of social stereotype. He argued that all perception was necessarily selective. The myriad stimuli impinging upon an individual's sensory apparatus are sorted into categories. The categories are to some extent culturally determined and the sorting process itself becomes largely unconscious and automatic. The categories are inevitably stereotypes in the sense that they obscure important differences among members of a group and exaggerate the differences among the groups.

Since Lippmann's seminal work, an immense literature on ethnic and racial stereotypes has accumulated. Although generalizing from these studies is difficult (Brigham 1971), several propositions pertinent to our argument can be stated at this time. First, selective perception as described by Lippmann (1930) does seem to be a universal fact of human cognition. People all over the world group phenomena into categories and exaggerate the differences among these categories (Levi-Strauss 1965; Needham 1978). Second, when these categories involve human beings, they may serve to define the boundaries and relations between groups. The perceived, exaggerated differences between two groups help to justify the behavior of people in one group toward those in the other. The exaggeration of stereotypes thus can militate against the in-group perceiving out-group traits in themselves or perceiving in-group traits in outsiders (Littlewood 1992; Fernando 1988; Shibutani 1970; Ehrlich 1973; Klapp 1972; Barth 1969; Berreman 1972; DeVos and Romanucci-Ross 1975). To be sure, research has shown that a trait praised in the in-group can be used prejudicially against outsiders (the stereotypical competitiveness and success of Jews in business for example); but the insiders invariably feel that the outsiders express this trait unfairly or in unseemly ways (Allport 1958; Glassner 1979).

These general statements about ethnic stereotypes suggest two propositions about stereotypes of mental illness: (1) if popular images of mental illness act like ethnic stereotypes in demarcating an in-group–out-group boundary, we should expect these images to be greatly exaggerated; and (2) passing from one group to another occurs in some situations with relative ease, but when the dominant group considers the subordinate group distinctly inferior, crossing over becomes difficult, if not impossible (Fernando 1988; Ehrlich 1973; Goffman 1964; Barth 1969; Eidheim 1969; Glassner 1979; Brigham 1971). Since insanity is by definition a grossly inferior condition, we should expect the threshold for redefining an in-group person as mentally ill to be very high. In fact, available evidence suggests that public images of mental illness remain extremely distorted and that crossing the boundary between sanity and insanity is problematic (Townsend and Rakfeldt 1985).

Exaggeration

The most consistent elements in our images of the mentally ill are violence and dangerousness. This is true of attitudes measured with abstract instruments as well as content analyses of media images. For example, an analysis of upstate New York *TV Guide* program listings (Townsend 1979) revealed that 54 percent of all allusions to mental health topics for 1976 portrayed the mentally ill as markedly bizarre and/or dangerous. Persons labeled "mentally ill," "psychotic," or "psychopathic" were depicted as appearing and behaving in obviously strange ways: disheveled or bizarre costume, catatonic stupor, glassy eyes, maniacal laughter, homicidal tendencies. In fact, 24 percent of all allusions suggested a direct link between mental illness and homicidal behavior. Research indicates that the situation is similar in West Germany and has changed little in either country in the last thirty years (Townsend 1978, 1979; Townsend and Rakfeldt 1985; Loring and Powell 1988; Lindsay and Paul 1989). Empirical data on the behavior of ex–mental patients strongly contradict these images. Extensive studies of dangerousness have shown that crime rates among ex–mental patients are no higher than among corresponding persons in the general population. In fact, the reverse may be true. Recent increases in arrest rates among ex–mental patients are apparently attributable to the increasing tendency to channel persons with arrest records into the mental health system (Townsend and Rakfeldt 1985; Lindsay and Paul 1989; Steadman, Cocozza, and Melick 1978; Steadman 1980, 1982).

Another commonly recognized image of mental illness is that of the delusional personality, that is, people believe they are Napoleon, Christ, or some other famous figure (Nunnally 1961; Scheff 1966; Schneider and Wieser 1972). Among twenty-five thousand patients Rokeach (1964) found only a handful of such people: only three patients without brain damage consistently believed they were Christ, and there were no Napoleons, Caesars, Krushchevs, or Eisenhowers. The evidence thus suggests that two of the most common stereotypes, violence and delusional personalities, are inaccurate.

Crossing

Barth has argued that ethnic boundaries only emerge in situations where the categorizations have a self-fulfilling character: "With such a feedback from people's experiences to the categories they employ, simple ethnic dichotomies can be retained, and their stereotyped behavioral differential reinforced despite a considerable objective variation. This is so because actors struggle to maintain conventional definitions of the situation in social encounters through selective perception, tact, and sanctions" (1969, 30).

Selective perception and self-fulfilling prophecy allow ethnic boundaries to persist despite a flow of personnel across them and despite campaigns that demonstrate their obvious inaccuracy or unfairness (Barth 1969; Ehrlich 1973). The sanity-insanity boundary is similar. The studies I shall examine below suggest that popular and professional conceptions of mental illness share four specific traits with ethnic stereotypes: (1) they are exaggerated and serve to dichotomize between the in-group and the out-group; (2) they are maintained through selective perception; (3) they erect high thresholds for "crossing"; and (4) they persist despite the flow of individuals across boundaries and despite campaigns to alter them.

In a now classic study from 1955, Star (1962) found that, when presented with textbook examples of mental disorders, the public defined only the most bizarre disorders (such as paranoid schizophrenia) as mental illness. Cumming and Cumming (1957) used the same psychiatric descriptions to study public attitudes. Like Star, the Cummings discovered that the public harbored much narrower, more concrete conceptions than the professionals' more psychological, normative, and continuous criteria. Public images of insanity apparently functioned to dichotomize between sanity and insanity. Because these images performed important cognitive functions, they were not easily altered by campaigns. Indeed, the Cummings' efforts to alter public conceptions were met with heated resistance. A replication of the Cummings' study in the same location (D'Arcy and Brockman 1976) indicated that people's recognition threshold for mental illness had not changed substantially in the preceding twenty years. These studies suggest that the public's exaggerated images of mental illness reflect a cognitive dichotomy between sanity and insanity. Typically, people's behavior has to be "really crazy" for them to earn the title "mentally ill."

In a study that remains unexcelled for richness of detail, Yarrow et al. (1955) found that husbands had to breach wives' expectations repeatedly before they would finally be recognized as mentally ill. The wives repeatedly rationalized and normalized their husbands' symptomatic behavior because of the unpleasant and threatening consequences of redefining the behavior as symptoms of mental illness. After the "recognition" occurred, the wives tended to redefine past behaviors as symptoms of the incipent disorder. The husbands' behavior became qualitatively different in their eyes. Other studies have produced similar results (Sampson et al. 1962; Silver 1955; Bakwin 1963; Smith et al. 1963). More recently, Townsend and Rakfeldt (1985) found that in patients' first contacts with the mental health system, patients harbored extremely negative images of the mentally ill and mental hospitals, and they continued to use definitions of mental illness that excluded them. This use of stereotyped images of insanity and mental hospitals as contrast conceptions, however, was more problematic for the patients who had been admitted to state mental hospitals than for those who had been diverted to other forms of treatment. Apparently the threshold for crossing the sanity-insanity boundary is high for in-group members. When an individual has been designated as "normal," he or she must repeatedly exhibit deviant behavior to be reclassified by the family, self, or other in-group members.

Ethnic stereotypes share important similarities with the stereotypes of mental illness. A person's actions, appearance, or behavior is often less important in how individuals will be perceived than the labels or categories attached to them. For example, when presented with pictures of faces that varied in skin tone from whitest to blackest, subjects attributed stereotypes to the faces according to the experimenter's random labeling of them as Black or White. Thus, a relatively Black face, if labeled White, elicited White stereotypes (Secord 1959). Naturally, there were some exceptions to this tendency. Most subjects would not attribute White stereotypes to the blackest faces (or the converse) but did follow the suggestion effects of the label attached to the intermediate faces. It is interesting to note, however, that a small group of subjects were so prejudiced that they sometimes followed the label regardless of the objective appearance of the stimulus. Similar results were achieved by changing the ethnic surnames attached to faces in the pictures (Razran 1950). We shall see later that mental health care professionals exhibit a similar tendency: a label previously attached by another professional or someone in the community appears to be a powerful determinant of how a clinician will perceive a prepatient.

Reentry

The role of stereotypes after initial labeling is less clear than in the initial stages. Smith et al. (1963) found that the incidents preceding rehospitalization increased in apparent dangerousness and disruptiveness. This suggested a raised threshold for rehospitalization, but it is not clear from the study whether this difference was actually behavioral or the result of a lowered cognitive threshold, that is, the second "last straw" was perceived as being more disruptive than the first (although not in reality). Some authors have suggested that labeling lowers the recognition threshold to the point where virtually any behavior could be perceived as a symptom. This seems to be particularly true in the context of the mental hospital (Goldman et al. 1970; Rosenhan 1973). In the community, however, it appears that crossing or recrossing the sanity-insanity boundary is more due to "negotiation" (Edgerton 1966, 1969). Some families may come to see the relative's problem as psychiatric, but many do not categorize him or her as "crazy."

This argument is consistent with the evidence indicating that some families refuse to define the patient as "mentally ill" even after extensive treatment. Lewis and Zeichner (1960) found that 16 percent of the families in their sample persisted in such denial, while family attitudes ranged from sympathetic understanding to overt hostility. Greenley (1972, 1979), found that rehospitalization correlated negatively with the family's desire to have the patient at home. Family attitudes that were significantly related to the number or readmissions included: keeping the patient at home would be like having a ten-year-old child around, would create a financial burden for the family, and would reinforce dislike of the patient. These correlations remained significant even when Greenley controlled for severity of symptoms. Similarly, Townsend and Rakfeldt (1985) reported that some families tolerated what others would not. Families who could empathize, or at least sympathize, with the patient's situation typically did not classify the patient as a member of the stereotyped mentally ill. Instead, like the patients themselves, they created a new category: someone who has problems or is "sick" but is not really "crazy."

It thus appears that the sanity-insanity boundary is maintained by the same mechanisms as ethnic boundaries: exaggerated stereotypes and selective perception. In both situations people struggle to maintain conventional definitions by selectively perceiving and by rationalizing their categorizations. In this way their stereotypes can exist side by side with their actual experience with a member of the out-group. In ethnic and racial prejudice, this process of rationalization allows the bigot to like some members of an out-group because "they're not like the rest" (Allport 1958; Ehrlich 1973).

Professional Conceptions

In the preceding section I argued that the public's initial tendency to diagnose mental illness is conservative. The public's initial recognition threshold (at least for family members) is high in part because they do think of mental illness in stereotyped terms. This high threshold becomes particularly significant when one considers that initial recognition does occur in the community. Representatives of the mental health system usually see the prepatient only after lay persons or non-psychiatric professionals in the community bring the prepatient to their attention (Yarrow et al. 1955; Mechanic 1962; Townsend 1979; Townsend and Carbone 1980; Cleary et al. 1990; Redman et al. 1991). This means that the mechanisms of social control are set in motion before the mental health professional sees the offender, and the public's high recognition threshold acts as a kind of conservative filter, repeatedly normalizing deviant acts until the last straw is reached.

Numerous authors have argued that psychiatrists and the courts act as filtering agents of social control once the public's recognition threshold has been exceeded. It is then their task to protect society from further disruption (Mechanic 1962; Scheff 1966, 1975; Szasz 1963, 1970). If this is true, then psychiatrists cannot employ the same recognition criteria as the public; otherwise they, like the public, would tend to normalize most of the deviant behavior and send the deviants back to the community. Logically, if psychiatrists are to perform their social control functions, compared to the public they must have rather broad criteria for recognition.

Broadness

In the late 1960s and early 1970s, several studies of diagnosis supported the notion that American psychiatrists had relatively broad criteria for the recognition of psychosis. Kendell et al. (1971) matched groups of British and American psychiatrists who viewed videotapes of patient interviews. Agreement was high in the major diagnoses of patients who exhibited classic, textbook symptoms. In contrast, the tapes that were chosen specifically to represent nonpsychotic disorders caused serious disagreement. The American audience tended predominantly to diagnose schizophrenia (69–85 percent) whereas the British shunned this category (2–7 percent). This glaring difference was not caused by semantics but rather by psychiatrists' actually perceiving different symptoms in the patients' behavior. One patient, for example, was rated by a majority of the Americans as showing delusions, passivity, and thought disorder. Only about 7 percent of the British psychiatrists gave similar responses. The author concluded that the diagnosis "schizophrenia" was used so freely in America as to be virtually meaningless.

Temerlin (1968) had a professional actor portray an ideal, normal man in an audiotaped clinical interview. Before hearing the tape, each group of experimental subjects heard a prestigious confederate remark that the man appeared neurotic but was really psychotic. Control subjects heard that the man was perfectly healthy. Of the experimental subjects, 60 percent of the psychiatrists, 28 percent of the psychologists, and 11 percent of the graduate students diagnosed psychosis. In contrast, all control subjects agreed unanimously that the man was not psychotic. Thus, in the Kendall and Temerlin studies, American psychiatrists seemed to have a perceptual set to assign a labeled "out-grouper" to the most extreme outgroup, and the broadness of their criteria allowed them to do so. Like the experiments in ethnic stereotyping (Secord 1959; Razran 1950), the label attached to a person played a more important role in determining what qualities were attributed to that person than the individual's actual appearance or behavior.

Some researchers would claim that widespread use of DSM-III has increased reliability and validity of psychiatric diagnosis to the point that influence of nonpsychiatric factors has been minimized if not eliminated, and findings like those of Kendall and Temerlin are no longer valid (Spitzer et al. 1980; Kass et al. 1983; cf. Kleinman 1988a). As we saw previously, however, initial "diagnosis" of mental health problems is typically made by lay persons in the community, or by nonpsychiatric professionals. For example, Bart and Grossman (1976) cite the following results from a sample of 250 questionnaires collected and analyzed by the Woman in Midstream group. Although only about 60 percent of the sample sought medical treatment for organic symptoms of the climacteric from their family physicians or gynecologists, 75 percent received estrogen therapy. For 11 percent no treatment was prescribed, and for 9 percent psychiatric therapy was recommended. The most alarming finding was that 55 percent received prescriptions for psychotropic medications.

In a pioneering study of symptom variation, Donovan (1951) found that the method of taking clinical history places disproportionate emphasis on the symptoms to which the physician directs the patient's attention. The author, over a period of several months, repeatedly interviewed women who were diagnosed by physicians as suffering from "menopausal syndrome." Of these women, 95 percent appeared to be highly suggestible and had had a series of similar complaints *before* menopause. Donovan concluded that symptoms of emotional stress occurred with menopause only if there had been a past history of emotional problems, and that considerable variability appeared in the reporting of symptoms in different interviews with the same woman.

Actually, all symptoms of disease that become organized into illness behavior do so through a process of negotiation. The impact of sociocultural factors, however, on this "construction of clinical reality" (Kleinman et al. 1978; Kleinman 1988a, 1988b) is most pronounced when symptoms are relatively amorphous and ambiguous. Certainly, this is true of mental disorders (Edgerton 1969; Rushing and Esco 1977; Rushing 1978; Townsend 1978, 1979, 1980). Most psychosomatic and psychological symptoms are nonspecific and amorphous (Strauss et al. 1979), and in many respects resemble symptoms of some of the folk illnesses described in medical-anthropological literature: headaches, dizziness, fatigue, anxiety, insomnia, general aches and pains, indigestion, depression (Madsen 1964; Kleinman 1988a, 1988b; Kleinman et al. 1978). When general complaints such as these are not tied to any demonstrable organic cause, they are especially vulnerable to the impact of social factors that shape illness behavior. These studies suggest that amorphous complaints and malaise produced by psychocultural factors become organized through clinicians' selective perception and broadness of criteria into psychiatric syndromes, and nonpsychiatric as well as psychiatric professionals play an active, albeit inadvertent, part in recruiting women into these roles (Kleinman 1988a, 1988b; Townsend and Carbone 1980). The two studies that follow suggest that primary-care physicians continue to play crucial roles in this process (Redman et al. 1991; Cleary et al. 1990).

A study of diagnoses made by primary-care physicians in Wisconsin compared the results of the General Health Questionnaire (GHQ) and the Schedule for Affective Disorders and Schizophrenia-Lifetime Version (SADS-L), with patients' medical records (Cleary et al. 1990). More women than men were diagnosed as having mental health problems. Using the GHQ as a measure of the tendency to self-report problems and the SADS-L data as a measure of physician-diagnosed psychiatric symptoms, the thesis that women are more likely to report symptoms and that this accounts for the frequently documented finding that women are more often diagnosed as having mental problems than are men, was not substantiated. Rather, patients with more severe psychiatric symptoms (as measured by the SADS-L) who used the clinic more frequently were more likely to be identified by their primary-care physicians as having mental problems. Using the SADS-L data as the criterion for "actual" psychiatric symptoms, recognition of psychiatric symptoms by primary-care physicians was poor: correct positives and negatives for women comprised only 35.7 percent, and for men only 26.7 percent. But women had significantly higher false positive rates (19.0 percent) than men did (10.7 percent). The authors conclude that some women without psychiatric problems may be receiving inappropriate attention, whereas men with psychiatric problems are less likely to receive needed psychological attention or referral from their primary-care physicians.

A study in New South Wales, Australia, yielded even more dramatic evidence of gender bias in primary-care physicians' diagnoses (Redman et al. 1991). In a sample of 1,913 patients, males and females showed equal levels of psychiatric symptoms when assessed by the GHQ; fifty-six doctors, most of whom were male, diagnosed more female than male noncases (as assessed by the GHQ) as having psychiatric symptoms; 77 percent of the doctors who diagnosed more than twenty cases ascribed a higher proportion of false positives to women. A second study of male and female interns yielded similar findings, but only male interns diagnosed a higher percentage of female noncases as having mental problems. The authors propose that female interns are more feminist in their sex-role attitudes than the male interns and are, therefore, less likely to harbor and be influenced by sexist stereotypes. High scores on the GHQ signified greater symptomatology. There were fewer false positives and negatives for high scorers, and there was no gender difference in the proportion of false positives for high scorers. These findings thus also support the view that nonclinical factors like gender, race, and social class have their greatest impact when symptoms are less discrete and severe and more ambiguous (Townsend 1978, 1980; Townsend and Rakfeldt 1985; Redman et al. 1991).

Loyal supporters of DSM-III might argue that when it is used by experienced psychiatrists, systematic bias such as that found in the diagnoses of primary-care physicians is improbable, if not impossible. To test this claim, Loring and Powell (1988) had 488 psychiatrists, comprising equal numbers of Blacks and Whites, and males and females, diagnose two actual cases that had previously been diagnosed as undifferentiated schizophrenia. Equal numbers of subjects read that the cases were either Black or White, or male or female, or received no information at all on the sex and race of the cases. Approximately equal percentages of the four groups chose the modal diagnosis, that is, the category that had previously been assigned these cases in real life: undifferentiated schizophrenia. The control subjects had no information on the cases' gender or race and their concordance rate was superior to those of the experimental groups, and alternative diagnoses assigned to the control cases showed no distinctive pattern.

In the alternative diagnoses assigned to the cases labeled by gender and race, however, systematic gender and racial bias appeared. In general, subjects were more accurate (that is, more likely to assign the modal diagnoses) when diagnosing cases that coincided with their own race and gender. The authors had predicted this result in terms of common experience and empathy: that greater familiarity with clients' experience and social position would lead to greater accuracy in interpreting the meaning of deviant acts. The one exception to this finding was the tendency of White female psychiatrists to assign the alternative diagnosis, brief reactive psychosis, to White female patients. The authors speculate that in this case, greater familiarity led to greater empathy (and perhaps greater sympathy) and caused the White female psychiatrists to assign a diagnosis that is less severe, that is a reaction to psychosocial circumstances rather than the manifestation of biological predispositions and that, therefore, has a better prognosis. Apart from this finding, the heterogeneity in diagnoses is suggestive.

As alternative diagnoses for female cases, male psychiatrists tended to assign depressive disorder for Axis 1 and histrionic disorder for Axis 2, suggesting that male clinicians continue to endorse the stereotype of women as having emotional problems (Chesler 1972; Kaplan 1983; Kass et al. 1983; Fabrega et al. 1990; Cleary et al. 1990). Black male patients tended to receive paranoid schizophrenia as the modal alternative diagnosis from all four groups—although of the four groups, Black male psychiatrists were the least likely to assign this category. This finding supports the view that members of an in-group are less likely to view other members in stereotyped terms (Townsend, 1978, 1979; Townsend and Rakfeldt, 1985). Paranoid schizophrenia contains elements of suspiciousness, dangerousness, and violence. Both male and female Black cases tended to receive paranoid personality disorder as the Axis 2 alternative diagnosis, whereas the modal diagnosis was dependent personality disorder. In contrast, when Black psychiatrists evaluated same-sex White patients, they chose either the modal diagnosis or less severe disorders.

The authors suggest that, compared to their alternative diagnoses for same-sex Black cases, this finding may indicate that Black psychiatrists internalize White standards during their medical training. If this is true, in terms of our model of stereotypes, these Black psychiatrists are using (perhaps unconsciously) White standards as their reference group, and the Black cases as contrast conceptions—albeit not to the same extent as do their White peers. Loring and Powell conclude that although the use of DSM-III has probably reduced the effects of race and gender bias, it has not eliminated them. Some significant effects remain and, even with carefully drawn standards, psychiatric diagnosis is to some degree still a subjective activity.

The results of these studies are not merely of academic interest. Some diagnostic differences carry weighty implications. A person labeled "psychotic" is much more likely than a nonpsychotic to be involuntarily committed; to be treated with major tranquilizers and shock therapy (ECT); to have his or her legal rights and responsibilities suspended.

The breadth of clinicians' recognition criteria probably springs from several sources, not just the suggestion effects of prior labeling. First, family and community members see a prepatient in a social context and are therefore more likely to observe coping strengths and assets as well as disordered behavior. Mental health professionals usually see the prepatient in a clinical context and are thus less likely to observe aspects that militate against a diagnosis of mental illness. Second, clinicians are trained to look for pathology. Because no demonstrable organic pathology exists for the functional mental disorders to validate diagnosis, there are fewer objective checks than in other clinical fields on the professional's tendency to look for pathology (Townsend 1980; Townsend and Rakfeldt 1985; Kleinman 1987). This may explain why, before DSM-III, large-scale psychiatric screening of the public turned up so many unreported "psychotics" (for example, Srole et al. 1962; Beiser 1971). Unquestionably, the systematic use of stringent diagnostic criteria can produce acceptable levels of reliability in research settings (Kendell 1975; Kleinman 1988a). In everyday clinical practice, however, breadth of criteria and selective perception continue to allow nonclinical factors to influence diagnosis and treatment.

A third reason American psychiatrists may have relatively broad recognition criteria for mental pathology is their basic assumption about normality. Beiser points out a common assumption: in the absence of symptoms, a person should be happy, productive, and competent (1971, 254). This assumption ignores the reality that any normal life involves some setbacks, some unhappiness, some depression. A comparison (Townsend 1978) of American and German ideology suggests that Americans tend to assume a more idealistic view of life than do Germans, and these basic ideological differences also appeared in American and German mental health professionals' conceptions of mental illness. Thus, harboring this assumption about normality, American professionals may be particularly liable to perceive pathology in normal people.

Selective Perception

Apparently, both public and professionals maintain their conventional definitions of situations through selective perception and rationalization. But compared to the public's relatively high initial threshold for recognition (at least for in-group members), professionals' thresholds appear to be lower, particularly if labeling by other mental health professionals has already occurred. In the 1970s, researchers who had themselves admitted as patients to mental hospitals corroborated this view (Rosenhan 1973; Goldman et al. 1970). Compared to the public, psychiatrists were able to perceive their stereotyped images in a much broader range of behaviors. The following examples indicate that some recently trained clinicians still maintain their definitions of out-groups through selective perception, rationalization, and behavioral sanctions.

Waisberg and Page (1988) had 45 male and 38 female psychotherapists evaluate case studies: experimental subjects read cases that exhibited gender inappropriate symptoms, (that is, males evinced emotional disorders and females exhibited antisocial disorders). Cases described as exhibiting gender inappropriate symptoms were evaluated as more psychologically disturbed by subjects, but this difference was strong only for male patients described as depressed. The authors concluded that Chesler's (1972) thesis—females' gender nonconformity is perceived as more threatening than males' and is therefore punished more strenuously— was not supported. Waisberg and Page argue, however, that recent research does support Broverman's original finding that women are perceived by professionals as intrinsically more maladjusted (Broverman et al. 1970).

The effects of selective perception, broadness of criteria, and stereotyping emerged in Townsend and Rakfeldt's (1985) investigation of first-admission patients. The interviewer, Jaak Rakfeldt, observed the admission of a 43-year-old woman who had had one previous, short admission and was reluctant to enter the hospital. She also was very much opposed to taking medication. After the admitting room doctor had asked the routine questions, the patient was admitted to the hospital. The doctor then grappled with how to diagnose the patient according to the standard nomenclature. The following dialogue ensued:

DOCTOR: [looking through DSM-III)] : Let's see . . . what do we have here? Which type of schizophrenia is she? [He discussed the matter with an attendant who had been helping with the admission procedure. He then looked over at the researcher and asked] What do you think?

RESEARCHER: She seems to know who she is, where she is, and when all this is happening. Also, her brother said she has been "slightly odd since she was fourteen," and has, according to her brother, had those strange thoughts for years. Perhaps, with the new classification in the DSM-III, she could be defined as a Schizotypal Personality Disorder—you know, like a characterological problem.

DOCTOR: But if it's a personality disorder, she should be out there [he gestured with his hand pointing out the window] not in here. People with personality disorders are out there. And how can I give her Thorazine [which he had already prescribed], if she is a characterological problem? This [medication] is for schizophrenia.

RESEARCHER: Well, those are just my thoughts.

On the admission papers she was diagnosed as "schizophrenia, undifferentiated, subchronic" (DSM-III 295.91), and the phenothiazine was administered. This woman was certainly not more symptomatic than many others who were observed or interviewed and who were not admitted, but unlike those others, she lacked community supports such as family and friends. For example, the researchers observed a young man who refused threatment at Crisis Residence although his family and girlfriend reported that he had recently become verbally abusive and had experienced auditory hallucinations. He finally agreed to receive outpatient treatment from a local psychiatrist. Thus, although this patient exhibited some definitive symptoms of schizophrenia, he was not hospitalized, whereas the middle-aged woman with less obvious symptomatology but with a previous hospitalization was admitted. These cases support the thesis that family supports and history of previous hospitalizations often are more potent determinants of disposition than symptomatology (Lamb and Talbott 1986; Talbott 1974; Greenley 1972; Strauss and Carpenter 1972; Leff 1976; Mendel and Rapport 1969; Harder et al. 1990).

In the case of the 43-year-old woman, the impact of the labeling process became evident when, after the decision had been made to commit and to medicate the patient, the diagnostic label was then used to justify this action. Furthermore, the psychiatrist used contrast conceptions when he stated that persons who are not psychotic should be "out there," but if someone is in the hospital, then "they must be psychotic." Finally, there did not appear to be great concern about stigma and disruption to this person's life. Perhaps because her life was already disrupted and she had previously been hospitalized, the admitting psychiatrist may not have considered these issues important. This is in marked contrast to the orientation and methods of the staff interviewed in a Crisis Residence Center (Townsend and Rakfeldt 1985). Ironically, the patient stated during the routine interview that a major part of her problem was that she had been "depressed about not being with her husband." She added that "after I was in the hospital [she had experienced one very brief mental hospitalization several years earlier] he [her husband] said he was afraid of me. He said he didn't want to be with me."

The case of institutionalized patients may have particular relevance for the study of stereotypes of powerless groups. Lindsay and Paul (1989) note that poor, uneducated persons who lack family and community supports still predominate in state and county hospitals despite deinstitutionalization (Kiesler 1980; Kiesler et al. 1983). Blacks are overrepresented in custodial institutions, and more so in acute admissions and readmissions in urban settings. Furthermore, Black patients are even more disproportionately represented among involuntary commitments. Compared to other admitted groups, Black patients tend to have slightly lower socioeconomic levels and are assigned more severe diagnoses. Otherwise, Blacks show no consistent differences from other groups that would account for these overrepresentations.

Lindsay and Paul's extensive review (1989) revealed that empirical investigations offer little evidence that the state's use of coercive power for involuntary commitments was justified by committed patients' having more severe symptoms. The criterion of dangerousness may have been consistently applied: that is, those individuals committed under this standard appeared to have committed more violent or dangerous acts. But the evidence that the criterion of grave disability had been consistently applied was singularly unconvincing. Moreover, even the best of these studies were marked by sloppy methodology and lack of controls, and they presented no explanation or justification of racial differences in the rates of involuntary commitment. The lack of cogent evidence to justify involuntary commitments is particularly critical in view of the increasing number of tort liability cases resulting from errors in commitment decisions, and because of current pressures to broaden the criteria for involuntary commitment, with consequent increases in the proportion of involuntary admissions and perhaps in overall admissions as well (Lindsay and Paul 1989, 179; see discussion of Lamb and Talbott 1986, below).

Even voluntary commitments are frequently not so voluntary. One study showed that in a majority of voluntary admissions, the individuals were already under some form of official custody and were faced with the threat of involuntary commitment proceedings as the principal alternative. When individuals decide on voluntary commitment, they waive certain constitutional rights, often without full cognizance, and frequently during all these proceedings they are living under heavy medication (Gilboy and Schmidt 1971). Lindsay and Paul point out that in studies of the justification of involuntary commitment, patients who sign in voluntarily under duress represent false negatives, whereas patients whose involuntary commitments cannot be justified on the basis of their symptomatology (false positives) "represent a serious error in the assessment/decision-making process, an error in which racial or other biases are suspect" (1989, 175).

Examining the records of 19,400 adult patients in Los Angeles County treated between 1983 and 1988, Flaskerud and Hu (1992) found that patients in lower socioeconomic levels had fewer sessions with their primary psychotherapist, received fewer prescriptions for psychotropic medications, and were less likely to be treated by professionally certified psychotherapists. Black race or ethnicity correlated with fewer sessions with the primary therapist, but Blacks received more treatment with psychiatric medications, despite the fact that Blacks were overrepresented in the lower socioeconomic strata. Receiving less psychotherapy and more medication is associated with poor prognoses, recidivism, and chronicity. In the Loring and Powell study (1988), male and female Black patients received paranoid personality disorder as the modal, alternative, Axis 2 diagnosis, and Black males received paranoid schizophrenia as the modal, alternative, Axis 1 diagnosis. The tendency to stereotype Black patients with these more threatening diagnoses, and then give them more drugs but less psychotherapy, may help to explain Blacks' overrepresentations among admissions, readmissions, and in particular, involuntary commitments. Furthermore, as Adebimpe has noted, even if it could be shown that symptomatic differences between Blacks and Whites were "merely" the effects of social class—something which has not been demonstrated—the overrepresentation of Blacks in the lowest socioeconomic groups means that any problems associated with belonging to those classes will afflict even larger numbers of Blacks, and clinicians and society have the responsibility to analyze and ameliorate those conditions (Adebimpe 1981, 284; see also review of Harder et al. 1990, below).

Social Control

In the 1970s, British psychiatrists apparently had much narrower conceptions of psychosis than did American psychiatrists (Kendall et al. 1971). One possible explanation for this discrepancy concerns our mental health care system's social control function. If this system functions to control (and help) a broad range of deviants, including geriatric cases, indigents, and otherwise helpless people, then American professionals must have extremely broad criteria for mental illness. Insofar as some other countries have better welfare systems, fuller employment, and less sexist, racial, and class exploitation, they can afford stricter criteria for "mental illness." Some evidence points in this direction (Townsend 1978; Taube and Redick 1973; Braginsky et al. 1969; Stearns and Ullman 1949).

In the United States, criteria for commitment and definitions of mental illness have fluctuated with the availability of public funding and with the public's awareness of (or annoyance with) mentally disordered individuals. As resources became scarce, and civil libertarian pressure for reform mounted in the 1970s, statutory and policy revisions narrowed the criteria for commitment and treatment. Agencies frequently manipulated labels and categories to avoid taking on patients with a bad prognosis, and an increasing number of patients were "dumped" on other agencies (Robbins et al. 1977). For example, the criminal justice and mental health systems both manipulated labels to channel repeaters into each other's system (Steadman et al. 1978; Lamb and Grant 1982, 1983). Similarly, mental helath agencies redefined or more strictly defined certain conditions (chronic brain syndrome, for example) to shift chronic patients to nursing homes and other agencies (Hoyer and Tars 1978). By the early 1980s, several states had consciously adopted policies to divert patients from hospitals and back into the community (Townsend and Rakfeldt 1985).

Townsend and Rakfeldt's (1985) interviews with crisis staff and mental health officials in upstate New York revealed a strong awareness of the problem of institutionalism. These professionals realized that state hospitals function as havens for people who have few options in mainstream society. These "chronics" are often less symptomatic than first-contact patients, many of whom are acting out or suicidal, but the former group wants to be in the hospital—or at least in some refuge—and will produce the necessary behaviors to be admitted (Braginsky et al. 1969). Mental health officials particularly feared that inflation and rising unemployment rates would contribute to a sharp increase of young, unemployed males in the mental health system. Interviews with three male repeaters showed that they matched the official definition (or stereotype) of young chronics: relatively young males with no marketable skills, a history of drug and/or alcohol abuse, and no strong ties to family and friends. These men were transient and looked to the hospital as a last resort (Braginsky et al. 1969). As one of these men remarked, the hospital gave him a roof over his head and he could work there, go to the gym, and make enough to buy soap, cigarettes, and razor blades. Another noted that the hospital was superior to jail in most respects, but it worried him that he could not smoke in the hospital when he wanted to.

Our model of stereotypes suggests that professionals maintain their definitions of those who have crossed the boundary not only by selective perception and rationalization but also by behaving in such a way as to "fulfill the prophecy." Merely appearing at an admissions unit thus often constitutes prima facie evidence that the patient probably needs hospitalization. An interview with a top-level mental health planner and policy analyst supported this view (Townsend and Rakfeldt 1985). This official noted that a study conducted in upstate New York indicated that 80 percent of the people who appeared at an admissions service were admitted, regardless of what alternatives existed in the community. He concluded, "This finding seems to say that if you locate an admissions service in a hospital, there is a good chance people will be admitted." Another administrator explained that the primary policy initiative had become management in the least restrictive setting: Don't admit patients if they can be handled in day care, don't treat them in day care if you can handle them in clinic, and don't get them into the mental health system at all if they can be managed in the community. Evidently, statements of mental health staff and administrators—and indeed the entire diversion policy of New York state in the early 1980s—constituted a relatively explicit acknowledgment that treatment, in and of itself, within the mental health system contributed to recidivism and chronicity, and that, therefore, the best intervention was often the least possible intervention (New York State Office of Mental Health 1982).

Attempts such as New York state's diversion policy to reform the mental health system enjoyed only limited success. Bagby and Atkinson (1988) conclude that, in general, attempts to reform commitment procedures by reducing medical discretionary authority and replacing it with evidentiary and objective criteria have met with substantial resistance from the psychiatric community. In several states, tightening diagnostic and commitment criteria produced only brief reductions in admission rates, which then steadily climbed back until they reached or exceeded their prereform levels. In some jurisdictions, tightening criteria merely increased the number of patients committed without adequate evidence, and for extralegal reasons such as "lacks insight" and "refuses treatment" (Bagby and Atkinson 1988; Hasebe and McRae 1987).

The American Psychiatric Association has proclaimed that policies of deinstitutionalization and diversion to the community have set adrift a vast population of mentally ill indigent and homeless (Lamb and Talbott 1986). As the authors remark, "Society has a limited tolerance for mentally disordered behavior" (1986, 499). Consequently, to meet the needs of these unfortunates, and to protect their relatives and the community, the entire mental health system must be greatly expanded, including the criteria for voluntary and involuntary commitments. The authors note that many indigent patients, especially the young, tend to drift away from their families and supervised residences because they are "trying to escape the pull of dependency," or, if they still have goals, because they find an inactive, low-pressure lifestyle extremely depressing, or because they want more freedom to drink or use street drugs. Once they are on their own, they typically stop taking their medications. Therefore, adequate "psychiatric and rehabilitative services must be available and must be provided assertively through outreach services when necessary" (500), with "easy access to short- and long-term inpatient care when indicated" (499). Evidently, the American Psychiatric Association now wants to reacquire the "young chronics" we identified earlier—exactly those patients that New York state officials wanted to exclude in the early 1980s.

The stigmatizing of disadvantaged economic, ethnic, and racial groups, and their relegation to public institutions in the United States has a long and unseemly history (Rothman 1971; Prudhomme and Musto 1973). In the past, stereotypes of mental illness have not only functioned like ethnic stereotypes, at times they actually were ethnic stereotypes. For example, Protestant New Englanders frequently labeled Irish immigrants "degenerate" or "mentally ill" and in the mid nineteenth century the Irish became the predominant population in Worcester, Tewksbury, and other state hospitals in the Northeast (Rothman 1971).

Several authors have noted that contemporary mental hospitals in America tend to serve the same populations as the old almshouses of the nineteenth century (Miller 1965, 1967; Braginsky et al. 1969). Stearns and Ullman's (1949) investigation of one such institution revealed that over a period of ninety-four years the inmates had not changed much—only society's label for them had. Before, they were merely helpless and poor; now they had become mental patients. Stearns and Ullman list the characteristics that made recent immigrants particularly vulnerable to such labeling: they have come to this country usually without funds and are sought out only as unskilled laborers; they speak a foreign dialect or language; when unemployment increases, they are the first to lose their jobs; they have few resources in family or friends. On examining the contemporary patient population, the authors concluded that most of the patients were there for the same reasons: they lacked family, friends, and the skills and connections that would enable them to cope in the outside world. It should be noted that these same traits characterize today's urban poor, particularly poor Blacks, and may help to explain the reported correlations among living in poverty, being Black, and having chronic mental illness (Pierce et al. 1985; Lamb and Talbott 1986; Lindsay and Paul 1989; Harder et al. 1990).

In an earlier study, Turner and Gartrell (1978) argued that the frequently reported correlation between low socioeconomic status and poor psychiatric outcome was a selection artifact. People's social competence

allegedly determines their length of stay in hospitals, and their social position and resources have no impact on outcome when one controls for
social competence. The authors' measure of social competence (derived
by means of some rather dubious statistical procedures) is a person's social mobility (controlling for education and point of origin). Thus, the
authors concluded that social status, good family connections, and work
performance themselves do not help to determine outcome but, rather,
arise as a consequence of conditions within individuals. These conditions
are describable as psychopathology on the one hand and social competence on the other (1978, 378).

There are several serious problems with this interpretation. First, the
literature just reviewed would suggest that diagnoses used in research
settings may already contain bias introduced by the processes of steretyp-
ing. Most researchers, including Turner and Gartrell, attempt to control
for bias by having a "blind" evaluator rate the psychiatric interview material. But the original interviewers were not blind, nor were the patients'
original clinical evaluators. Indeed, it is doubtful whether anyone can
ever be totally blind to a respondent's gender, race, ethnicity, or poverty
(Adebimpe 1981; Fernando 1988; Littlewood 1992; Loring and Powell
1988). This suggests that the bias introduced by selective perception may
affect not only the makeup of the original population but also subsequent
research procedures.

A second objection to Turner and Gartrell's conclusion is that some
extremely elegant studies have documented the relevance of family desire
and social status to patient outcome (Greenley 1972, 1979; Steadman and
Cocozza 1974). These studies controlled for various measures of positive
social functioning and found that family desires nevertheless remained a
potent determinant. Their broader measures of social competence seem
more convincing than Turner and Gartrell's rather narrow, abstruse, and
possibly artifactual measure. Furthermore, Rushing (1978) demonstrated
that, controlling for other significant variables, lower social status correlated with involuntary commitment. People with more resources are able
to avoid being committed, their symptoms being equal.

A third problem with Turner and Gartrell's argument is their insis-
tence on locating the determinants of outcome exclusively within individuals. Earlier we saw that psychiatric diagnosis can operate like ethnic stereotypes in defining social relations between groups, including
relationships of power. The attempt to locate the causes of deviance and
social "failure" exclusively within individuals preempts an examination
of these relationships of power and possible sociocultural determinants
of human misery (Caplan and Nelson 1974). The assumption embodied
in such thinking is convenient for those already in power and very much

in the American grain. The assumption is that people can "make it" if they really try, regardless of external circumstances (Arensberg and Niehoff 1975; Hsu 1972; Townsend 1978). A corollary of this assumption, clearly embodied in Turner and Gartrell's definition of social competence, is that people who are not upwardly mobile—that is, do not have a more prestigious occupation than their fathers—are somehow inferior to those who do. This seems a rather arbitrary, but very American, value judgment. It is quite possible that, viewed from another perspective, some of those behaviors that contribute to upward mobility might be considered selfish, stress-producing, alienating, or otherwise undesirable (Hsu 1972; Henry 1963). The emphasis on self-reliance and upward mobility, however, is deeply entrenched in American ideology and social policies. A comparison of Germany and America (Townsend 1978) demonstrated that these values also permeate American popular and professional conceptions of mental health. It is not surprising, therefore, that these values should also crop up in American mental health policy and research.

At first glance, the findings of Harder et al. (1990) appear to support Turner and Gartrell's (1978) argument regarding social competence. In a longitudinal study of first-admission patients, Harder et al. (1990) found that social competence was a powerful predictor of psychiatric outcome. As in numerous prior studies, patients' social class emerged as a significant predictor for outcome functioning and level of health or sickness. But psychotic and schizophrenic symptoms increased disproportionately among Blacks even when the influence of patients' social class was statistically controlled. Of all predictor variables, patients' IQs showed the strongest correlations with all outcome measures and with the increases in symptomatology between the initial and follow-up surveys. Patients' gender, age, and amount of interim life-event stress were not significant predictors of outcome. The authors concluded that a general "social competence factor"—comprising premorbid marital adjustment, social functioning, and IQ—predicts psychiatric outcome across the entire spectrum of severe disorders. The authors speculate that a higher degree of chronic environmental stress, as opposed to specific life events, may account for Black patients' greater increases in symptomatology.

To their credit, Harder et al. (1990) do not attempt to locate the causes of poor people's greater recidivism and symptomatology solely within individuals—unlike Turner and Gartrell (1978). Harder et al. also opine that Blacks may suffer from greater chronic environmental stress, which was not controlled in their measures. The authors used Hollingshead's two-factor index to control for social class. Although this measure is adequate for some research purposes, it is probably too crude to differentiate and control for psychocultural factors that might explain Black patients' disproportionate increase in symptoms. It is also possible that a relatively small percentage of Blacks in higher socioeconomic levels in the sample precluded valid statistical control of this factor. Finally, the authors' conclusions ignore a long history of criticism of IQ tests as culturally and socioeconomically biased. Fernando, for example, argues that researchers and clinicians continue to use IQ and personality tests without consideration of cultural and racial bias because such tests confirm their everyday observations and substantiate their stereotypes (1988, 137).

Conclusion

Evidently, institutionalized patients have particular relevance for the study of stereotypes of powerless groups. In both cases the stereotypes held by the dominant group may prescribe not only how they will act toward the subordinate group, but also how they will allow the subordinate group to act (Fernando 1988; Glassner 1979). Thus, if White slaveowners thought that Blacks were lazy, shiftless, and childlike, the slaveowners' own behavior may have contributed to the fulfillment of that prophecy (Elkins 1961). Similarly, if hospital staff expect female patients to suffer from emotional problems, and Black patients to be paranoid and potentially violent, their own treatment of the patients may help to fulfill their prophecy. There is considerable evidence, in fact, that patients become institutionalized at least partially because they are often rewarded for adjustment to hospital routine rather than for normal, extra-institutional behaviors (Goldman et al. 1970; Barton 1959; Wing 1962; Braginsky et al. 1969; Townsend 1976; Townsend and Rakfeldt 1985). The evidence that we have examined here suggests that stereotypes of race, gender, and mental illness significantly affect this process.

REFERENCES

Adebimpe, Victor. 1981. Overview: white norms and psychiatric diagnosis of black patients. *American Journal of Psychiatry* 138:279–81.
Allport, Gordon. 1958. *The nature of prejudice.* New York: Anchor.
Arensberg, C. M., and Niehoff, A. H. 1975. American cultural values. In *The Nacirema: readings on American culture,* ed. J. Spradley and M. Rynkiewich. Boston: Little, Brown.
Asnis, G. M., et al. 1977. A survey of tradive dyskinesia in psychiatric out-patients. *American Journal of Psychiatry* 134:1367–70.
Aviram, U., and Segal, S. 1973. Exclusion of the mentally ill. *Archives of General Psychiatry* 29:126–31.
Bagby, R. M., and Atkinson, L. 1988. The effects of legislative reform on civil commitment admission rates: a critical analysis. *Behavioral Sciences and the Law* 6:45–61.

Bakwin, R. M. 1963. Attitudes of parents of mentally ill children. *Journal of American Medical Women's Association* 18:305–8.

Bar-Levav, Reuven. 1976. The stigma of seeing a psychiatrist. *American Journal of Psychotherapy* 30:473–482.

Bart, P. and Grossman, M. 1976. Menopause. *Women and Health* 1:3–11.

Barth, Fredrick. 1969. *Ethnic groups and boundaries.* London: Allen and Unwin.

Barton, Russell. 1959. *Institutional neurosis.* Bristol: John Wright.

Bassuk, E. L., and Gerson, S. 1978. Deinstitutionalization and mental health services. *Scientific American* 238:46–53.

Beiser, M. 1971. A study of personality assets in a rural community. *Archives of General Psychiatry* 24:244–54.

Berreman, G. 1972. Social categories and social interaction in urban India. *American Anthropologist* 74:567–86.

Bittner, Egon. 1967. Police discretion in emergency apprehension of mentally ill persons. *Social Problems* 14:278–92.

Braginsky, B. M., Braginsky, D., and Ring, K. 1969. *Methods of madness: the mental hospital as a last resort.* New York: Holt, Rinehart, and Winston.

Brems, C., and Schlottmann, R. 1988. Gender-bound definitions of mental health. *Journal of Psychology* 122:5–14.

Brigham, John C. 1971. Ethnic stereotypes. *Psychological Bulletin* 76:15–38.

Brooks, Garland P. 1971. The behaviorally abnormal in early Irish folklore. *Papers in Psychology* 5:5–13.

Broverman, I. K., et al. 1970. Sex-role stereotypes and clinical judgments of mental health. *Journal of Consulting and Clinical Psychology* 34:1–7.

Caplan, N. and Nelson, S. 1974. Who's to blame? *Psychology Today* 8:99–104.

Carpenter, W. T., McGlashan, T. H., and Strauss, J. 1977. The treatment of acute schizophrenia without drugs: an investigation of some current assumptions. *American Journal of Psychiatry* 134:1–20.

Chauncy, Robert. 1975. Comment on the labeling theory of mental illness. *American Sociological Review* 40;248–52.

Chesler, Phyllis. 1972. *Women and Madness.* Garden City: Doubleday.

Cleary, Paul, et al. 1990. The identification of psychiatric illness by primary care physicians: the effect of patient gender. *Journal of General and Internal Medicine* 5:355–60.

Cocozza, J., and Steadman, H. 1978. Prediction in psychiatry: an example of misplaced confidence in experts. *Social Problems* 25:253–77.

Cohen, E., Harbin, H., and Wright, M. 1975. Some considerations in the formulation of psychiatric diagnosis. *Journal of Nervous and Mental Disease* 160:422–27.

Crocetti, G., Spiro, Herzl, and Siassi, Iradj. 1974. *Contemporary attitudes toward mental illness.* University of Pittsburgh Press.

Cumming, E., and Cumming, J.

    1957. *Closed ranks: an experiment in mental health education.* Cambridge: Harvard University Press.

    1972. On the stigma of mental illness. In *Rebellion and Retreat,* ed. S. Palmer, pp. 449–61. Columbus, Ohio: Merril.

    1976. Changing public recognition of psychiatric symptoms? Blackfoot revisited. *Journal of Health and Social Behavior* 17:302–10.

D'Arcy, Carl, and Joan Brockman. 1976. Changing public recognition of psychiatric symptoms? Blackfoot revisited. *Journal of Health and Social Behavior* 17:302–10.

Davis, Kingsley. 1959. The myth of functional analysis as a special method in sociology and anthropology. *American Sociological Review* 24:757–72.

Dawidoff, Donald J. 1975. Commitment of the mentally ill in New York: some comments and suggestions. *Journal of Psychiatry and Law* 3:79–95.

DeVos, G., and Romanucci-Ross, L. 1975. Ethnicity: vessel of meaning and emblem of contrast. In *Ethnic identity*, ed. G. Devos and L. Romanucci-Ross. Palo Alto: Mayfield.

Donovan, J. C. 1951. Menopausal syndrome: a study case histories. *American Journal of Obstetrics and Gynecology* 62:1281.

Edgerton, Robert B.
    1966. Conceptions of psychosis in four East African societies. *American Anthropologist* 68:408–25.
    1969. On the "recognition" of mental illness. In *Changing perspectives in mental illness*, ed, S. C. Plog and R. B. Edgerton, pp. 49–72. New York: Holt, Rinehart, and Winston.

Ehrlich, H. J. 1973. *The social psychology of prejudice*. New York: Wiley.

Eidheim, H. 1969. When ethnic identity is a social stigma. In *Ethnic groups and boundaries*, ed. F. Barth. London: Allenand Unwin.

Elkins, S. 1961. Slavery and personality. In *Studying personality cross-Culturally*, ed. B. Kaplan. New York: Row, Peterson.

Ennis, B., and Siegel, L. 1973. *The rights of mental patients: the basic ACLU Guide to a mental patient's rights*. New York: Avon.

Erikson, Kai. 1967. Notes on the sociology of deviance. In *Mental illness and social processes*, ed. Thomas J. Scheff. New York: Harper and Row.

Fabrega, Horacio, et al. 1990. Females and males in an intake psychiatric setting. *Psychiatry* 53:1–16.

Felix, R. H. 1967. *Mental illness: progress and prospects*. Columbia University Press.

Fernando, S. 1988. *Race and culture in psychiatry*. Worcester: Billing and Sons.

Fischer J. 1969. Negroes and Whites and rates of mental illness: reconsideration of a myth. *Psychiatry* 32:428–46.

Flaskerud, J. and Hu, Li-tze. 1992. Racial/ethnic identity and amount and type of psychiatric treatment. *American Journal of Psychiatry* 149:379–84.

Foucault, M. 1965. *Madness and civilization: a history of insanity in the Age of Reason*. Trans. Richard Howard. New York: Pantheon.

Fracchia, J., Canale, D., Cambria, E., Ruest, E., and Sheppard, C. 1976. Public views of ex-mental patients: a note on perceived dangerousness and unpredictability. *Psychological Reports* 38:495–98.

Friedberg, J. 1975. Let's stop blasting the brain. *Psychology Today* 9:18–20.

German, J. R., and Siner, A. C. 1977. Punishing the not guilty: hospitalization of persons acquitted by reason of insanity. *Psychiatric Quarterly* 49:238–54.

Gilboy, J., and Schmidt, J. R. 1971. "Voluntary" hospitalization of the mentally ill. *Northwestern University Law Review* 66:429–53.

Glassner, Barry. 1979. *Essential interactionism*. London: Routledge, Kegan Paul.

Goffman, Erving. 1964. *Stigma*. Englewood Cliffs, N.J.: Prentice Hall.

Goldman, A. R., Bohr, R. H., and Steinberg, T. A. 1970. On posing as mental patients: reminiscences and recommendations. *Professional Psychology* 2:427–34.

Gove, W. R. 1975. The labelling theory of mental illness: a reply to Scheff. *American Sociological Review* 40:242–48.

Gove, W. R., and Fain, T. 1973. The stigma of mental hospitalization: an attempt to evaluate its consequences. *Archives of General Psychiatry* 28:495–500.

Greenley, J. R.
    1972. The psychiatric patient's family and length of hospitalization. *Journal of Health and Social Behavior* 13:25–37.

1979. Familial expectations, posthospital adjustment, and the societal reaction perspective on mental illness. *Journal of Health and Social Behavior* 20:217–27.

1981. Family symptom tolerance and rehospitalization experiences of psychiatric patients. In *Research in Community and Mental Health*, ed. R. Simmons. Greenwich, Conn.: JAI.

Halpert, H. P. 1969. Public acceptance of the mentally ill. *Public Health Reports* 84 (January): 59–64.

Handel, Janet. 1973. Breaking fears of mental illness. *Journal of Emotional Education* 13:133–39.

Harder, D. W., et al. 1990. Predictors of outcome among adult psychiatric first-admissions. *Journal of Clinical Psychology* 46:119–28.

Hasebe, Tad, and McRae, John. 1987. A ten-year study of civil commitments in Washington State. *Hospital and Community Psychiatry* 38:983–87.

Hempel, Carl. 1959. Logic of functional analysis. In *Symposium on Sociological Theory*, ed. Llewellyn Gross. New York: Row, Peterson.

Henry, Jules. 1963. *Culture against man*. New York: Random House.

Hoyer, F. W., and Tars, S. E. 1978. Problems and issues facing the gerontological practitioner in the community mental health center. Paper presented at the 86th Annual Meeting of the American Psychological Association, Toronto, August.

Hsu, R. L. K. 1972. American core value and national character. In *Psychological Anthropology*, ed. F. Hsu. San Francisco: Schenkman.

Jaeckel, Martin, and Wieser, Stefan. 1970. Das Bild des geisteskranken in der Öffentilichkeit. Stuttgart: Georg Thieme Verlag.

Journal of Criminal Law and Criminology. 1975. The "crime" of mental illness: extension of "criminal" procedural safeguards to involuntary civil commitments. *Journal of Criminal Law and Criminology* 66:255–70.

Kaplan, Marcia. 1983. A woman's view of DSM-III. *American Psychologist* 38:786–92.

Kaplan, Marcia, et al. 1990. Psychiatrists' beliefs about gender-appropriate behavior. *American Journal of Psychiatry* 147:910–12.

Kass, Frederick, et al. 1983. An empirical study of the issue of sex bias in the diagnostic criteria of DSM-III axis II personality disorders. *American Psychologist*, July, pp. 799–801.

Katz, M. M., Cole, J. O., and Lowery, H. A. 1969. Studies of the diagnostic process: the influence of symptom perception, past experience, and ethnic background on diagnostic decisions. *American Journal of Psychiatry* 125:109–19.

Kendell, R. E. 1975. *The role of diagnosis in psychiatry*. Oxford: Blackwell.

Kendell, R. E., Cooper, J., Gourley, A., and Copeland, J. 1971. Diagnostic criteria of American and British psychiatrists. *Archives of General Psychiatry* 25:123–30.

Kety, S. S. 1974. From rationalization to reason. *American Journal of Psychiatry* 131:957–63.

Kiesler, C. A. 1980. Mental health policy as a field of inquiry for psychology. *American Psychologist* 35:1066–80.

Kiesler, C. A., et al. 1983. Federal mental health policymaking: an assessment of deinstitutionalization. *American Psychologist* 38;1292–97.

Klapp, Orrin E. 1972. *Heroes, villains, and fools*. San Diego: Aegis.

Kleinman, A.
1988a. Rethinking psychiatry. New York: Free Press.
1988b. The illness narratives. New York: Basic Books.

Kleinman, A., et al. 1978. Culture, illness, and care: clinical lessons from anthropologic and cross-cultural research. *Annals of Internal Medicine* 88:251–58.

Lamb, H. R., and Grant, R. W.
1982. The mentally ill in an urban county jail. *Archives of General Psychiatry* 39:17–22.

1983. Mentally ill women in a county jail. *Archives of General Psychiatry* 40:363–68.

Lamb, H. R., and Talbott, J. 1986. The homeless mentally ill. *Journal of the American Psychiatric Association* 256:498–501.

LaPiere, R. T. 1934. Attitudes vs. actions. *Social Forces* 13:230–37.

Leff, J. P. 1976. Schizophrenia and sensitivity to the family environment. *Schizophrenia Bulletin* 2:566–74.

Levinson, D. J., and Gallagher, E. B. 1964. *Patienthood in the mental hospital*. Boston: Houghton-Mifflin.

Levi-Strauss, Claude. 1965. *The raw and the cooked*. New York: Harper and Row.

Lewis, Verl S., and Zeichner, Abraham N. 1960. Impact of admission to a mental hospital on the patient's family. *Mental Hygiene* 44:503–10.

Lindsay, K., and Paul, G. 1989. Involuntary commitments to public mental institutions: issues involving the overrepresentation of blacks and assessment of relevant functioning. *Psychology Bulletin* 106:171–83.

Lippmann, Walter. 1930. *Public opinion*. New York: Macmillan.

Littlewood, R. 1992. Psychiatric diagnosis and racial bias: empirical and interpretative approaches. *Social Science and Medicine* 34:141–49.

Loring, Marti, and Powell, Brian. 1988. Gender, race, and DSM-III: a study of the objectivity of psychiatric diagnostic behavior. *Journal of Health and Social Behavior* 29:1–22.

Madsen, W. 1964. *The Mexican Americans of South Texas*. New York: Holt, Rinehart, and Winston.

Mattes, J., Rosen, B., and Klein, D. 1977. Comparison of the clinical effectiveness of short vs. long stay psychiatric hospitalization. *Journal of Nervous and Mental Disease* 165:387–94.

Mechanic, David. 1962. Some factors in identifying and defining mental illness. *Mental Hygiene* 46:66–74.

Melick, M. E., Steadman, H., and Cocozza, J. 1979. The medicalization of criminal behavior among mental patients. *Journal of Health and Social Behavior* 20:228–37.

Mendel, W., and Rapport, S. 1969. Determinants of the decision for psychiatric hospitalization. *Archives of General Psychiatry* 20:321–28.

Mendelsohn, F., Egri, G. and Dohrenwend, B. 1978. Diagnosis of nonpatients in the general community. *American Journal of Psychiatry* 135:1163–67.

Miller, Dorothy.
    1965. Worlds that fail: retrospective analysis of mental patients' careers, Part I. California Mental Health Research Monograph, no. 6. Sacramento: California State Department of Mental Hygiene.
    1967. Retrospective analysis of posthospital mental patient's worlds. *Journal of Health and Social Behavior* 8:136–40.

Millon, T. 1975. Reflections on Rosenhan's "On being sane in insane places." *Journal of Abnormal Psychology* 84:456–61.

Murphy, Jane M. 1976. Psychiatric labeling in cross-cultural perspective. *Science* 191:1019–28.

Nagel, Ernest. 1961. *Structure of science*. New York: Harcourt, Brace.

Needham, Rodney, ed. 1978. *Right and left: essays on dual symbolic classification*. University of Chicago Press.

New York State Office of Mental Health. 1982. *Five year comprehensive plan for services to the mentally ill persons in New York*. Albany: New York State Office of Mental Health.

Nunnally, Jum C. 1961. *Popular conceptions of mental health*. New York: Holt, Rinehart, and Winston.

Olmsted, D., and Durham, K. 1976. Stability of mental health attitudes: a semantic differential study. *Journal of Health and Social Behavior* 17:35–44.

Pasamanick, B. 1963. Some misconceptions concerning differences in the racial prevalence of mental disease. *American Journal of Orthopsychiatry* 33:72–86.

Pierce G., et al. 1985. The impact of broadened civil commitment standards on admissions to state mental hospitals. *American Journal of Psychiatry* 142:104–7.

Prudhomme, C., and Musto, D. F. 1973. Historical perspectives on mental health and racism in the United States. In *Racism and mental health*, ed. C. V. Willie, B. M. Kramer, and B. S. Brown, pp. 25–57. Pittsburgh: University of Pittsburgh Press.

Rabkin, J. G.
1972. Opinions about mental illness: a review of the literature. *Psychological Bulletin* 77:153–71.
1974. Public attitudes toward mental illness: a review of the literature. *Schizophrenia Bulletin* 10:9–33.

Razran, G. 1950. Ethnic dislike in stereotypes. *Journal of Abnormal and Social Psychology* 45:7–27.

Redman, S., et al. 1991. The effects of gender on diagnosis of psychological disturbance. *Journal of Behavioral Medicine* 14:441.

Robbins, E. S., et al. 1977. Transfers to a psychiatric emergency room: a fresh look at the dumping syndrome. *Psychiatric Quarterly* 49:197–202.

Rokeach, M. 1964. *The three Christs of Ypsilanti*. New York: Knopf.

Rosenhan, D. L.
1973. On being sane in insane places. *Science* 179:250–58.
1975. The contextual nature of psychiatric diagnosis. *Journal of Abnormal Psychology* 84:462–74.

Rothman, D. J. 1971. *The discovery of the asylum: social order and disorder in the New Republic.* Boston: Little, Brown.

Rushing, W. 1978. Status resources, societal reactions, and type of mental hospital admission. *American Sociological Review* 43:521–33.

Rushing, W., and Esco, J. 1977. Status resources and behavioral deviance as contingencies of societal reaction. *Social Forces* 56:132–47.

Sampson, H., Messinger, S., and Towne, R. 1962. Family process and becoming a mental patient. *American Journal of Sociology* 68:88–96.

Scheff, Thomas.
1966. *Being mentally ill*. Chicago: Aldine.
1975. A reply to Chauncey and Gove. *American Sociological Review* 40;252–57.

Schneider, U., and Wieser, S. 1972. Der Psychischkranke in den Massenmedien: Egenbnisse einer systematischen Inhaltsanalyse. *Fortschritte der Neurologie Psychiatrie und ihrer Grenzgebiete* 40:136–63.

Schrag, Peter. 1978. *Mind control*. New York: Pantheon.

Secord, P. 1959. Stereotyping and favorableness in the perception of Negro faces. *Journal of Abnormal and Social Psychology* 59:309–15.

Shibutani, Tamotsu. 1970. On the personification of adversaries. In *Human nature and collective behavior*, ed. T. Shibutani. Englewood Cliffs, N.J.: Prentice Hall.

Silver, A. 1955. The home management of children with schizophrenia. *American Journal of Psychotherapy* 9:196–215.

Smith, K., Pumphrey, M. W., and Hall, J. S. 1963. The "last straw": the decisive incident resulting in the request for hospitalization in 100 schizophrenic patients. *American Journal of Psychiatry* 120:228–33.

Spiro, Melford. 1961. Social systems, personality, and functional analysis. In *Studying personality cross-culturally*, ed. Bert Kaplan. New York: Row, Peterson.

Spitzer, R. L. 1975. On pseudoscience, logic in remission, and psychiatric diagnoses: a critique of Rosenhan's "On being sane in insane places." *Journal of Abnormal Psychology* 84:442–52.

Spitzer, R. L., et al. 1980. DSM-III: the major achievements and an overview. *American Journal of Psychiatry* 28:128–32.

Srole, L., et al. 1962. *Mental health in the metropolis: the Midtown Manhattan study.* New York: McGraw Hill.

Star, S. A. 1962. The public's ideas about mental illness. Paper presented to the Annual Meeting of the National Association for Mental Health. Indianapolis, 5 November 1955.

Steadman, Henry J.

1972. The psychiatrist as a conservative agent of social control. *Social Problems* 20:263–71.

1980. The right not to be a false positive: problems in the application of the dangerousness standard. *Psychiatric Quarterly* 52:84–99.

1982. A situational approach to violence. *International Journal of Law and Psychiatry* 5:171–86.

Steadman, Henry J., and Cocozza, Joseph J.

1974. Careers of the criminally insane: excessive social control of deviance. Lexington, Mass.: Lexington Books.

1977–1978. Public images of the criminally insane: a case of selective reporting and false perceptions. *Public Opinion Quarterly* 41:523–33.

1978. Public perceptions of the criminally insane. *Hospital and Community Psychiatry* 29(7):457–59.

Steadman, H. J., Cocozza, J. J., and Melick, M. E. 1978. Explaining the increased crime rate of mental patients: the changing clientele of state hospitals. *American Journal of Psychiatry* 135:816–20.

Stearns, A. W., and Ullman, A. D. 1949. One thousand unsuccessful careers. *American Journal of Psychiatry* 11:801–9.

Strauss, J. S., and Carpenter, W. T., Jr. 1972. The prediction of outcome in schizophrenia I: characteristics of outcome. *Archives of General Psychiatry* 27:739–46.

Strauss, John S., et al. 1979. Do psychiatric patients fit their diagnoses? Patterns of symptomatology as described with the biplot. *Journal of Nervous and Mental Disease* 167:105–13.

Stumme, Wolfgang. 1973. Das Bild vom Psychischgestörten und seinem Therapeuten in den Massenmedien. *Praxis der Psychotherapie* 18:193–99.

Szasz, Thomas.

1963. *Law, liberty, and psychiatry.* New York: Macmillan.

1970. *The manufacture of madness.* New York: Harper and Row.

Talbott, J. A. 1974. Stop the revolving door: a study of readmissions to a state hospital. *Psychiatric Quarterly* 48:159–67.

Taube, C., and Redick, R. 1973. *Utilization of mental health resources by persons diagnosed with schizophrenia.* Rockville, Md.: Biometry Branch, NIMH.

Temerlin, Maurice K. 1968. Suggestion effects in psychiatric diagnosis. *Journal of Nervous and Mental Disease* 147:349–53.

Townsend, J. M.

n.d. *Media images of mental illness: an analysis of T.V. Guide descriptions for 1976.* Unpublished manuscript.

1976. Self-concept and the institutionalization of mental patients: an overview and critique. *Journal of Health and Social Behavior* 17:263–71.

1977. Self-concept and the institutionalization of mental patients: a reply to Henley. *Journal of Health and Social Behavior* 18:442–44.

1978. *Cultural conceptions and mental illness: a comparison of Germany and America*. Chicago: University of Chicago.

1979. Stereotypes of mental illness: a comparison with ethnic stereotypes. *Culture, Medicine, and Psychiatry* 3:205–29.

1980. Psychiatry versus societal reaction: a critical analysis. *Journal of Health and Social Behavior* 35:68–78.

Townsend, J. M., and Carbone, C. 1980. Menopausal syndrome: illness or social role—a transcultural analysis. *Culture, Medicine, and Psychiatry* 4:229–48.

Townsend, J. M., and Rakfeldt, J. 1985. Hospitalization and first-contact mental patients: stigma and changes in self-concept. *Research in Community and Mental Health* 5:269–301.

Turner, R. J., and Gartrell, J. W. 1978. Social factors in psychiatric outcome: toward the resolution of interpretive controversies. *American Sociological Review* 43:368–82.

Waisberg, Jodie, and Page, Stewart. 1988. Gender role non-conformity and perception of mental illness. *Women and Health* 14:3–16.

Wallace, Anthony F. C. 1972. Mental illness, biology, and culture. In *Psychological Anthropology*, ed. F. L. K. Hsu. San Francisco: Schenkman.

Weiner, B. 1975. "On being sane in insane places": a process (attributional) analysis and critique. *Journal of Abnormal Psychology* 84:433–41.

Wicker, A. W. 1969. Attitudes vs. actions: the relationship of verbal and overt behavioral responses to attitude objects. *Journal of Social Issues* 25:41–78.

Wing, J. K. 1962. Institutionalism in mental hospitals. *British Journal of Social and Clinical Psychology* 1:38–51.

Yarrow, M. R., Schwartz, C. G., Murphy, H. S., and Deasy, L. C. 1955. The psychological meaning of mental illness in the family. *Journal of Social Issues* 11:12–24.

PART II
Individuals and Families

Racism and African American Adolescent Development

DOLESCENCE is one of the most challenging and consequential periods along the developmental course. Mastery of adolescent tasks gives young people a reasonable chance to successfully address life tasks—to achieve in school at a level that will make desirable future employment possible, to earn a living and take care of self and family, to live in a family successfully and rear children adequately, to find personal satisfaction and meaning, and to be motivated to be a responsible citizen. Racism adds a powerful adverse dimension to this period for African American young people in particular, although Latino and Native American young people are also adversely affected; and other minorities, and to a more limited extent and in a different way, even young people from socially powerful ethnic and racial groups can be adversely affected as well.

The key developmental task of adolescence is to establish a stable, positive identity. Historical and current structures in American life, however, generate beliefs, attitudes, values, and ways that make it difficult for African American young people to establish a positive personal identity. Without family and social network promotion of conditions that counter the societal message, a negative personal identity can develop and contribute heavily to mental health problems and problem behaviors. Societal mechanisms operate to blame troublesome behaviors on the victims, making matters worse (Ryan 1976, 5).

The processes contributing to these outcomes are difficult to elucidate. For whatever reason—but probably to justify our society's high value of individuality—behavioral sciences focus more on intrapsychic determinants of behavior than on institutional and/or societal structures. Indeed,

151

in psychiatry there is no significant body of literature dealing with the concept of power, in spite of the fact that power disparities affect almost all relationships and behavior—between parent and child, between other relatives and individuals, between people of different social and economic status (to name just a few). Political, economic, and social structural forces generate these power disparities.

The behavioral sciences that do examine structural forces generally do not adequately explore the mechanisms through which such forces affect the development of individuals. As a result, a force as powerful as racism is often not considered in the context of political, economic, and informational policy; nor is it considered how racism can affect child growth and development (Ryan 1976, 22). In this chapter I will briefly review the definition of racism; its root and function; degree of presence; its forms; its historical and current consequences for American life; and its effects on child development in general, and on the adolescent development of African American youth in particular.

Racism

Racism is a low-level social and psychological adaptive mechanism. A racist perspective is rooted in personal anxiety and insecurity and is used by groups to deal with psychological and social insecurities much as individuals utilize psychic defenses and adaptive mechanisms to deal with anxiety. The racist attitudes of individuals affect all institutions, and in turn, individuals are affected by institutional racism. American society has promoted and rewarded racism by enabling members of the group in control (Whites) to obtain economic, social, and psychological advantages at the expense of the group with less control (Blacks and other minorities). White racism is pervasive, affecting every aspect of American life. Black and other minority individuals can also hold racist attitudes, but as groups, they lack significant political, economic, and social power, and as a result, racist attitudes among individuals in these groups have little effect on American institutions and structures. Actually, minority racism occurs largely in response to the expression of White racism, or the quest among Whites to gain and maintain economic, social, and psychological power and advantage (Pinderhughes 1989, 89).

Racism is manifested in at least four major forms and is transmitted from generation to generation as a cultural value similar to patriotism and religion. I. A. Newby, in his book *Jim Crow's Defense*, described three different forms of racism or three major groupings of White racism—extremist, moderate, and reformers (Newby 1965). Newby described extremists as people and institutions that are openly hostile and who endorse repressive policies to maintain White superiority. Moderates are convinced of the innate inferiority of Blacks but urge understanding and reason. The reformer, consciously and unconsciously, accepts the concept of Black inferiority but explains it away as a product of environment. The reformer usually supports basic rights of Blacks—the ballot and economic opportunity—as long as White supremacy and control can be maintained. To this classification, I would add another group, one that acknowledges racial differences without a value judgment, and that favors equal opportunity but occasionally manifests racist behavior as a result of growing up in a society that is permeated by racist attitudes and behaviors.

Racism and American History

America was formed as a reaction to the wealth, power, and control of a Western European oligarchy; as an effort of the masses to improve their poverty-stricken lot; and also to achieve religious freedom. The frontier condition of the new land permitted and promoted full expression of a fierce and almost spiritual commitment to individuality, independence, and freedom from control of authority of any kind. The value of the individual—the common person—had been affirmed by religious concepts that had grown out of the Protestant Reformation. And the theory of predestination—prosperity as a mark of God's favor and poverty as a punishment for sin—became part of the cultural fabric of the new land. Despite these values, however, cheap labor was needed to produce individual and national wealth. This led to a system of slavery.

Slavery, as a contradiction of the American cultural heritage, had to be justified. Africans were vulnerable. First, the African slave—unlike the European indentured servant—was different in appearance, culture, and particularly in religion. Because of these differences, pulpits and papers across the land were able to justify the enslavement of "African heathens" for their own salvation. But as Africans were born into the new religion, the old justification did not work. At that point, educational institutions joined pulpit and paper in proclaiming the inferiority of Africans. They were said to be less than human and undeserving of freedom. These assertions were a way of justifying the practice of slavery, leaving no moral blemish on the enslaver, the slaveholder, or those who condoned slavery (Gould 1981, 31–32, 35).

Extreme poverty and powerlessness generate feelings of inadequacy and insecurity among human beings; many of the European settlers had experienced these conditions for a long time. Some were among the most marginal and troubled people in Europe; some were even criminals. Thus, the potential for scapegoating others was great. Nineteenth-century notions suggesting survival and success of the intellectually and physically fittest, and the greatest rewards for those who applied themselves, strengthened rationalizations for the exploitation, scapegoating, and abuse of Blacks by these groups. Also the nature of Protestant religion required that individuals repress aggressive, sexual, or "dark" impulses. Dark skin, or Blackness, and cultural differences made African people a target for projecting evil upon them and served to intensify the scapegoating tendency in America (Frazier 1962, 112). Finally, a competitive economic system was being established in the land. The caste-like social system that emerged to contain and control Africans worked to the competitive benefit of poor, uneducated Whites. Thus, many supported the repression and scapegoating of African slaves, and later African American citizens, without needing any rationalization (Comer 1972).

The experience of Africans during slavery—and afterward during the caste-like system characterized by exclusion and abuse—led to behaviors that were then used to further justify slavery and the caste system after slavery (Frazier 1957, 257–62). After the intensification of the Civil Rights Movement in the 1960s, this process was modified but continues in more subtle and sophisticated ways even today. The troublesome behavioral reactions of many Africans and African Americans is entirely understandable, and it is here that the behavioral sciences fail society most completely. The psychological and social consequences of adverse political, economic, and social structural forces cannot fully be appreciated with our present behavioral science emphasis on intrapsychic dynamics and with the lack of emphasis on the effect of social conditions on families and child development. Thus, most Americans cannot fully appreciate the power of these adverse conditions.

Racism and the African American Experience

Human beings are social animals. In their quest to survive and thrive, they create social systems consisting of beliefs, attitudes, values, and customs—culture. Culture provides individuals and groups with a sense of belonging, meaning, purpose, identity, and security that protects against the insecurity of the unknown, isolation, and meaninglessness (Rosaldo 1984, 137–57). Relationship experiences within families, within kinship groups, social networks, religious, educational, governmental, and other systems provide individuals with opportunities to achieve a sense of adequacy and worth. Slavery disrupted West African culture and eliminated the mechanisms that meet the most basic and most important human needs (Park 1969, 117).

A slave culture was imposed. Slavery in America was a system of enforced dependency, inferiority, lacking hope for an improved future. The Black slave was dependent on the White master for the most fundamental needs: food, clothing, and shelter; a sense of adequacy, worth, and value. The latter psychosocial needs were satisfied only when the slave met the needs and expectations of the master, not of the self, family, or group. No matter how intelligent, hard working, or socially skilled the slave happened to be, he or she was still considered inferior to a White. The slave, or slave parent, was not preparing the self or the children for a higher future status. These conditions existed for African slaves at a time and in a surrounding society that valued independence, personal adequacy, and the opportunity for a better future.

These conditions promoted among slaves a behavior seeking immediate gratification rather than the delay of gratification to achieve a future goal. The slaves' conditions promoted, on the one hand, identification with the more powerful, and on the other, often negative feelings and identification with less powerful people like the self or other Blacks. The conditions also promoted aggressive acting up and acting out behavior toward other Blacks among some, and apathy, depression, and hopelessness among others. These situations led inevitably to the "Uncle Tom," "honey child," "bad nigger," and "Sambo" sterotypes (Elkins 1970, 131–53).

Largely for purposes of control, the masters permitted their slaves to participate in religious activities, usually Protestant. Religion became a powerful organizing force. After slavery, many Blacks combined the aesthetic attributes of African culture with the ideology of the Protestant church, creating the Black church (Frazier 1962, 112–15; Park 1969, 118–19). After slavery, the church was the only institution independent of White control. It was the source of a belief system in which Africans could experience a sense of belonging and adequacy independent of a master, and of Whites in general. Thus, the Black church was an important adaptive mechanism. As a result of the church, Blacks who lived under better conditions of slavery, as well as free Blacks, were able to establish some sense of adequacy and worth despite negative social conditions. Nonetheless, the overall experience of separation from the instrumental and organizational aspects of aesthetic components—and what one anthropologist calls "Africanisms"—survives and still exists today.

After slavery, Blacks attempted to make satisfactory adaptations to a whole new series of traumatic circumstances. Despite working at the lowest level of the job market as agricultural laborers and domestics, heads of households were able to take care of themselves and their families and meet all adult tasks and responsibilities—live in families, rear children, and carry out responsible adult behaviors, including citizenship behaviors, as far as possible without political rights and social opportunities. The communal nature of small rural towns where most Blacks lived and the presence of the Black church enabled most families to function reasonably well.

Before 1900, even as late as 1945, most heads of households did not need an education to earn a living. Between 1900 and 1945, the heavy industrial era, most Americans received the education needed to function in the late industrial era between 1945 and 1980, and the post-industrial era after 1980. Because of the generation-to-generation transmission of beliefs, attitudes, values, knowledge, and ways, families with reasonable education levels before the 1940s were better able to prepare their children to be educated in the subsequent generations (Comer 1980). But during the period between 1900 and 1945, approximately four to eight times as much money was spent on the education of a White child as on the education of a Black in the eight states where 80 percent of the Black population was located. Where Blacks were disproportionate in number, the disparity was as great as twenty-five times. The same disparity existed in higher education (Comer 1988, 212–16).

In addition, educated and uneducated Blacks alike were closed out of the political and economic mainstreams. Educated Blacks became a professional class, not an economic class (Frazier 1962, 42–43). Knowledge, skills, and contacts important in mainstream politics and business could neither be established within the Black community nor transmitted from generation to generation. There was no network of Black political and economic leaders who could work together to create the push-pull phenomenon as it occurred among immigrant groups before the middle of the century—political and economic opportunities pulling the masses into the mainstream and families pushing and supporting the development of their children so that they could take advantage of these opportunities. As a result, Black community identification with constructive, powerful elements and people of the societal mainstream was nonexistent or negative. The sense of adequacy and belonging created within the Black community was not affirmed within the larger society. Blacks could have only a limited sense of opportunity within the larger society. Blacks had to seek adequacy, belonging, and protection through a struggle against barriers created by political, economic, and social structures and by people in the larger mainstream society who should have been a major source of these psychosocial benefits.

Racist social policies that led to the undereducation of Blacks before the 1950s were greatly harmful to Blacks and the society after the 1950s. In the 1940s technology began to push large numbers of Blacks out of rural, Southern areas into urban areas both North and South. Without political and economic power, high levels of racism remained and closed Blacks out of high-paying, low-skilled jobs made possible for other under-educated groups through union activities (Ogbu 1988, 175–78). Also, the supportive nature of the church and the communal nature of small-town rural areas were lost or weakened by urbanization. Many families that once functioned successfully in the rural South began to function less well in the urban North (Franklin 1988, 23–26).

Families functioning effectively among all groups began to reduce family size in urban areas. Among families having more difficulties, fam-ily size remained relatively unchanged (Moynihan 1970, 387, 389). Be-cause of the more traumatic social history, a disproportionate number of Black families were not coping well. In Western European countries, coherent, comprehensive family policies were established to help families succeed better in industrial economies (Frazier 1966; Kamerman and Kahn 1981). Such policies were not developed in the United States, how-ever, in part because of racist attitudes and politics. As a result, the growth population not only among Blacks but in general has been great-est among the least well functioning, more often poor families. More and more Black families came to live under economic and social stress. Such families are less able to provide their children with the kind of develop-ment that will allow them to achieve well in school and to have a reason-able chance to succeed in an economy that requires increasingly higher levels of education. Blacks gradually became more vulnerable to the im-pact of an underground economy of drugs and crime. In the 1950s only 22 percent of all Black families were single-parent families (Comer 1988). And not only were Black communities reasonably safe, they were warm-hearted, communal-spirited, and supportive of creativity and hard work. Today, single-parent families number more than 50 percent, and many low-income communities are disorganized and dangerous (Comer 1988).

Parents made numerous heroic efforts to prepare and support their children for success in school despite the many difficulties. There were similar heroic efforts on the part of church and school people to provide Blacks with a sense of adequacy and education in spite of the barriers. The church ultimately became the vehicle that promoted and supported the intensified civil rights movement. Eventually the civil rights move-ment dismantled the legal structures and weakened the accompanying beliefs, attitudes, values, and ways that served to maintain segregation.

Despite these heroic efforts on the part of Blacks, however, education and media sources even now tend to ignore or underplay their signifi-cance. They often focus on problems among Blacks and glamorize the roles played by Whites in promoting Black rights more than those played by Blacks. A Black success or hero image has never been permitted or promoted in American culture. Since "the enemy" was and is White racism, heroic Black efforts against racism reflect poorly on Judeo-Christian democratic "survival and well-being of the fittest" notions that many Whites need in order to maintain a positive sense of self and group. Simultaneously, the adverse effects of conditions of the past are denied. Ignoring the adverse effects of past conditions permits social policy makers to blame the victims and allows many Americans to avoid taking moral or social responsibility for adverse conditions among Blacks (Ryan 1976, 20). This situation prevents effective corrective policies.

To social policy makers, laymen, and too many behavioral scientists, notions of the survival of the fittest and the like explain away the difficulties among a disproportionate number of Blacks. Many of these notions are the products of an immigrant experience that paralleled the rising tide of economic fortune in the country. The illusion that individual success was due only to individual effort is seductive under these circumstances. The role played by public policies—good public schools, home loans, low and no taxes until the 1940s, veterans' benefits, and many others whereas Blacks were still living under caste-like conditions in the South—are too easily ignored. Difficult past and present conditions produced adverse effects on family and child functioning and development for many, adversely affecting Black adolescent development.

Racism and Child Development

A child is born as a poorly regulated bundle of biological energies, urges, and needs, with the potential of becoming a fully developed adult, capable of meeting all adult tasks and responsibilities—learner, worker, family member, child rearer, and citizen who takes satisfaction and enjoys meaning in life. The newborn, however, is totally dependent on adult caretakers for survival and initial development—usually parents, particularly the mother. Through expanding sets of interactive relationships with other people, self-regulation of the biological systems and intrapsychic development takes place.

Families are enmeshed in primary social networks or groups of friends, kin, and institutions in which they are more or less accepted. Through the caretaking function, an emotional attachment and bond develops between parent and child. Children imitate, identify with, and internalize the beliefs of their parents as they engage in a variety of everyday activities, from the content and ritual of eating to the expression of religious beliefs. Parents are the carriers of the attitudes of their primary social network and transmit them to the children as they provide care. The complete dependency of children and their way of learning gives the parents the ability to channel aggressive energies that can be destructive to them and the people around them into the energies of learning, work, and play. Through mediating the experiences of their children, parents also help them grow along all the critical developmental pathways—physical, social interactive, psychoemotional, moral, linguistic, and intellectual-cognitive.

Erik Erikson theorized that developing children identify with the traits, habits, ideas, and occupations of the meaningful people around them, obtaining identity fragments. And through activities in their primary social network, children who are developing well achieve a sense of mastery and a sense of competence, confidence, adequacy, and efficacy—in sum, a perception of being able. They also develop a sense of being worthwhile and belonging. Through the mastery of social and psychologcial tasks in all the preadolescent developmental stages and the genuine, enthusiastic, consistent approval of the important people around them, their ego identity is strengthened and they are likely to do well in elementary school. Adolescence is the stage, however, when the positive ego identity can be established (Erikson 1963, 239–40).

Continued desirable development is not guaranteed because adolescents are threatened by the rapid, confusing physical and psychological changes from within and the challenging social demands around them, and they need significant support from meaningful others. Without such support, difficult or delinquent behavior—eventually even illness—is possible. With continued support, culturally acceptable growth and achievement is likely. With support, an integration of inner drives and identity fragments takes place in the social world in a way that can prepare a child for the future. A positive identity protects against feelings of inferiority, of inadequacy, or of being evil or "bad."

For full adolescent and continued successful development, these psychosocial benefits need to be achieved beyond the family and primary social network. These include the secondary social networks of school and other institutions, and the tertiary social networks of political, economic, and social institutions where families perhaps may have a strong sense of belonging and may be valued. Erikson wrote, "An individual feels isolated and barred from the sources of collective strength when he (even though only secretly) takes on a role considered especially evil, be it that of a drunkard or a killer, a sissy or a sucker, or whatever colloquial designation of inferiority may be used in his group" (Erikson 1963, 36). The same isolation occurs for the group in relation to the larger society.

The problem in this science- and technology-based age is that the number of ways youths from any group can be successful have been reduced. Even before the actual requirement of a high level of education for desirable employment, the devaluation of anything but academic learning and white-collar work posed a problem for many youths. The opportunities are now even more limited, creating a higher level of anxiety and a more intense fear of failure and feelings of inferiority and evil. These are heightened by the strong historical-cultural prohibition of evil, and the notions that ability is genetically determined and a sign of favor and that achievement is a matter of will, not influenced by experience or practice and support.

This situation increases the need for average- and low-status groups to identify with high-status or more powerful individuals and groups to feel more successful, powerful, and strong themselves—sometimes even when such identification is detrimental. The increased scapegoating of Blacks after a decade of improved conditions in the 1960s is largely related to economy-generated insecurities. As a result, African American children, even those who grow up in well-functioning families and social networks, receive a mixed message from conditions and powerful information systems within the larger society: "You are Americans entitled to all the rights and privileges of all other Americans if you earn them. But if you and your group doesn't have them, it's your fault. You either have not worked hard enough, or you are inadequate, inferior, bad, and evil."

When Blacks are successful, the message is modified: "You are different, exceptional, like us—the most successful segment of the White community." The image of White America does not include average, low-level, and negative achievers. Thus, when Blacks achieve in significant numbers or in areas held to be beyond the group capacity, it is threatening; and most problematically, it does not change the negative perception of the group or of Blackness. A successful Black secretary was walking to lunch with a White secretary from her office when they encountered several groups of Blacks behaving in ways the White secretary considered undesirable. She made several comments about "nigger" behavior. When her colleague reminded her that she was Black, the White secretary said, "Oh, I'm not talking about you or your kind." Despite the success of African American football quarterbacks and coaches in the highly symbolic and visible professional leagues, the perception that Blacks are not capable of coaching or taking other leadership positions still has not changed. The fact that Black students achieve honors at colleges and universities across the country still does not save all Black students from the perception that they are not bright until they prove otherwise. The African American community, then, is the designated scapegoat for shortcomings in the society in the same way that a vulnerable child is often designated as the "sick" person in a family that is not functioning well.

Ironically, legal segregation fostered the existence of African American institutions such as powerful churches, elementary, secondary, and post-secondary schools, health organizations, strong civil rights organizations, and businesses, all of which created a visible mainstream leadership group with the clear mission of improving the status and opportunities for the group. This promoted a reasonable degree of cohesion in a group that has powerful divisive forces related to multiple origins in Africa, a loss of the instrumental aspects of African cultures, different and dependent conditions during slavery, and the like. A church-centered Black community served as a "substitute society" and provided the psychosocial benefits the larger society refused. It anchored and protected Black families and enabled many to function well and to adequately support the development of their children. Without an economic base, however, the Black community could not neutralize the effects of past racism and poverty, eliminate contemporary barriers to opportunity, or create wider opportunities for group, family, and individual development and success. As more Blacks were closed out of the changed economy, family and social problems grew.

The elimination of legal segregation—while absolutely necessary to destroy the powerful symbols of Black inferiority and low status—led to a diffusion of leadership and power. It also led to great uncertainty about the nature of the forces maintaining difficult community conditions, and to uncertainty about goals and strategies. Desegregation without full, enthusiastic membership in the larger society has made group cohesion and a positive group identity more difficult to achieve. In a renewed effort to avoid any responsibility for difficult conditions in the Black community, powerful voices within the larger society have mounted an intensified, very effective campaign of "blaming the victims," even labeling legitimate complaints pathological, ("victim behavior," for example). These developments have weakened the chances for young people to gain strength from membership in a group that is effectively addressing harmful attitudes and behavior exhibited by the larger society.

Because identification with a low-status group is not innately helpful, some Blacks are identifying with the powerful (initially conceptualized as identifcation with the aggressor) and joining in the scapegoating of their own. Such behavior is encouraged and rewarded by those in the larger system who wish to maintain the status quo. Self- or group criticism can be useful, but it is harmful when it does not acknowledge the effects of powerful economic and social factors. Identification with the powerful among some Blacks buttresses false assumptions of superiority among some Whites and interferes with the development of more healthy adaptive responses on their part. This then prevents the development of social policies that can effectively address undesirable conditions in the Black community and the larger society.

As a result of racist social policies concerning job and educational opportunities in the past, which is now true for many, Blacks are disproportionately poor and under attack. Poor people under attack more often have inadequate housing and health care, inadequate nutrition, and more often live under conditions with environmental hazards, safety problems, and psychological stress. All of these conditions adversely affect development. Parents living under severe economic and psychosocial stress are unable to give their children the kind of childrearing experiences that promote adequate self-regulation of biological systems. This often interferes with personal control and the ability to concentrate, learn, and manage the social environment. This, in turn, interferes with development along all the critical developmental pathways—social-interactive, psychoemotional, moral, speech and language, intellectual-cognitive. Inadequate development in these areas leads to poor school learning and often problems with confidence, self-worth, adequacy, and efficacy. Because of social policies based on race, Black children more often go to poorly functioning schools. Thus, even when the children develop adequately, they are less likely to obtain the quality of education needed to succeed as adults. Even when they obtain such an education in the early years, the identification process in late pre- and early adolescence can interfere with their academic and social performances in later years.

Racism and Identity

African American adolescents from families under the greatest stress are least likely to master social and psychological tasks in each developmental period and to achieve good ego functioning and related successes in school. For many, with few other opportunities for life success, this leads to what some call perpetual adolescence: irresponsibility; a lack of discipline; uneven, unpredictable, sometimes contradictory behavior; and the inability to take hold, follow through, and achieve in the mainstream social world. Meeting adult tasks, work, family, and citizenship at a high level is unlikely.

Denied success and the opportunity to achieve a positive identity in the mainstream, however, these adolescents will seek it elsewhere. They often have little choice but to identify with people, places, ideas, and activities that further limit their opportunities—teen pregnancy and low-level aspirations lead to antisocial activities, delinquency, drug use, and crime. These activities are characterized as typical Black behaviors by the society. A positive racial identity is then difficult to achieve, and the negative overall identity leads to feelings of inferiority, inadequacy, or being evil or bad, and sometimes even to psychological illness, particularly depression.

Some adolescents reject opportunities and related behaviors in the mainstream institutions, label them as White behavior, and deride Blacks who are participating in the mainstream as "acting White." Clothing, music, language, and other aspects of lifestyle substitute for substance. This self-protective or defensive effort proves ultimately inadequate. Nonetheless, because achieving a positive Black identity in America is a problem, the charge of "acting White" creates confusion and puts pressure on those Black adolescents with greater opportunities.

African American young people from better-functioning families and social networks have a better chance to establish good ego functioning and success in school. Nevertheless, achieving a positive racial identity, a critical aspect of overall identity, can remain a problem. In a variety of direct and indirect ways, they experience past history and present environments in which the most powerful people are White and favored, people like themselves are of lower status and lower apparent success, and these outcomes are continually being justified through negative messages and images of Blacks and positive images of Whites. Without powerful sources of group affirmation and the presence of neutralizing, corrective images, the desire to identify with the powerful and reject the Black self—at an unconscious level, inferior, bad, evil—is great.

Elaine Pinderhughes points out that African American culture values affiliativeness and interdependence, which are greatly different from the mainstream society's values of autonomy and independence. Achieving a positive racial identity requires an integration of Black culture and mainstream culture. This increases the possibility of confusion, conflict, and because Blacks are less powerful, negative racial identity (Pinderhughes 1989, 160–61). Nonetheless, successful Black families and social networks provide Black children with self-and race-affirming models and messages and the skills needed to relate to both worlds. Many young people achieve a positive cultural and racial identity. Many, however, do not recognize the need to give special attention to this effort. As a result, some achieve social success without a positive racial-cultural identity. Early school success is likely in both situations but may deteriorate during later years if there is no strong, positive cultural-racial identity as a well-integrated component of overall ego identity.

Black adolescents tend to respond in several ways—with varied outcomes for their identity, their performance, and their psychological health. Some reject race and culture and attempt to exist as individuals. Some remain marginal in both Black and White cultures. Some reject their

Blackness and identify with White culture only, and even identify with the powerful, which carries with it negative perceptions of Blacks. One such adolescent wrote, "Help. I am a White man trapped in an ugly Black skin." Some develop a strong, pro-Black posture with a rejection of all things White. All these responses require denial and rejection in one way or another (of the self, the group, and others). The denial mechanism is never completely effective and requires a great deal of psychic energy. Persons who deny all collective culture, Black or White, deny themselves the collective strength such affiliation provides. This can create an enormous sense of isolation, constriction, and insecurity. Marginality leads to overall ineffectualness, without full expression here or there.

Rejection of the racial self and culture, and that of others, also carries a psychic price: related anger, hostility, and the need for self-limiting projection of bad, evil, and incompetence. African American youngsters who reject their group experience self- and group hatred, low self- and group esteem. When they identify with the powerful and the dominant culture's generalized perceptions of Blacks, they experience a sense of defect, a sence of being dumb, bad, and evil. They have an uncritical need to be accepted and "made whole" by White people. This makes them vulnerable to exploitation, abuse, and self-defeating behaviors. Often they act out the stereotypes needed by some in the larger culture. "White is right," "Uncle Tom, Clown," "Good Time," and the Black policeman who harasses and intimidates Blacks and caters to Whites are problematic expressions of such rejection and identification.

Also, human beings appear to have an unconscious self-harming impulse that is not expressed when personal identity is positive and ego functioning is adequate. Conversely, with negative identity and poor ego functioning the impulse can be turned inward against the self or outward as a projection of the negative self. In the most troublesome social environment this can be manifest in self-destructive addiction and provocative behaviors, or violent or murderous acts against others. And in environments with better conditions and opportunities, the impulse can manifest itself in success-undermining behaviors, from poor school performance to inappropriate sexual behavior.

African American adolescents who reject Whites and White culture (more correctly, White-dominated mainstream culture) and who strongly, and often indiscriminately, embrace Blacks and Black culture address one major problem but create another. There is a need to counter the negative, but they lose the psychic strength of being involved in becoming, if not belonging, through modification of the mainstream culture. They lose the claim to a right to belong and participate fully. Also, behind the overidentification there is sometimes an underlying fear of

Black inadequacy and/or a sense that "We can't win." This requires an overcompensation in the rejection of Whites and an exaggeration of Black goodness. Young people with this orientation from otherwise well-functioning families are most vulnerable and often give up constructive behavior in the face of "acting White" charges. The diffusion of Black community power in the last few years and the historic inability of the African American community to systematically counter the negative message of the larger society have contributed to this response.

A racial-cultural identity that does not require denial or rejection of the self or others, and that provides group appreciation and belonging in the group and larger society—and the related collective strength—is most economical and useful from a psychic standpoint. This requires, however, a significant degree of, or potential for, acceptance of the African American group in the larger society so that the culture of the group and that of the larger society can be integrated with limited conflict, confusion, anxiety, and maladaptive behavior. This is possible today in that there is a growing understanding of the fact that civilization now requires both interdependent and independent functioning, both affiliativeness and autonomy.

Many Black families help their young people manage and achieve a reasonable integration of cultures—albeit still a duality—and establish a positive racial identity in spite of the high level of racism. This occurs through a particular perspective, and by providing systematic experiences, interpretations, and support within their primary social networks, in school, and in the larger society. Such families provide their young people with this same perspective through successful childrearing. This requires affirmation of their race and the best of both cultures while the children are young and the parents are still the dominant source of understanding and psychosocial comfort for the child. Such parents provide their children with information and experiences that help them understand the social conditions they encounter and the forces working to maintain racism. They provide them with the skills to minimize the damaging effects of racist attitudes and acts. This nurturing often leads to some personal and/or group-based effort to modify the larger society to facilitate African American belonging and opportunity on just terms. Such young people are best able to establish a positive racial identity and full adolescent and adult development.

Often the historic achievements of friends, kin, and the segment of the African American community from which such families draw their frame of reference or experience a feeling of belonging enables them to feel adequacy, reject the negative message of the society, and hold a positive racial identity. Then they do not perceive a monolithic White American group in unalterable opposition to Black rights. They usually will identify with the just and responsible people, beliefs, attitudes, values, and ways within the larger, mainstream society. They will value the essence of Black culture without demeaning Whites and without an uncritical need for association. Such young people are best able to establish a positive racial identity along with full adolescent and adult development.

Even under the best of circumstances, however, establishing a positive African American identity is difficult because the negative social forces in society remain powerful. Those negative forces are being fueled by economic and social insecurity in the larger society. Nevertheless, this analysis suggests what is needed: When a group experiences rejection from the larger social collective, the group must create powerful forces within that have high visibility and are engaged in obvious, tangible efforts to reduce the political, economic, and social structures representing obstacles to mainstream opportunities. The group must provide members with a sense of adequacy, belonging, and psychosocial protection. Simultaneously, the larger society must be visibly working to create a system of inclusion, opportunity, and belonging rather than exclusion, denial, and scapegoating.

For historical reasons, cohesive force within the Black community has always been minimal. Ironically, it has been strengthened, in part, by denial and by the common need to overcome the structures that supported segregation abuse. With the elimination of legal segregation, and some positive changes in beliefs and attitudes, the clear need to create powerful adaptive structures within the Black community was not apparent. Even where the need was recognized, a history of largely autonomous functioning—especially in the important, influential area of religion—made a collaborative effort difficult. Instead of being able to retool and address community building, the civil rights groups, already tired and weakened by the effects of their own success (including legal integration), had to fight a steady erosion of Black gains since the mid 1970s.

In the vacuum, numerous spontaneous, fragmented individual and group efforts have emerged to meet the needs of African American youths for a positive sense of identity as individuals and as members of the group. Some recognize that young people's confusion and their difficulty in establishing a positive racial identity interfere with the ability to meet their developmental tasks and, in time, life responsibilities. The growing custom of Kwanzaa celebrations; plans to establish African American boys choirs; and the establishment of schools for African American boys, Saturday Schools with an emphasis on self- and group appreciation, specialized scouting, and the like, all reflect needs to support African American youth development by helping to establish a positive racial identity. The desire of the Children's Defense Fund to establish a Black Child Crusade, a Black church, a fraternity and sorority, and some civil rights' groups programs to promote Black youth excellence; the Legal Defense Fund's interest in understanding and addressing education problems; Black educators' efforts as individuals and organized associations; and numerous, varied contributions by successful Black students, young adult professionals, diverse professionals, and others—all these are strong indications of the desire among African Americans to help their own.

These efforts need to be systematically studied, based on sound theoretical and empirical knowledge, enlarged, coordinated, and disseminated so that they touch and give psychological support to more young people. Existing organizations with long-standing, widespread meaning within the community must be developed into a powerful structure that can give protection, support, and direction from within, and simultaneously connect the group and individuals to mainstream political, economic, and social structures. The current individual and small-group effort cannot keep up with the powerful forces of exclusion in the larger society, and the harmful activities that young people create for themselves, or get drawn into. In the absence of unusual family and community support, and in the absence of reasonable access to mainstream opportunities and the related sense of belonging, fragmentation increases.

Unfortunately, powerful organizing structures cannot exist within the modern African American community without significant help from powerful people and institutions belonging to the larger society. Legislation, financing, opinion influencing, and the like—among all groups—are determined largely by the institutions of the larger society. Thus, policy makers within the larger society must understand that their best interests are served not by weakening the organizing structures of the African American community, but by strengthening them and facilitating their ability to interact constructively with the organizing institutions—economic, educational, and social—of the larger society. At present, the economic and social vitality of large segments of the Black community suffers because such linkage (particularly economic integration) with the larger society does not exist. Psychological and social problems arise that interfere with family functioning, child development, the establishment of positive racial identities among many, and school and life difficulties—all complicated by the emergence of an underground economy in the absence of access to the mainstream economy.

Organizing institutions and forces that provided for their members' psychosocial protection and constructive interaction with the larger society developed among many groups without the need of special mechanisms. This occurred because of the existence of greater innate cohesive forces and greater opportunities in agricultural and industrial economies. New immigrants who managed to do well were usually a part of organizing, supportive systems in the old country; they faced less exclusion and abuse than even many mainstream African Americans, and they often had ties to earlier immigrants who facilitated their entry into the American mainstream. Again, the rising tide of affluence and various social programs that carried most other groups to modest successes are experienced as the result of individual effort and not as resulting from structural forces. The reality that social problems exist among any group other than African Americans receives less, fleeting, or no attention from the rest of society.

These subtle but extraordinary differences, perceptions, and adaptive responses make it difficult to convince the larger society that the Black experience has been peculiar, unfair, and unmanageable for many without special programs and approaches; and that the entire society—and not just Blacks—is in jeopardy as a result. This is part of the justification for programs such as affirmative action, business contract set-asides, race-based scholarships, and many other activities designed to overcome the effects of the reality that the Black social experience has been particularly traumatic. Societal policies effectively excluded the Black community from the opportunity structure during the critical national development period from the 1900s through the 1960s. Unless society finds a way to facilitate African American community development so that its structures can promote a broader base of well-functioning families and adequate individual development and opportunity in the larger society, White society and African American society will continue to deteriorate.

I therefore offer a modest proposal in this context and in a hopeful spirit:

The African American experience was the social and psychological equivalent of the destruction created by an atomic bomb attack. Whereas America rebuilt Germany and Japan, the aggressors, the society has never made a meaningful effort to compensate for the harmful effects of illegal and immoral treatment of its own people.

I suggest that a significant percentage of the federal taxes paid by African Americans be used to establish an endowment as an—economic base—and other structures in the community that would then work to promote constructive interactions with mainstream economic, governmental, informational (education and media), and social structures—to provide African Americans with psychosocial protection and a sense of adequacy and belonging and, where necessary, to furnish the African American community's own members with the experiences and competencies needed for successful mainstream functioning. Governance and management systems would be created to build on community-adaptive efforts for the full spectrum of African Americans. These activities would be designed to strengthen the community and the society as an integrated whole.

Such an approach would be a unique, relatively painless, and justified form of social reparation. Reparations have a precedent in this country and other civilized societies. The United States paid reparations to the Aleuts (Hattis 1992) and to the Japanese (Thornburgh 1990) for their internment during World War II. Germany paid reparations both to the Israeli government and to individual Jews. Reparations would enable African Americans to help themselves. They would largely overcome the perception that programs designed to compensate for the effects of past abuse take something away from Whites. Reparations would be a legitimate structural intervention with the capacity to bring about the kind of large-scale structural changes in the larger society that are needed but difficult to accomplish even when there is considerable will to do so. They would, in time, improve our economic competitiveness in the way that a significant investment improved the economies of Germany and Japan. Such an approach could create the kind of conditions in the African American community and society that would enable a majority of young people to achieve a positive racial identity during their overall development.

We must continue to adjust existing institutions so that they can become more fair and effective. The quantum leap that society needs to achieve in race relations, youth development, educational gains, and economic development cannot be achieved by settling for business as usual, however. There are too many divisive attitudes and practices that can be overcome only by structural changes. An America that reaches the twenty-first century without having taken significant steps toward the necessary structural and psychosocial changes will have reached a point of no return and will have no chance of returning to stronger forms of prosperous, diverse, open, democratic society.

REFERENCES

Comer, J. P.
    1972. *Beyond Black and White*. New York. Quadrangle Books.
    1980. *School power*. New York: Free Press.
    1988. *Maggie's American dream*. NAL Penguin Inc.
Elkins, S. M. 1970. Slavery and Negro personality: personality types and stereotypes. In

Americans from Africa. Vol. 1: Slavery and its aftermath, ed. P. I. Rose, pp. 131–53. Chicago: Atherton Press.

Erikson, E. H. 1963. *Childhood and society*. New York: W. W. Norton.

Franklin, J. H. 1988. A historical note. In *Black families*, ed. H. P. McAdoo, pp. 23–26. Beverly Hills, Calif.: Sage Publications.

Frazier, E. F.
    1957. *Race and culture contacts on the modern world*. New York: Alfred A. Knopf.
    1962. *Black bourgeoisie*. New York: Collier Books, Macmillan Publishing Company.
    1966. *The Negro family in the United States*. Chicago: University of Chicago Press.

Gould, S. J. 1981. *The mismeasure of man*. New York: W. W. Norton.

Hattis, R. 1992. Forgotten internees. *The Progressive* 56:16.

Kamerman, S. B., and Kahn, A. J. 1981. *Child care, family benefits, and working parents*. New York: Columbia University Press.

Moynihan, D. P. 1970. The Negro family. In *Americans from Africa. Vol. 1: Slavery and its aftermath*, ed. P. I. Rose, pp. 387–89. Chicago: Atherton Press.

Newby, I. A. 1965. *Jim Crow's defense*. Baton Rouge: Louisiana State University Press.

Ogbu, J. U. 1988. Black education: a cultural ecological perspective. In *Black families*, ed. H. P. McAdoo, pp. 175–78. Beverly Hills, Calif.: Sage Publications.

Park, E. R. 1969. The Negro conflict and fusion of cultures with special reference to the Negro. *The Journal of Negro History* 4:117–19.

Pinderhughes, E. 1989. *Understanding race, ethnicity, and power*. New York: Free Press.

Rosaldo, M. Z. 1984. Toward an anthropology of self and feeling. In *Culture theory*, ed. R. A. Sheweder and R. A. Levine, pp. 137–57. Cambridge: Cambridge University Press.

Ryan, W. 1976. *Blaming the victim*. New York: Vintage Books.

Thornburgh, D. 1990. Making amends. *U.S. News and World Report*, October 22, p. 19.

Joyce A. Ladner and Ruby M. Gourdine

Transracial Adoptions

THE resilience of the African American family, in spite of racism and discrimination, is possibly one of history's most profound sociological phenomena. The strength and flexibility of the African American family structure have enabled the African American community to nurture children whose natural parents were not physically or psychologically available for them (Hill 1972; Billingsley and Giovannoni 1972; Staples 1978). Yet one of the most controversial issues today is the efficacy of this family system. Many people view it as pathological and question its viability. Frequently cited indicators of the precarious predicament of the African American family include: over one-half of the children live in single-parent, female-headed households; the poverty rate for single- and two-parent African American families is greater than that of the wider community; and high pregnancy rates exist for African American teenagers (Alan Guttmacher Institute 1988; Moore 1990; Burnham 1985).

The problems that these families face permeate several systems and institutions. The statistical data used to describe them are also used to determine practices for child welfare service delivery systems. Many African American social work professionals assert that some practices of the child welfare system disrupt rather than aid such families (National Association of Black Social Workers [NABSW] 1991). African American children represent a significant proportion of the children awaiting foster care or adoptive placement. This situation has caused a mounting controversy about transracial placement—the practice of placing non-White children in the custody of White parents.

This chapter examines the history, politics, policies, and practices that have kindled the controversy surrounding transracial adoptions. The authors also blend the themes of racism, mental health, and transracial adoption.

Statement of the Problem

In 1972, the National Association of Black Social Workers (NABSW) opposed the placement of African American children in White homes. This opposition virtually stopped transracial adoptions in the United States (Simon and Altstein 1977). Generally, White families adopting across racial lines have disagreed with the NABSW's position and have resented scrutiny of their motives for adopting (Simon and Altstein 1977; Ladner 1977). The escalating number of African American children who are removed from their natural families and placed in foster care by the child welfare system has rekindled the debate about the validity of transracial adoptions. Further, the drug epidemic and the need for protective custody are cited as reasons for removal of children from their homes (American Public Welfare Association [APWA] 1987; National Adoption Information Clearinghouse [NAIC] 1991). Punitive policies of child welfare agencies imposed upon these families have also contributed to the high number of children in the foster care system. Agencies contend that there are too few African American families willing to adopt the waiting children.

The assumption that there are too few African Americans available to adopt is based upon several misconceptions:
- They do not adopt
- They do not meet the child-rearing standards of adoption agencies
- They suffer from too many social pathologies
- Caucasians make better parents because of their social class advantages
- African American families do not have adequate resources to adopt.

The following can be cited as reasons for African Americans' opposition to transracial adoption:
- Transracial adoption dilutes the culture of African American families
- Transracial adoption is used to assimilate African American children into White culture, thereby causing the children to be alienated from their racial group
- Agencies place African American children with White families because no White infants are available for adoption
- African Americans and Native Americans have suffered historic dis-

crimination and thereby do not wish to have their offspring taken from them.

Ladner (1977) explains the factors influencing the opposition and support for transracial adoptions:

The controversy and politics of transracial adoption often overshadows its more intimate aspects. Opponents of transracial adoption have biases which are based upon their general opposition to social integration, and the historic racial discrimination in the United States. The proponents are often unwilling to ask the serious question about all facets of the African American adopted child's welfare. So convinced are they that any parent who voluntarily assumes such a serious responsibility toward a child can only be a sincere humanitarian, they consider it as an irrelevant and unkind act to question the motives of such people—to question what kind of parents they are or to question whether the child's interests are fully being served.

NABSW's opposition is based on the assumption that institutional racism has had a devastating impact on African Americans. According to NABSW, the family should also be regarded as a political entity. Thus, the viability of the family is jeopardized when its children are placed with non-Blacks (Ladner 1977).

Whereas White families have adopted non-White children to meet the same personal needs as those who adopt in-racial children, some also perceive their deed as a social benefit, given these children's needs for permanent homes. Some admit they considered transracial adoption only after they realized a white infant was not available (Ladner 1977; Grow and Shapiro 1974). Such families appear comfortable with their personal decisions and challenge the NABSW's politicalization of the issue. Their high level of comfort frustrates those who adhere to the NABSW position because it is a reflection of their perceived reality—whatever Whites want, they get, including African American children. Therefore, the NABSW takes the position that African Americans are denied choice as well as the right to be self-directing and self-determining. For them, access to economic and political power in America continues to be tantamount to having the ability to exercise determination of how one lives in this society. When a particular group lacks these powers, it then becomes unlikely that the policies they support will be implemented. Thus, the impacted group feels powerless to effect decisions and policies that affect their personal lives and communities.

"It is difficult to separate personal values from professional knowledge and to distinguish both of these from the societal values embedded in law" (Goldstein et al. 1986, 10). Child placement laws are society's response to the "success" or "failure" of a family in providing its children with an environment that adequately serves their needs (Goldstein et al. 1986). Legal adoption does not guarantee that the adopting adults will become the psychological parents or that the adopted child will become a wanted child. These outcomes depend largely on the parents' motivations for adoption (Goldstein et al. 1979, 22).

Thousands of African American women served as nannies for White children and proved that they were capable of rearing these children. However, these nannies did not become the psychological parents of their charges. It is logical to assume that White parents can raise Black children. What is less clear is what are those factors that can facilitate their capacity to become psychological parents?

Review of the Literature

The first transracial adoptions in this country occurred in the 1940s, with the momentum increasing in the 1950s and diminishing in the 1960s. The number of transracial adoptions increased again in the mid 1960s but dropped in the 1970s (Simon and Altstein 1977; Ladner 1977).

Simon and Altstein (1977) and Ladner (1977) acknowledge that transracial adoptions were not the result of deliberate agency programming to address the shortage of homes for African American children. Rather, these agencies placed non-White children with White families because there was a shortage of adoptable healthy White infants. Increased use of contraceptives and the availability of legal abortions reduced the number of healthy White infants available for adoption. Hence, agencies initiated transracial adoptions to serve White parents who were willing to accept non-White children. Ladner (1977) found that a majority of the children adopted by White parents were of mixed ancestry.

The number of intercountry adoptions also rose in response to the large numbers of children orphaned by wars and political upheaval in Southeast Asia (Simon and Altstein 1977). The numbers of immigrant children available for adoption increased dramatically from 1961 to 1974. During this period, the United States admitted 33,237 immigrant children. At least 65 percent of these children were identified as non-White. Simon and Altstein (1977) confirm that these children were admitted for the purpose of adoption.

The most notable increase in Asian adoptions occurred among Vietnamese children whose numbers were estimated to range from eight hundred thousand to 1.5 million (Simon and Altstein 1977). These children were either homeless or orphaned as a result of the Vietnam war. There were tremendous efforts by charity groups to provide homes for these

children, but the placement of these children was not without controversy. Part of the controversy was political because of the damaging
image of the war; other aspects included bafflement by citizens why more
emphasis was given to placing Vietnamese children than to placing
American children. This act of Christian charity was conceived by some
as an alternative to the dwindling supply of White children available for
adoption (Simon and Altstein 1977).

Political changes in the communist bloc countries in the 1980s have
made many Romanian children available for adoption. Again, war and
political disruption have left many children homeless, orphaned, or in a
needy state. Americans have responded by attempting to arrange their
adoption. They are viewed as being akin to the original (that is, White)
immigrants, from which America was built. For an example, an article in
the May 23, 1991, issue of the *Washington Post* reported that American
and Western European families have been attempting to adopt Romanian
children in response to the low number of White infants available in the
United States. Further, some families are so desperate that they have cir-
cumvented adoption placement and immigration laws (*Washington Post,*
May 23, 1991).

Agency Requirements

Traditionally, adoption agencies' exclusive policies and practices, such
as the use of matching criteria and worthiness scales, made it difficult
for African Americans to adopt. Matching, which was the cornerstone of
adoption policies in the United States, is the practice of placing children
in families with similar physical characteristics and social circumstances
(Simon and Altstein 1977). In 1959 the Child Welfare League of America
(CWLA) recommended that agencies discontinue using background and
characteristics as major criteria for determining adoption placements unless they actually facilitated adoptions (Simon and Altstein 1977). It was
the CWLA's position that the opportunity should exist for the child to
develop his or her capabilities, and not meet unrealistic expectations of
adoptive parents (Simon and Altstein 1977). The matching referred to
here was related to physical characteristics. White parents adopting African American children tended to select biracial or light-skinned children
(Ladner 1977). Traditionally, adoption agencies' use of worthiness scales
resulted in the exclusion of African American families from the adoption
process (Simon and Altstein 1977; Ladner 1977). Typical criteria for worthiness scales included: two-parent family, nonworking mother, a bed-
room for each child, and home ownership. These criteria were implemented to determine the suitability of the adoptive applicant. Hill (1972)
asserts that formal adoption agencies did not cater to non-Whites, and

African Americans had to develop their own network of informal adoption for their children. This informal adoption network among Black families served to tighten kinship bonds, since many African American women were reluctant to put their children up for adoption (Hill 1972, 6). According to the North American Council on Adoptable Children (NACAC 1991), many minority families still support the notion of informal adoption and question why a formal process is necessary.

The child welfare system removes a disproportionate number of African American children from their families of origin because of the inability of these families to provide adequately. Historically, the child welfare system has not made effective attempts to reunite these children, often allowing them to languish in foster care. As a result, many African Americans view the child welfare system with suspicion. This suspicion is a manifestation of a healthy paranoia that has developed over generations in response to racial discrimination. On the other hand, some of the White parents who adopt Black children feel they must "rescue" these children whom they feel no one else would adopt. Often the altruistic efforts of one group are viewed as intrusive by another group (Kadushin 1972). Agencies serving African American children tend to have a higher proportion of African American social workers. Further, studies have revealed a direct correlation between a social worker's race and his or her attitude toward transracial adoption. African American social workers reject transracial adoptions more often than do White social workers (Simon and Altstein 1977).

Two phenomena helped dispel the myth that African Americans do not adopt: the hiring of African American social workers by adoption agencies and the development of programs that recruited prospective adoptive African American parents. The presence of minority staff may be seen as proof that the agency is interested in working with minorities. Additionally, these staff are used to train non-minority staff about issues sensitive to minorities. Thus, it appears that agencies employing minority staff do better in recruiting and maintaining minority families (NACAC 1991). The issue of preferential service to White families for African American children emerged again in the 1990s. In an interview, Mae Best, director of Black Homes for Black Children in Washington, D.C., stated:

Many traditional adoption agencies continue to place transracially, not because African American families are not available, but rather for their own survival. That is, typically African American families are available for healthy children from birth to four or five, yet, the African American families may not be considered as the placement of choice for these children. A major barrier to same race placement in traditional agencies is the charging of fees. African Americans either cannot afford the fees or feel that paying for children is against their moral code. (Telephone interview, February 20, 1992)

Best represents a cadre of minority persons who have demonstrated through their outreach efforts that African Americans do adopt, despite the many barriers they face.

Data

It was not until 1982 that a mandatory system of reporting child welfare data, the Voluntary Cooperative Information System (VCIS), was instituted. It is coordinated by the American Public Welfare Association (APWA). The data the APWA compiles is not comprehensive because fewer than fifty-two jurisdictions participate. Therefore, APWA cautions the user of these statistics to view the data as rough estimates (APWA 1991). The VCIS report uses 1987 data, the most current available, derived from the submission of data from forty jurisdictions. These figures show a steady increase since 1982 in the number of entrants to substitute care. APWA (1991) estimates that by the end of 1987, 300,000 children were in substitute care. Of that number 43,000–45,000 children will have adoption as their permanency plan. In 1987 an estimated 18,000 to 20,000 children had their adoptions finalized. Table 6.1 describes the entrants into substitute care by race and ethnic status.

For African American children over the five-year period there is an increase in entrants from 26.7 to 30.7 percent. Black entrants enter at a higher rate as compared to their total population. As shown in table 6.2, the most common reasons cited for removal of children were protective service reasons, followed by parent condition or absence. It can be assumed that economic and social conditions may contribute to the child's removal.

TABLE 6.1. Race and ethnicity of children who entered substitute care for fiscal years 1983–1987

	Race/Ethnicity					Number of	% of
	White	Black	Hispanic	Others	Unknown	States	Sub. Care
FY 83	56.4%	26.7%	10.3%	4.5%	2.1%	29	57.0%
FY 84	59.8	22.9	10.2	5.3	1.8	28	62.8
FY 85	57.7	24.0	10.2	5.7	2.4	31	70.0
FY 86	56.0	25.9	9.4	5.0	3.7	33	81.0
FY 87	49.9	30.7	10.8	4.7	3.9	24	71.1

SOURCE: APWA 1991.

TABLE 6.2. Reasons children entered substitute care for fiscal years 1984–1987

	Protective Services	Status Offense	Child Disability	Parent Conditions/ Absence	Relinquish- ment of Parental Rights	Other State- Defined Reasons	Unknown	Number of States Included	% Total of Substitute Care Population
FY 84	55.7%	9.9%	2.3%	17.0%	1.4%	9.3%	4.4%	25	42.9%
FY 85	58.9	9.5	2.0	16.4	1.2	9.0	2.9	21	27.6
FY 86	53.6	11.4	1.5	17.5	1.9	8.1	6.0	21	40.9
FY 87	49.8	12.8	2.1	21.0	1.5	8.8	4.4	19	61.9

SOURCE: APWA 1991.

Table 6.3 depicts children who left care, by race and ethnic group, whereas table 6.4 depicts the reason the children left care. Black children exited the system at a slower rate than other groups. It will be interesting to note the rate of entry and exit as the data begin to reflect the current social crises in the United States (that is, data for 1988–1991). According to table 6.3, more African American children left the system than in previous years. One must note that again the exit rate is slower than the entry rate. However, in table 6.4 fewer children left for adoption since 1985. The majority of children who left care were reunited with their parents or relatives.

Organizational Positions on Transracial Adoptions

National Association of Black Social Workers

The National Association of Black Social Workers (NABSW) was organized in 1968 to confront the issues of racial discrimination and the em-

TABLE 6.3 Race and ethnicity of children who left substitute care for fiscal years 1983–1987

| | Race/Ethnicity | | | | | Number of States Included | % Total of Substitute Care Population |
	White	Black	Hispanic	Others	Unknown		
FY 83	60.7%	23.0%	9.4%	5.0%	1.9%	29	51.9%
FY 84	61.4	22.1	8.9	5.6	2.0	28	59.0
FY 85	58.7	24.6	8.9	5.8	2.0	31	66.5
FY 86	57.7	26.1	8.3	4.6	3.3	33	80.1
FY 87	55.4	26.5	9.7	5.2	3.2	26	57.3

SOURCE: APWA 1991.
NOTE: Sixteen states were able to provide data for all five years included in the table.

TABLE 6.4 Outcomes for children who left substitute care for fiscal years 1982–1987

	Reunited/ Placed with Parent/ Relative	Adopted	Majority Age/Eman- cipated	Other Outcomes	Unknown	Number of States Included	% Total of Substitute Care Population
FY 82	49.7%	10.4%	33.4%	a	6.5%	17	39.6%
FY 83	56.3	11.5	9.4	20.3	2.5	28	51.3
FY 84	62.4	9.9	9.3	16.3	2.1	31	57.3
FY 85	65.3	8.8	9.0	13.5	3.4	30	59.6
FY 86	58.8	7.3	7.9	19.4	6.3	33	76.5
FY 87	62.5	8.5	9.9	13.4	5.7	23	36.7

SOURCE: APWA 1991.
a. For FY 1982 data, the category "Other Outcomes" was included in "Majority Age/Emancipated."

powerment of its members. In 1972 at its annual conference, the NABSW presented a position paper in opposition to transracial adoption. Their position was so controversial that its impact is still debated today in child caring agencies. The NABSW challenged child welfare agencies to address the particular needs of Black families and children. The position of the Black social workers on transracial adoption stated:

The National Association of Black Social Workers has taken a vehement stand against the placement of Black children in white homes for any reason. We affirm the inviolable position of Black children in their Black families where they belong physically, psychologically, and culturally in order that they receive the total sense of themselves and develop a sound projection of their future. (NABSW, Position Statement on Transracial Adoptions, September 1972)

The debate continued and the controversy began to focus on the lack of Black families available to adopt. In response, the NABSW updated its position on transracial adoption by observing that:

As the National Association of Black Social Workers (NABSW) is dedicated to the preservation of the Black family, it strongly supports and endorses the fact that there exist in the black community, resources to provide suitable homes for those black children in need of permanency. NABSW fully rejects any position that will continue a policy of institutional racism that leads to the destruction of the Black family and ignores the inherent rights of the black child to his birthright. As an organization, NABSW supports and advocates for the placement of black children in racially and ethnically congruent homes. (NABSW, Position Paper on Transracial Placements, February 1983)

The counter position taken by some advocates of transracial adoption is that such placements involve only those African American children for whom homes are not found. However, the NABSW argues that little attention is given to the reasons these children linger in foster care, and that many Black families would adopt these children if they were freed for placement between the age of birth and five. Thus, NABSW reaffirmed its position against transracial placement and challenged child welfare agencies to revamp its policies and practices to focus on family preservation rather than on removal of children from their biological parents (NABSW 1991). Family preservation seeks to keep families together through the use of intense intervention strategies. If more resources are available on the front end of services, then perhaps the entry into substitute care by minorities can be minimized.

The NABSW brought transracial adoption to the forefront of the American Child Welfare concerns. Transracial adoptions practiced (initially) without scrutiny from the public and the implication for African

American children and other children of color had not been debated. Because the stand against transracial adoption is so controversial, it continues to carry with it great pain and emotional distress. Further, NABSW opposed transracial adoptions because it was not primarily a practice to salvage Black children from the effects of foster placements or institutionalization. Rather, these adoptions were used to fulfill the needs of childless White couples, affected by the dwindling pool of available healthy White infants. Therefore, NABSW viewed transracial adoption as an activity instituted to meet the needs of White prospective adoptive parents, rather than to provide an optimal solution to the plight of African American children in foster care. Transracial adoptions were also considered by a small segment of radical Black social workers as a demeaning, blatant attempt by Whites to further render Black people impotent (Simon and Altstein 1977). These views have been echoed by the Native Americans who opposed Native American children being adopted by White families (Fanshel 1972). Given the history of these two groups in the United States, it is not surprising that their responses are similar. NABSW's and the Native Americans' protests forced adoption and child welfare agencies to revamp their policies and procedures.

North American Council on Adoptable Children

The North American Council on Adoptable Children (NACAC) conducted a study on Barriers to Same Race Placement. The purpose of this study was not to solve the debate about transracial adoptive placements, but to look at the policies and procedures of public and private agencies across the country (NACAC 1991). A total of eighty-seven agencies in twenty-five states was surveyed. Seventeen of the agencies surveyed were specialists in placing minorities. The study was not random and consisted of forty-two questions. This survey is useful for it enumerates the barriers to same race placements. The most frequently noted barriers, according to the study, are listed below.

- *Institutional Racism.* Many of the respondents indicated that adoption is a microcosm of our racist society; therefore, White middle-class attitudes dominate adoption as they dominate other institutions in this country.
- *Lack of People of Color in Managerial Positions.* Many of the boards of directors and agency heads remain predominantly White. These people are more interested in maintaining the status quo.
- *Fees.* Fees can create psychological and financial barriers. The Black community strongly opposes the "purchasing of children." This feeling goes back to their beliefs about slavery as an institution in

this country. Additionally, the fee structure can be exorbitant. Agencies claim fees are for the purchase of services, not children.

- *Adoption as Business Mentality/Reality.* The reliance on a fee structure for services has caused agencies to place transracially for mere survival, not necessarily for their position for or against the practice of placing transracially.
- *Communities of Color Historical Tendencies toward Informal Adoption.* Black and Hispanic families are from strong informal extended families and do not necessarily understand the need for the formal adoption process.
- *Negative Perceptions of Agencies and Their Practices.* The agency process alone is intrusive. This is a part of the perception of how social services are delivered by public and private agencies.
- *Lack of Minority Staff.* There is a lack of minority line staff as well. The presence of minority staff appears to signal something positive to the minority potential adopter.
- *Inflexible Standards.* Workers appear to hold fast to what an acceptable family looks like.
- *General Lack of Recruitment Activity and Poor Recruitment Techniques.* To be blunt, most agencies are poor recruiters of minority families.
- *Word Not Out.* Most minority families are not aware of the problem. Until the minority community understands the scope of the problem, they will not adopt en masse. (NACAC 1991)

Table 6.5 reviews the percentage of same race placement by race (Black and Hispanic) and the average fees charged for placement. The South has a particularly high fee rate, considering its perceived economic status in the United States. Additionally, the table shows the percentage of Black children placed out of state. The South, by far the most often,

TABLE 6.5. Regional comparison of traditional non-specializing agencies

Same Race Placements	South	East	Midwest	West
Black	90/248(36%)	84/154(55%)	203/357(57%)	38/47(81%)
Hispanic	18/64(28%)	1/22(50%)	4/12(33%)	17/70(24%)
Average fees charged	$6,659	$4,445	$5,079	$6,684
% of Black children placed out of state	26%	1%	3%	4%
% of agencies with formal written policies on racial matching	17%	43%	50%	33%

SOURCE: North American Council on Adoptable Children 1991.

uses this practice of out-of-state placements. This is interesting because it is also assumed that the majority of the Black population is in the South and East. The East, however, had an almost negligible out-of-state placement rate. The East and Midwest do best in terms of policy on racial matching.

The NACAC study shows that public agencies placed in same race placements 85 percent of the time, compared to minority specialist agencies, which placed 91 percent in the same race home. Traditional agencies placed in same race homes only 47 percent of the time.

NACAC (1991) has been involved in the debate on transracial adoptions since the NABSW presented the original position paper. The NACAC board issued a statement in 1991, which stated that "placement of children with a family of like ethnic background is desirable because such families are likely to provide the children with skills and strengths that counter the ill effects of racism." While supporting same race placements, NACAC acknowledged that older handicapped children may have to be placed transracially rather than languish in foster care (NACAC 1991, 37).

NACAC has also recognized that the current furor over transracial adoption has been caused by the admission that some agencies place transracially for financial reasons. To that end, NACAC's position is recognizing that fees charged prospective adoptive families present barriers to the most culturally appropriate placement for children in need of adoption, and NACAC advocates that all child placing agencies have, as a goal, working to develop alternative funding sources to cover all costs related to adoption services by working with other private and public sectors (NACAC 1991, 38).

NACAC's position statement strongly supports same race placements. Their study assists agencies in dealing with the barriers to same race placements and lends itself to commitment to task. They have provided data that minorities do adopt. Agencies must now commit to place these children with available minority families.

National Adoption Information Clearinghouse

The National Adoption Information Clearinghouse (NAIC) provides a fact sheet to agencies that are attempting to recruit African American families to adopt Black children. This effort is made because of the approximately 36,000 children needing adoption services, one-half of whom are African American (NAIC 1991). NAIC also attributes the problem of the large numbers of African American children in substitute care to the crack epidemic in urban areas. There can be no doubt that the crack epidemic has recently increased the number of children in substitute care.

Yet, one also must note that, for most children, the demographic data consistently cites poverty as a major cause of the high rate of children removed from their homes of origin.

According to NAIC (1991), the 1960s and 1970s were a transitional period for African American families who had serious concerns about the agency requirements and the cost. After the passage of the Adoption Assistance and Child Welfare Act of 1980, federal monies became available for adoption services (NAIC 1991). Recognizing that attitudes needed to change if minority families were to be recruited, many agencies sought to structure their agencies to be more inviting to clientele who once were excluded. NAIC has assisted in this process by publishing and distributing materials to agencies to assist in their efforts to recruit African American families.

Child Welfare League of America

The Child Welfare League of America (CWLA) sets standards for its member agencies. These standards are developed based upon current knowledge of the developmental needs of children and tested ways to meet those needs (CWLA 1988). Several of their standards are especially pertinent to the discussion:

Adoption of American Indian Children. In 1978, the U.S. Congress passed the Indian Child Welfare Act to protect the best interests of Indian children and promote the stability of Indian Tribes. The CWLA recommends that agencies seek legal counsel before entering into an Indian adoption (CWLA 1988, 13–14).

Resources for older, handicapped, and racial or ethnic minority group children. CWLA's standard is as follows: "Special efforts should be made to find adoptive families for children who have special needs or are members of minority racial or ethnic groups. The child welfare agency and the community should recognize that the placement of these children requires a commitment to skilled and trained staff members who reflect the cultural and ethnic groups to be served" (CWLA 1988, 64).

The CWLA proposes a continuum of services such as family preservation, placement with a relative, or placement in community, prior to alternative placement options. This progression of placement options is gaining support in the child welfare profession. Although organizations have made attempts to encourage same race placements, the reality is that independent agencies make the final decision as to same race placement. Therefore, many agencies articulate verbal and written support for same race placement, but their practices do not necessarily reflect their verbal or written policies.

Mental Health Issues in African American Families

According to Boyd-Franklin (1989) "educating their children about the realities of racism in this country while simultaneously teaching them to strive to 'be all that they can be,' is one of the most difficult tasks for all African American families" (p. 25). Parents must help children to develop self-awareness and a healthy racial identity. Parents must also give children enough information about the types of problems they are likely to encounter in their environment so that they are prepared to function as productive members of their communities. This preparation prevents children from becoming immobilized and bitter in response to racism (Boyd-Franklin 1989). This point is at the heart of the controversy about transracial adoption. NABSW questions the ability of White families to impart strategies that help their African American children deal with racism. Many White families contend that they raise their African American children as human beings, not limited by their racial background, thereby deemphasizing cultural heritage (Ladner 1977; Simon and Altstein 1977; Grow and Shapiro 1975).

While there is cultural diversity among African Americans, there are four main areas that are unique to the experience of people of African descent: the African legacy, slavery, racism and discrimination, and the victim system (Hines and Boyd-Franklin 1982; Boyd-Franklin 1989, 7). Boyd-Franklin (1989) states that the African legacy involves traditions of family kinship and collective unity. Racism and discrimination are difficult for those who have not experienced these practices to understand. The victim system is a circular feedback process that exhibits properties such as stability, predictability, and identity, which are common to all systems that affect the African American community (Pinderhughes 1982, 109).

Some social scientists believe that the significance of race is declining in the society and that social class may be a more prominent factor in determining the condition of African Americans (Wilson 1980). Others argue that race continues to be the most powerful variable in determining the life chances of African Americans (Glasgow 1981). Lack of access to education, employment, housing, health care, and other opportunities to relegate African Americans to an "underclass position" that is difficult to escape. Additionally, some social scientists believe that African Americans' ability to survive is based on their instinctive reactions to the subtle manifestations of racism (Boyd-Franklin 1989). NABSW contends that White parents cannot impart these instinctive reactions to Black children.

Many African Americans turn to the church in response to the intensity of racism and the concomitant mental health problems. The church eases the pain of racism and supports African Americans' strong sense of religion and spirituality (Hill 1972; Boyd-Franklin 1989). Gary (1978) argues that racism is the most critical mental health problem faced by African American people. Whereas NABSW believes African Americans provide the best home environments for the psychological development of Black children, most proponents of transracial adoption interpret this vital issue as less important. However, older children who are adopted or removed from their original homes, regardless of the reason, feel pain because of that removal and may have difficulty understanding their roles in society in contrast to their White parents' role. Goldstein et al. (1979) state:

Children may also be deeply attached to parents with impoverished or unstable personalities and may progress emotionally within this relationship on the basis of mutual attachment. While the tie is to adults who are "unfit" as parents, unbroken closeness to them, and especially identification with them, may cease to be a benefit and become a threat. In extreme cases this necessitates state interference. Nevertheless, so far as the child's emotions are concerned, interference with the tie, whether to a "fit" or "unfit" psychological parent, is extremely painful. (19–20)

Family preservation efforts have grown because the best knowledge indicates that agencies can serve children best when they remain with their family of origin. Further, Goldstein, Freud and Solnit (1979) state that the continuity of relationships, surroundings, and environmental influence are essential for a child's normal development. Often, professionals in their zeal to rectify problematic family situations do not consider the child's need to be with his or her parents, family, or community. Child placement laws must be revamped to protect the mental health of the child with the welfare system. Mental health is one means toward maximum human growth and development (Gary and Jones 1978). This has relevance for the practice of transracial adoption because successful adoption requires that a family provide an opportunity for a child to grow and develop mentally, physically, and emotionally. Raising children who are mentally healthy is a difficult task for most families, and the stress of racism and poverty makes this task even more difficult.

In fact, racism is a major source of stress for African Americans. Staples (1978), Knowles and Prewitt (1969), and Willie et al. (1973) have shown that racism significantly influences the delivery of social and health services to African Americans. Further, other stressful phenomena in the African American community—such as family instability, child abuse and neglect, inadequate nutrition, poor physical environment, and poverty—are clearly linked to race and discrimination in American society (Gary 1978, 31).

Adoption policies and practices have also been influenced by racism. Adoption agencies were not created to serve African American families and their depiction in the social science literature. Nobles (1974) calls this phenomenon "conceptual incarceration," which means that the agencies use criteria based on White middle-class values to assess the appropriateness of African American families for adoption. Staples (1978) theorizes that the African American family is a sanctuary that has buttressed individuals from the pervasiveness of White racism, provided needed support systems that are unavailable in predominantly White institutions, and nurtured and socialized African American children. According to Staples (1978), people who are detached from their cultural roots cannot resist the forces of oppression, racism, and class exploitation. Minimizing the significant connectiveness resulting from cultural experience is a great disservice to children adopted by White parents. White parents who are unable to teach African American children to be Black and proud in a White racist society should not adopt these children. If a White parent's motive for adopting an African American child is to rescue the child from his Black heritage, the child's mental health should take precedence over a White parent's desire to adopt (Rosser 1978).

Transracial Adoption Studies

Research has been conducted to determine the effects of placing African American children in White homes. Grow and Shapiro (1974) studied 125 cases of transracial adoptions. They selected these cases from a pool of fifteen agencies in diverse communities with the families who volunteered to participate. The study has two major limitations: (1) the instrument used was not tested for validity or reliability; and (2) since the children in the study were very young, long-range projections could not be made. However, they concluded that African American children placed in White homes fared well. They acknowledged some problems with integration and racism but attributed more of the bias to the professionals handing the adoptions. However, they admitted that lighter-skinned African American children tended to be placed in "the better homes." There is a question of whether the lighter-skinned African American child was considered "the better child."

Some key findings of the Grow and Shapiro (1974) study are listed below:

- Almost half of the parents reported that their child had been subjected to some type of cruelty, usually name-calling or heckling, and occasional physical abuse. (What is not clear is what strategies the families used to assist the child, and if they needed any agency help for the resolution of the problems.)

- Over half (55 percent) of the families expressed little or no concern with racial background. (This is a key area of concern for NABSW— the lack of concern by White families about societal racism.)
- The study concluded that the disruption rate for these transracial adoptions was comparable to the disruption rate for all adoptions. (The reasons for the disruption of these adoptions remains unclear. What constituted a successful transracial adoption was also unclear.)

In a follow-up study on transracial adoptions, Grow and Shapiro (1975) studied the views of the adoption workers as well. The researchers reported the following significant findings:

- Of the thirty-three families in the study, the vast majority described their neighborhoods as predominantly or totally White. (There were no attempts to provide an integrated environment.)
- Approximately 12 percent of the participants indicated that the transracial adoption was a second choice, and that they would have preferred a White baby.
- Most of the children placed in these homes were considered biracial.
- The social workers placing the children were typically married White women between 25 and 45 years old.
- The children's average age when placed with these families was four months old. Whereas the researchers concluded that African American families were not available for these children, these authors (Ladner and Gourdine) also assumed that White families were given preference for adopting these children over African American families.
- Generally, the adoption workers in this study agreed that transracial adoption is an acceptable practice and a better alternative for African American children than indeterminate foster care.

On the other hand, they acknowledged the risks; that more exploration was needed; and that heavier demands for authenticity be made on the adoptive families (Grow and Shapiro 1975). They unanimously agreed that the African American child's heritage be maintained in his White adoptive home. However, there was no discussion concerning how an agency would assess the maintenance of a child's heritage.

In related work, David Fanshel (1972) conducted a study of the placement of Indian children in White homes. His findings are important because the adoption of Indian children by Whites parallels the placement of African American children with White parents. Children placed in White homes were from tribes in eleven different states. They had a broad range of physical characteristics. They came from family situations affected by the oppression of poverty and the meanness of daily living. Their adoptive parents viewed these children as the "Real" Americans—a special appeal not available to other minority children (Fanshel 1972).

As with the African American children placed in White homes, some of these White parents preferred not to acknowledge the children's racial differences, particularly if they were biracial. During the era in which Lyndon Johnson was president of the United States, the Native American was portrayed as the forgotten American. This evaluation affirms that "the loss of a people's children might well be seen as the ultimate indignity to endure" (Fanshel 1972, p. 25). Fanshel also found that many of the Native American children appeared to be doing well in their White adoptive homes. However, he concluded that more of these placements should not be encouraged:

It seems clear that the fate of most Indian children is tied to the struggle of Indian people in the United States for survival and social justice. Their ultimate salvation rests upon the success of that struggle. Whether adoption by white parents of the children who are in the most extreme jeopardy in the current period—such as the subjects of our study—can be tolerated by Indian organizations is a moot question. It is my belief that only the Indian people have the right to determine whether their children can be placed in white homes. Reading a report such as this one, Indian leaders may decide that some children may have to be saved through adoption even though the symbolic significance of such placements is painful for a proud people to bear. On the other hand, even with the benign outcomes reported here, it may be that Indian leaders would rather see their children share the fate of their fellow Indians than lose them in the white world. It is for the Indian people to decide. (1972, 341–42)

Fanshel's insights indicate his understanding of the plight of disadvantaged, politically impotent people and the right of these people to be self-determining. The studies previously mentioned lacked this insight, even though they acknowledged that in-race placements were preferable.

Ladner (1977) conducted a study of White Americans who adopted African American children. This researcher examined the lives of the families and the reactions of extended family and community members. The purpose of her research was to clarify the motivations of parents who adopt across racial boundaries. She raised a methodological concern about the ability of an African American sociologist to be objective in researching White subjects. This methodological concern should also be addressed by White researchers studying transracial adoptions. The topic is so sensitive that opponents and supporters of transracial adoptions have difficulty maintaining objectivity. The study was conducted in Georgia, Missouri, Washington, D.C., Maryland, Virginia, Connecticut, and Minnesota, and 136 parents were selected from the rosters of the Open Door Society, Council on Adoptable Children, and organizations that promoted transracial adoption. The researcher interviewed each set of parents in an informal setting. The limitation of this approach is that it was a one-shot study, allowing little opportunity for validation. This study, like the others, relied on parents' perceptions of the success of the placement and did not obtain feedback from the children, who in many cases were in their formative years. Some significant findings based on the interviews with adoptive families follow:

- A small number of parents who were interviewed felt that African American identity is more important than any considerations of the universal assumption that "all people are the same."
- Some parents did not concede that they had adopted a "Black" child but emphasized that he or she was part White, biracial, or a human being.
- One parent stated that people have no right to make children the objects of social issues.
- Parents who felt the identity issue was unimportant usually lived in all-White communities and were rearing their mixed race children as Caucasians.
- An adult who had been adopted by a White family said "he failed to develop the 'survival skills' that the black social workers mention so prominently.

Ladner's conclusions and recommendations include:

- If an extensive search for an African American family is unsuccessful, then transracial adoption might be considered.
- White parents who adopt African American youngsters must also be willing and able to identify not only with their African American children but also with African Americans generally.
- To adopt an African American child means that these parents have forfeited their rights to be regarded as a White family.
- Parents cannot insulate their children from societal forces.
- The future of transracially adopted children is inextricably linked to the future of the American people.

Future Directions

The NABSW reaffirmed its position opposing transracial adoptions at the 1991 annual conference in Atlanta, Georgia, almost two decades after

issuing its original position paper on this practice. African American social work professionals continue to question the effects of transracial
adoption on African American children. A new dimension of the controversy involves White foster parents who are applying to adopt non-White
children. Cable (1991) states that a permanent placement with a capable,
loving family regardless of race is better for a child than a situation where
serial placements will occur. Cross (1989) observes that 50 percent of the
children in the United States waiting to be adopted are children of color.
Yet, the history of child welfare agencies reveals inequitable, exclusionary,
and discriminating policies for these children and their families. The federal government recently conducted a survey that assessed current practices by adoption agencies to increase adoptions by minority group families and to identify obstacles to minority adoptions (Meyer 1989). The
survey included the District of Columbia and four states with large urban
populations of African Americans and Hispanics. The survey's findings
follow:

- Most agencies serving a substantial number of African American
  and Hispanic foster children have incorporated special techniques
  to recruit families.
- Most minority families report predominantly positive experiences
  in trying to adopt a child.
- A mismatch exists between the types of children waiting and the
  preferences of waiting families.
- Foster parents are a valuable resource for minority adoption.
- There is a lack of systematic data on children.
- Existing practices to work with minority families were noted as best
  practices.
- Adoption agencies are finding minority parents for many minority
  children, but not enough families for older handicapped children.
- There are obstacles for minority families but no agreement on how
  to overcome these obstacles.
- Minority organizations are helpful in increasing public awareness
  of the need for homes for African American children.

McRoy (1989) describes the organizational and racial dynamics that
have led adoption agencies to continue conducting transracial adoptions
despite the controversy. McRoy asserts that since African American children and their families are viewed as powerless, services to them have
not been developed to meet their needs. The adoption agencies, especially
private ones, have always catered to White middle-class families. The
agencies charge fees, the White families have the money, so the agencies
must provide what they want. White agencies also blame African American families for not being available to adopt, but do not blame themselves

for inefficient recruitment strategies. The issue of transracial adoption has become mired in politics, as some White families have filed complaints that their civil rights are being violated when African Americans are given preference in adopting African American children (McRoy 1989). This resembles a power play in which Whites are not adopting children who wait, but are competing with available African American families for African American children. Lee succinctly states that:

Transracial adoptions are a form of cultural genocide and the practice stems from the great demand for children by childless white couples and the limited number of healthy white infants. They [NABSW] further note that these white families are not generally desirous of adopting older handicapped children, but healthy African American babies and African American families are available for them. (Lee 1987, 1–4)

Opponents of transracial adoptions have identified the following obstacles to African American efforts to adopt children:
- Racial composition of adoption agencies' staffs.
- Agencies' limited approvals of African Americans for adoption.
- The influence of powerful interest groups (fee-paying Whites).
- Agencies are prepared to work with White families and unprepared to work with African American families.
- Agencies blame African American families for not adopting, instead of recognizing their own exclusionary policies.
- African American families are screened out of the adoptions process.
- Private agencies focus their services on the fee-paying White families, not the children they place. (They may do this to avoid legal battles.)
- Agencies who place transracially do not do anything special to make sure African American children fare well in White homes.

It is unclear that any standards exist for placing an African American child in a White home (McRoy 1989). Indian advocates echo the same themes: "The great majority of the research indicates that Indian children would benefit from placements that closely identify with the child's ethnocultural and socioeconomic status. . . . Many adoption workers underestimate the importance of culture and heritage of Indians and the mental health of the adopted Indian youth" (Braden and Field 1991).

The NABSW promotes family preservation and supports efforts to combat the societal ills that face minorities and cause irreparable problems. The social services delivery system should solidify families and use its resources to enable families to solve their problems. If a family continues to be dysfunctional after supportive interventions have been tried, then adoptive placement should be considered.

The CWLA also recognizes the validity of family preservation: "Family foster care is an essential and valuable child welfare service. But it must be a part of a national policy of strengthening families to prevent the unnecessary separation of children from their families, supplemented by a full array of fully funded quality out-of-home care options, such as kinship care, treatment, foster care, group and residential treatment" (*NASW News*, May 1991). CWLA offers recommendations regarding foster care placements: (1) placement with a relative should be the first option for children requiring foster care; and (2) foster parents should be of the same cultural and ethnic heritage as the children placed with them.

Recommendations

One goal in improving the child welfare system is the preservation of the family. The disenfranchised suffer disproportionately because of the dire circumstances they experience, which contribute to their vulnerability. Therefore, more attention must be given to families on the front end of service delivery, in order to maintain and preserve family unity. Support for family preservation is not enough; advocacy to review and change child welfare policies is necessary. Another necessity is the monitoring of agencies that continue to place transracially when African American families are available.

The nuclear family, extended family, and community should be viewed as resources for children, and must be nurtured and developed to meet the children's best interests. Children are not detached from their families of origin, and they desire a sense of continuity and stability. Omission of this process implies a devaluation of African American culture.

Child placement agencies must make strong commitments and develop written policies on same race placements. Fee structures cannot be used as a pretext for posing barriers to placement. This allows the issues to become clouded. One implicit message is that wealthier parents make better parents. This is tantamount to the continued use of worthiness scales and adherence to policies that give preference to White families over African American families.

Racism and discrimination are difficult concepts to discern. Well-intentioned people's actions are sometimes misinterpreted by the minority group. The behavior of the majority members may be interpreted or observed as covert or overt, intentioned or non-intentioned racism against minority members. Majority persons need to develop a greater understanding of the attitudes, feelings, and behavior of minorities. Many minority expressions of racism are valid. Some are not. Same race placement should be the major goal of child welfare agencies, whenever possible.

Families who have adopted across racial boundaries should avail themselves of post-adoption services, and standards should be developed for these placements. Children of color should have the opportunity to maintain their cultural ties. Additionally, minority persons must become advocates for children of color and articulate the needs of African American children in their own communities.

Older, disabled populations of children pose additional concerns. The disability may be as much of an issue as the racial or ethnic group membership. The authors support a system that considers both issues. Training and staff development should be provided for the families and professionals who are interested in adoption of, or working with, children who have disabilities. Attempts to make same race placements should be a priority.

The authors concur with the notion that African American children should be in culturally congruent homes. They also advocate full reform in child welfare services and advocate that agencies not be remiss in making commitments to same race placement for all cultural groups. NABSW supports family preservation, revamping child welfare policies, and the placement of African American children in African American homes. CWLA supports a continuum of services beginning with family preservation and moving to adoption, preferably in racially congruent homes. NACAC supports same race placements and raises the issue of the placement of older handicapped African American children who are typically more difficult to place.

Most agencies support the recruitment of minority adoptive parents. What is less clear is their commitment to this process and the elimination of perceived preferential treatment to White families. Many barriers are subjective rather than objective measures of selection of families. Agency policies in child welfare are a microcosm of the larger society, which does not usually give just treatment, let alone preferential treatment, to African Americans. How can agencies with preferential practices ensure that African American families and African American children get the best services in terms of placement options? This is not a simple issue. The authors support a position that empowers African American families and communities to be self-determining and self-sufficient. If efforts are not made to rectify the current situation of child placement in the United States, the success of adoption for children of color can never be obtained. No reforms will be successful in child welfare unless the system becomes more family friendly. Efforts to revitalize the family system lie in the ability of the systems of government to acknowledge the importance of the integral relationship of family life to a successful society. This should be done by demonstrating commitment to the full citizenry of vulnerable children and their families who have yet to realize the American dream.

REFERENCES

Alan Guttmacher Institute. 1988. *United States and cross national trends in teenage sexuality and fertility behavior.* New York. (Unpublished data.)

American Public Welfare Association (APWA). 1991. *Characteristics of children in substitute and adoptive care: a statistical summary of the VCIS National Child Welfare Data Base.* Washington, D.C.: APWA.

Best, M. 1992. Telephone interview. February 20. Washington, D.C.

Billingsley, A. 1968. *Black families in White America.* Englewood Cliffs, N.J.: Prentice Hall.

Billingsley, A., and Giovannoni, J. 1972. *Children of the storm: Black children and American child welfare.* New York: Harcourt Brace Jovanovich.

Boyd-Franklin, N. 1989. *Black families in therapy: a multisystems approach.* New York: The Guilford Press.

Braden, J. M., and Field, K. 1991. Cultural issues in the adoption of Indian children: post legal. In *The Roundtable: Journal of the National Resource Center for Special Needs Adoption* 5(1).

Burnham, L. 1985. Has poverty been feminized in Black America? *The Black Scholar* 16(2):14–24. March–April.

Cable, R. O. 1991. Cross racial placements: what do we know? In *The Roundtable* 5(1).

Child Welfare League of America (CWLA). 1988. *Standards for adoption service.* Washington, D.C.: CWLA.

Cross, T. L. 1989. Cultural competence necessary to keep minority families in adoption process. *The Roundtable* 4(2).

Fanshel, D. 1972. *Far from the reservation: the transracial adoption of American Indian children.* Metuchen, N.J.: Scarecrow Press.

Gary, L. E. 1978. Mental health: the problem and the product. In *Mental health: a challenge to the Black community,* ed. L. E. Gary. Bryn Mawr, Pa.: Dorrance.

Gary, L. E., and Jones, D. J. 1978. Mental health: a conceptual overview. In *Mental health: a challenge to the Black community,* ed. L. E. Gary. Bryn Mawr, Pa.: Dorrance.

Gill, O., and Jackson, B. 1983. *Adoption and race.* New York: St. Martin's Press.

Glasgow, D. 1981. *The Black underclass.* New York: Vintage Books.

Glazer, N., and Moynihan, D. P. 1963. *Beyond the melting pot.* Cambridge, Mass.: MIT and Harvard Press.

Goldstein, J., Freud, A., and Solnit, A. J.
1979. *Beyond the best interest of the child.* New York: Free Press.
1986. *In the best interest of the child.* New York: Free Press.

Grier, W. and Cobbs, P. 1968. *Black rage.* New York: Basic Books.

Grow, L. J., and Shaprio, D.
1974. *Black children, White parents: a study of transracial adoption.* New York: CWLA.
1975. *Transracial adoption today: views of adoptive parents and social workers.* New York: CWLA.

Gutman, H. G. 1977. *The Black family in slavery and freedom, 1750–1925*. New York: Vintage Books.

Haley, A. 1965. *Autobiography of Malcolm X*. New York: Ballantine Books.

Hartman, A., and Laird, J. 1983. *Family-centered social work practice*. New York: The Free Press.

Hill, R. B.
1972. *The strengths of Black families*. White Plains, N.Y.: Emerson Hall.
1977. *Informal adoption among Black families*. Washington, D.C.: National Urban League.

Hines, P. M., and Boyd-Franklin, N. 1982. Black families. In *Ethnicity and family therapy*, ed. M. McGoldrick, J. K. Pearce, and J. Giordano, pp. 84–107. New York: The Guilford Press.

Kadushin, A. 1972. *Child welfare services*. New York: MacMillan.

Kamen, A. 1991. Adoption laws trap Americans in Romania: U.S. demands permits to leave. *Washington Post*, May 23, pp. 1, 16.

Keniston, K., et al. 1977. *All our children: the American family under pressure*. New York: Harcourt Brace Jovanovich.

Knowles, L. L., and Prewitt, K. 1969. *Institutional racism in America*. Englewood Cliffs, N.J.: Prentice Hall.

Ladner, J. A. 1977. *Mixed families: adopting across racial boundaries*. New York: Anchor Press.

Lee, E. 1987. Issue of color: white couples battle obstacles to adoption of nonwhite children. *Wall Street Journal*, February 27, pp. 1, 4.

McRoy, R. G. 1989. An organizational dilemma: the case of transracial adoptions. *Journal of Applied Behavioral Science* 25(2):145–60.

Meyer, A. S. 1989. Federal government surveys minority adoptions. *The Roundtable* 4(2).

Moore, K. A. 1990. *Facts at a glance*. Washington, D.C.: Child Trends.

Myrdal, G. 1972. *An American dilemma: the Negro problem and modern democracy*. New York: Pantheon Books.

NASW News. 1991. Foster-care blueprint: social work essential. Silver Spring, Md.: NASW. May.

National Adoption Information Clearinghouse (NAIC). 1991. *Adoption and the African American child: a guide for agencies*. Rockville, Md.: NAIC.

National Association of Black Social Workers (NABSW).
1968. *Our roots: position statement of the National Association of Black Social Workers*. San Francisco, Calif.: NABSW.
1972. *National Association of Black Social Workers position statement on transracial adoptions*. New York: NABSW.
1983. National Association of Black Social Workers Position Statement on Transracial Placement. Detroit, Mich.: NABSW. (Reprinted, 1985).
1991. *Preserving African American families: research and action beyond the rhetoric*. Detroit, Mich.: NABSW.

Nobles, W. N. 1974. Africanity: its role in Black families. *The Black Scholar* 5:10–17.

North American Council on Adoptable Children (NACAC). 1991. *Barriers to same race placement*. St. Paul, Minn.: NACAC.

Pinderhughes, E. 1982. Afro-American families and the victim system. In *Ethnicity and family therapy*, ed. M. McGoldrick, J. K. Pearce, and J. Giordano, pp. 108–12. New York: The Guilford Press.

Rosser, P. L. 1978. The child, young, gifted, and Black. In *Mental health: a challenge to the black community*, ed. L. E. Gary. Bryn Mawr, Pa.: Dorrance.

Simon, R. J., and Alstein, H. 1977. *Transracial adoption*. New York: John Wiley.

Staples, R. E. 1978. Black family life and development. *Mental health: a challenge to the Black community*, ed. L. E. Gary. Bryn Mawr, Pa.: Dorrance.

Willie, C. V., Kramer, B. M., and Brown, B. S., eds., 1973. *Racism and mental health*. Pittsburgh: University of Pittsburgh Press.

Wilson, W. 1980. *The declining significance of race*. 2d ed. Chicago: University of Chicago Press.

Teenage Motherhood

TEENAGE childbearing is a relatively recent issue on the public agenda. It emerged as a social problem in the United States in the 1970s when the overall birth rate among teenagers was declining. While the rate declined, however, the actual number of births to teens increased, owing to the number of adolescents in the population and a decline in births to older women. Approximately one million teenagers became pregnant every year during the 1970s, and more than half of them gave birth. Between 1985 and 1988, the number of births to teens fell below the half-million mark and then increased to 517,989 in 1989. Births to teens continued to rise in 1990, to 533,483. This is an increase of 61,402 over 1986 and represents increases in births to both Black and White teenagers (Moore et al. 1993). The reasons for the increase are not clear.

In the years after abortion was legalized, the proportion of teenage pregnancies terminated by abortion doubled from 20.1 percent in 1972 to 40 percent in 1982 (Hardy and Zabin 1991, 36). Given this increase in abortion by teens, it is logical to conclude that restrictions on abortion services to poor women may be a factor in the recent increase of teen births. However, according to Moore et al. (1992), no decline in the abortion rate or in contraceptive use among teens has been documented. One influence on the increase in births to teens, Moore suggests, is the increased proportion of teens who are sexually active. Though teens the world over have high rates of sexual activity, more abortions, pregnancies, and births occur among adolescents in the United States than in any other western industrialized country (Jones et al. 1986). However, numbers alone do not cause teenage childbearing to be perceived as a grave social problem in the United States. Rather, the causes are multiple: the sexual behavior of adolescents; the unmarried status of the majority of teen mothers; the relationship between early childbearing, welfare, and persistent poverty; the disproportionate number of teenage childbearers who are Black; and an increase in childbearing among White teenagers.

In this chapter I will discuss these aspects of adolescent motherhood in their social context. A number of factors attributed to teenage child-bearing are actually due to poverty and women's changing sexual and reproductive behavior. Further, effects of teenage childbearing have been based on the years immediately following birth when mothers have not completed high school and are most likely to depend on public assistance for support. Recent longitudinal studies show, however, that some nega-tive effects of teenage childbearing have been exaggerated. Portraying teenage pregnancy as an epidemic of children having children ignores particularly the historical and cultural context of childbearing and the convergence in sexual behavior of White teenagers and Black teenagers. Finally, the policy implications of longitudinal research and the views of those who think the problem has been overstated will be considered.

Sexual Behavior and Marital Status

Since the 1970s, the availability of contraception and abortion, rising divorce and remarriages, and the uncoupling of sex and marriage have had profound effects on family structure and sexual conduct. The Na-tional Center for Health Statistics reports that in 1988 over one million babies were born to unmarried mothers. In recent years growth in non-marital births has been greater for White women than for Black women. For example, the rate of childbearing for unmarried Black women was 88.9 in 1988, compared to 82.9 in 1980; whereas the rate for White women was 26.6 in 1988, compared to 17.6 in 1980. One researcher asks: "Can we effectively teach teenagers abstinence and skills for delaying the initiation of intercourse in a social climate where nonmarital sex is common and supervision and wholesome activities are absent?" (Dryfoos 1990, 74). This question suggests that the sexual behavior of teenagers is influenced by standards of sexual behavior in the general population, a lack of over-sight of teenage behavior by adults, and missing neighborhood recreation and services. Vinovskis observes that youth generally—not teenagers spe-cifically—were targets for instruction about the sins of premarital sex in nineteenth-century America. "Thus, the general societal attitudes toward premarital sex played a much larger role in determining how young people would be treated than any special view of adolescents" (1988, 20).

In the twentieth century, however, the tendency is to treat the sexual and reproductive behavior of female adolescents apart from the social context of sexual and reproductive behavior of older women. This is a mistake, for while the social and economic consequences of childbirth for older unmarried women are not the same as those for unmarried teenagers, the social context that shapes their behavior remains the same. The relative economic advantage of older women is likely to be less apparent to teenage girls than their reproductive behavior. Teenagers then may engage in sexual conduct similar to that of older women without considering the advantage of their relatively greater economic security and better education.

Among health professionals, age and marital status are key factors in predicting adverse outcomes for mothers and children. According to the National Center for Health Statistics, "Childbearing by unmarried women is typically associated with less favorable outcomes because high-risk women, particularly teenagers, tend to predominate among the mothers" (*Monthly Vital Statistics Report* 39 [Aug. 1990]:7). Nonetheless, social and economic factors are often more important than age. Recent research has shown that unfavorable outcomes are less related to age (except for teens 15 years of age and younger) than poverty, access to health care, and other environmental conditons (Makinson 1985). Further, the highest rate of nonmarital births is not among teens aged 15–17 years, whose rate is 26.5 births per thousand, but among women aged 18–19 and 20–24 years, at 52.7 and 56.7 births per thousand, respectively (*Monthly Vital Statistics Report,* 39 [Aug. 1990]:7). These statistics indicate that young teenagers have ample opportunity to observe women in age cohorts just above them having children while remaining unmarried. Teenagers are less apt to notice how they differ from these older child-bearers in advantages that stem from racial, economic, and social characteristics. Teenage mothers often are daughters of unmarried women who began childbearing as unmarried teenagers and who are still unmarried and having children.

Nonmarital sexual activity, then, is a common phenomenon that has greatly increased among women in recent decades. In 1988, for example, 52 percent of females between the ages of 15 and 19 engaged in premarital sexual intercourse, compared to 29 percent in 1970 (Moore et al. 1992). Nearly all (96 percent) of Black males and 76 percent of White males have engaged in premarital intercourse by the age of 19, compared to 79 percent of Black females and 76 percent of White females (Moore et al. 1992). As these data indicate, by age 20, three-quarters of all women are sexually experienced. Black females, however, are at higher risk of having a baby while teenagers, because they are more likely to engage in early unprotected intercourse than their White or Hispanic counterparts.

In past decades, teenage sexual activity occurred in the context of courtship with expectations that marriage would follow (Furstenberg 1991). Premarital conceptions were less visible because marriages usually occurred before births took place. Today 67 percent of all births to teenage women are nonmarital births. Changing standards toward premarital sex and the fact that marriage is no longer the routine response to unplanned pregnancy has consequences for the sexual and reproductive behavior of adolescents. A significant proportion of births to teens are to unmarried teenagers. In 1989, 92 percent of Black babies and 55 percent of White babies born to teenagers were born to unmarried mothers (Moore et al. 1992). Thus the fact that almost all Black teenage mothers and over half of all White teenage mothers are unmarried places teenage mothers in the center of the debate about the rising number of "mother-only households" and the growth in public assistance. In 1989, approximately 25 percent of all American children lived in households with one parent, usually the mother. Nonmarital births are second only to divorce and separation as a major cause of single parenthood.

Poverty, Welfare, and Early Childbearing

Unmarried teenage childbearing is associated with poverty and welfare dependence. Long-term welfare dependence has been linked to becoming a recipient of Aid to Families with Dependent Children (AFDC) while being a teenage mother (Moore et al. 1981). Any statement about length of time on welfare should be placed in context. The facts are that fewer than 10 percent of AFDC recipients have received aid for over ten years and only a fourth have been recipients for five or more years (Hacker 1992, 86). It is also known that most young mothers who become welfare recipients were from poor households before they had children (Bane 1986a). Thus poverty and welfare among teenage mothers are related to antecedent social and economic conditions.

Research on the long-term effects of teenage pregnancy and motherhood shows that family background, poverty, and environmental factors such as access to early prenatal care affect health and other outcomes for mothers and infants more than age (Furstenberg et al. 1987; Horwitz et al. 1991). The Furstenberg and associates (1987) longitudinal study of Black teenage mothers in Baltimore shows that, over time, they left welfare and became economically self-sufficient. Whereas they did not do as well economically as a comparison group of women who delayed childbearing until their twenties, they did earn adequate incomes. Another follow-up study of Black New Haven mothers who participated in one of the first comprehensive programs for pregnant teens in the 1960s found that 82 percent of the mothers were completely self-supporting twenty years later (Horwitz et al. 1991).

The claim is frequently made by human capital economists that early childbearers lack sufficient motivation for economic success. However, McCrate (1989) rejects the idea that teenage mothers do not value school or work as highly as women who are not early childbearers: "Rather, I hypothesize that they correctly anticipate smaller average economic rewards for postponing birth and focusing more exclusively on their schooling" (1989, 2). For example, Black teenage mothers have higher school completion rates than White teens, yet it is Black teen mothers who earn the least. McCrate concludes that for poor Black women, postponement of childbearing is not an effective strategy for gaining higher wages because discrimination and job segmentation are stronger factors than early childbearing in determining their chances in the labor market. McCrate's research suggests that we should pay more attention to the devastating effects of poor schools, the absence of neighborhood resources, and labor market discrimination on the lives of poor teenage mothers than we do to their age.

An analysis by Franklin and Smith (1991) of the effects of teen parenthood on poor women suggests that teen childbearers spend more time on welfare than any other group of mothers. In retrospect, according to these authors, the accepted wisdom of the 1960s—that "staying in school and getting a job" would lead to good economic outcomes for mothers with children—was overstated. Instead, they suggest, it would have been more realistic to advise teenagers to "delay childbearing, stay in school and get a job so that you can ensure your chances of marrying a man with a steady job" (1991, 26). This advice may have been as misleading as the advice it was to replace. It suggests a pattern that fits the life-course decisions of middle-class women who have more assurance that their investment in education and delay in childbearing will be rewarded by career advancement and marriage opportunities.

Poor Black women are having children early and remaining unmarried. They tend to stay in school or return to school, which leads to higher school completion rates for Black teenage mothers than for their White counterparts. Educational attainment does not get them jobs that lift them out of poverty, however. This is not surprising in light of the fact that a wide gap exists between incomes and earnings of Black and White families. In 1990, the median for all Black families was $21,423 compared to $36,915 for White families; while the median for Black women was $8,328 compared to $10,317 for White women (Hacker 1992, 94). Such wide disparities between Black and White median incomes suggest that structural inequality in the major sectors of society contributes to the poor economic status of Black families, and that high rates of nonmarital childbearing constitute only one contributing factor to the disproportionate number of Black women and children in poverty.

A common goal of programs for teenage mothers is to assist them to achieve self-sufficiency. Achieving self-sufficiency translates into leaving AFDC and getting a job that, after a transitional period, pays enough to permit the mother to buy health benefits and child care. It is rare, however, for teenage mothers to have the requisite education and work experience to get a job that pays much more than the welfare grant. Most of the research on teenage childbearing focuses on the years immediately following the birth of a child, when mothers are likely to be on welfare. Economic self-sufficiency may not occur until after several years on welfare have allowed young mothers to invest in education and job training (Furstenberg et al. 1987).

As stated earlier, a follow-up study of New Haven women aged 32–38 years who participated in a comprehensive program for teen mothers in the 1960s found them to be self-supporting twenty years after the index birth (Horwitz et al. 1991). The majority of the New Haven women remained unmarried, as did the women in Furstenberg's Baltimore sample. Marriage—often identified as the surest route out of poverty for women—is unlikely to be an option for Black women because of the joblessness among Black males and a shrinking pool of men of marriageable age (Wilson 1987). According to Hacker, even if the number of Black families with male earners increased, "emulating the white family structure would close only about half of the income gap" (Hacker 1992, 95). Of equal importance, perhaps, to the lack of available marriage partners and the lack of hope that economic security will come from marriage is Black women's cultural orientation toward marriage and children.

The cultural orientation of Black teenagers toward sexual behavior and childbearing is formed by the particular history of Blacks, changes in women's sexual behavior and reproductive patterns, and the harsh economic realities of inner-city life.

Cultural Orientation of Black American Teenagers

E. Franklin Frazier (1966) traced the roots of modern childbearing behavior among Blacks to survivals of African culture, the experience of slavery, conditions after emancipation, and family disorganization in the wake of migration from the American rural South to northern cities. Among African Americans, sex was regarded as natural, and women fulfilled their destiny through childbearing. This orientation was present during slavery, and its continuance was documented by Frazier in the late

1920s and the 1930s in high nonmarital birth rates and in the prevailing sentiment among the descendants of slaves that motherhood was more highly regarded than marriage. In the 1970s, researchers using ethnographic methods to study childbearing among Black teenagers described teenage motherhood as an accepted and natural route to adulthood and responsibility (Ladner 1971). Unmarried mothers in public housing relied on support networks of relatives and neighbors for the exchange of goods and child care (Stack 1974).

An ethnographic study of life in a northern urban Black community in the 1980s describes an elaborate pattern of sexual conduct that ends in nonmarital childbearing. According to the study, unsupervised girls from female-headed households engage in sex with the hope of getting a commitment from young men. The men, however, are loyal only to their peers, who require sexual prowess and fathering babies as proof of manhood. Girls seeking lasting commitment and material support become pregnant and have babies that provide them with status and a welfare check but not a male partner. The welfare check makes many young mothers attractive to unemployed males who in return for economic benefits provide companionship and sexual favors (Anderson 1990).

A Boston study found that Black teenage mothers did not seek lasting commitment and marriage, but that socialization to early motherhood occurred in single-parent households where teenage girls regarded their mothers as role models. Respondents were daughters of women who began having children when they were teenagers. Most of their mothers never married and had children by more than one partner. Adult supervision, after school activities, and neighborhood recreation were missing from the lives of the teenage mothers. Having babies was common among their peers and unmarried relatives in their twenties and thirties (Williams 1991).

Outside the family the majority of these young mothers had unsatisfactory school lives and little involvement with church or neighborhood organizations. Contact with hospitals, neighborhood health centers, and alternative schools began after pregnancy occurred. Ironically, pre- and postnatal care from consistent and caring adults in the adolescent clinics of two urban hospitals and from the instructors in alternative schools for pregnant teens were remembered by young mothers with a fondness not extended to relationships with public school teachers or other adults. Similarly, evaluators of the Johns Hopkins Adolescent Pregnancy and Parenting Program (APP) observed that, whereas services for pregnant teens and putative fathers were well utilized, they reached adolescents only after pregnancy (Hardy and Zabin 1991).

It is common for Black teenage mothers to live with their mothers, who exhibit a range of feelings about assuming the role of grandmother—from conflict about taking on a role associated with old age to enthusiasm about having a grandchild (Burton and Bengtson 1985; Williams 1991). The majority of adolescent mothers report that their male partners encourage them to have a baby rather than terminate a pregnancy (Williams 1991; Hardy and Zabin 1991). Thus, significant others in the Black teen mother's culture convey that having a baby is desirable. If the baby is healthy and school is uninterrupted, the teen mother may be accurate in her perception that in comparison with other women she knows, her life has not been adversely affected by having a baby. Some teen mothers report an increased sense of worth, responsibility, and purpose after having a baby (Williams 1991).

Anderson (1990) and Williams (1991) describe poor urban teenagers from mother-only families where early childbearing is common. But these studies present different motives for early motherhood. Teenagers described by Anderson are seeking lasting commitment from their partners and use their welfare checks to attract continued attention from males. The teenagers described by Williams show little interest in marriage while they are living with their mothers, who may receive welfare only for the teenager's baby. These differences remind us that there is no monolithic teen mother and that a variety of responses to pregnancy and motherhood exist between and within racial and ethnic groups.

An underutilized source of information about teenage motherhood is the teenage mother herself. Explanations for the prevalence of teenage childbearing that are uninformed by the teen mother's perspective are unlikely to increase understanding of the meaning of childbearing to teenagers. Similarly, suggestions by the National Research Council that sexually active teens become diligent contraceptive users or delay the onset of sexual activity, while well intended, ignore the context of daily life for many poor adolescents (see Hayes 1987, 7–8). Diligent contraception and delay in the onset of sexual activity would, of course, reduce the number of adolescents at risk of becoming pregnant and, thereby, reduce the number of births. However, unless accompanied by fundamental changes in family and community life, adequate schools, positive involvement by parents and other adults in the daily lives of children, and changes in peer group expectations, teenagers will lack the support and motivation necessary to postpone early sexual activity and childbearing.

During the 1970s, adverse health and education outcomes were attributed to early childbearing. Subsequent research showed that adverse health outcomes were associated with social and economic conditions rather than age per se (Makinson 1985). The magnitude and duration of economic dependency and the welfare costs associated with female-headed families and nonmarital teenage childbearing are also being re-examined.

Are the Effects of Teenage Childbearing Overstated?

In *Adolescent Mothers in Later Life*, Frank Furstenberg and colleagues (1987) presented longitudinal data from research on teen mothers begun in the 1960s showing that the adverse effects of teenage motherhood may have been overstated. Furstenberg found that teen mothers do not do as well as those who are later childbearers. Nevertheless, based upon a majority of those studied, they do "recover" and become economically self-sufficient. Now, A follow-up study of New Haven teen mothers in the 1960s provides more data on the economic recovery of mothers in later life. These longitudinal data, together with early ethnographic studies by Ladner (1971) and Stack (1974) and recent studies by Anderson (1990) and Williams (1991), provide a perspective on teenage childbearing that argues for studying its effects over the course of women's lives and in the context of cultural and economic conditions relevant to the group of teens being studied.

Ladner and Stack presented teen childbearing as an understandable survival strategy and adaptive response to disadvantage and poverty. Their findings were based on actual contact with Black mothers and poor Black adolescent girls whose behaviors are shaped by poverty and the culture of their families and neighborhoods. Geronimus (1987) has gone beyond the interpretation that teenage childbearing is adaptive and shaped by poverty to make the assertion that early childbearing may also be beneficial. Her research on infant mortality, for example, asserts that women who are economically and socially disadvantaged are at higher risk for bearing low-birthweight babies the longer they postpone childbearing. According to Geronimus's thesis, disadvantaged teenagers make the decision to begin childbearing to have healthier babies and to elicit maximum social and economic support from family members that may not be forthcoming if childbearing is delayed beyond the teen years.

Geronimus and Korenman (1991), using the National Longitudinal Survey of Young Women, studied sisters, one of whom was a teen childbearer and one who delayed childbearing into her twenties. They found that teen mothers were not substantially worse off than their sisters who delayed childbearing. Geronimus and Korenman's examination of cross-sectional studies on costs and benefits of early childbearing and their own findings—that the effects of teen births were significantly reduced when family background characteristics were held constant—led them to conclude that the negative effects of early childbearing had been overstated.

Other scholars have examined teenage pregnancy and childbearing from the perspective of the development and definition of social problems. According to Vinovskis (1988) and Nathanson (1991), teenage pregnancy was defined as an "epidemic" to elicit responses from policy makers and the public to favor solutions advanced by particular interest groups. For example, teenage pregnancy was defined by health professionals as a medical problem, which resulted in a redefinition of adolescent women's sexual morality "to depend on their contraceptive rather than on their sexual conformity" (Nathanson 1991, 71). Clearly, the nonconforming adolescents were poor, Black, and (Nathanson reminds us) associated with the stigma of unmarried mothers, illegitimacy, welfare dependence, and uncontrolled sexuality. Thus race, teenage pregnancy, morality, and welfare became intertwined.

In spite of the fact that nonmarital births are higher among older teens (aged 18–19) and women aged 20–24, increases in illegitimacy are often attributed to teenage childbearing. Further, the myth that women have babies to receive welfare continues to be believed, although research does not support this misconception (Bane 1986b). Bell's (1987) analysis of the latent consequences of AFDC eligibility criteria states that some rules "were barely disguised devices for disproportionately rejecting black and illegitimate children" (1987, 167).

A recent welfare reform effort in Wisconsin proposed to deny increased benefits to mothers who have a second child. According to national data, the majority of mothers on AFDC have one child, while only 30.6 percent have two children (Hacker 1992). The Wisconsin proposal is punitive and rests on the assumption that the motivation for childbearing is to obtain an increase in welfare income. Such policy proposals are not based on facts about the motivations and reproductive behavior of teenagers, the majority of whom report their pregnancies were unintended (Hayes 1987; Hardy and Zabin 1991). The promulgation of policies that ignore what is known about the complex, multifaceted issue of teenage childbearing may be encouraged by claims that teen childbearing leads to long-term welfare dependency and irreversible health consequences. Clearly, it is not helpful to inflate the effects of teenage childbearing, any more than it is helpful to claim there are no negative social consequences that flow from teenage childbearing. Persons who take either stance in the debate or who are characterized by others as inflating or deflating the effects of teenage motherhood may, in fact, contribute to a polarized debate that pays less attention to issues related to teenage motherhood and more attention to the parties to the debate.

In a discussion of Geronimus's and Vinovskis's views, Furstenberg (1991) doubts that medical personnel and service providers were guided by selfish motives that caused them to define teenage pregnancy for the benefit of particular interest groups. Furstenberg understands the reaction of health professionals and service providers in the context of demographic trends that led to an increased number of teens in the population at a time when teen pregnancy rates decreased and the absolute number of teen births increased. This increase had an impact on medical and other services because more pregnant and parenting teens sought care.

In addition, Furstenberg reminds us that the problem became more visible because teen mothers were not marrying as they had in the past. In relation to Geronimus's claim that infants of Black teen mothers have higher survival rates than infants of older Black women, Furstenberg cites studies that contradict her findings. He also finds no evidence that disadvantaged mothers believe that teenagers bear healthier babies than women in their twenties and base their reproductive decisions on this belief. Unlike some critics of scholars who believe that the problem of teenage pregnancy has been exaggerated, Furstenberg takes the views of the revisionist scholars seriously. Although he counters their claims, he expresses concern that their findings will confuse policy makers and cause service providers and funders to wonder: "Have we been mislead into believing that the reduction of teenage pregnancy and childbearing is a productive strategy for improving the chances of disadvantaged youth?" (Furstenberg 1991, 135).

Program and Policy Implications

Longitudinal data based on follow-up studies of Baltimore and New Haven teen mothers who participated in comprehensive programs during the 1960s indicate that teen mothers benefited from the programs. Furstenberg's participants who attended a special school for pregnant girls did better than a comparison group who attended regular school. Participants in Williams's study who went to alternative schools during the final months of pregnancy reported that their experiences in alternative schools were positive compared to their experiences in the public schools they had previously attended.

School-linked clinics that serve young teenagers have reduced teenage pregnancy rates and had other positive effects (see Hardy and Zabin's description of the Baltimore program). Such programs should be supported but not at the expense of programs that serve teenagers who are already parents. Helping teen parents to prevent subsequent births is a worthwhile goal, because teens having more births are far more disadvantaged than teens having a first birth (Hardy and Zabin 1991). The most significant difference between a group of Boston teen mothers of one child and teen mothers of similar ages with two children was their educational attainment (Williams 1991). The majority of mothers with two children were dropouts, whereas most of the mothers of one child were attending high school or post–high school programs. These examples show that programs for pregnant and parenting teens are worthy of support.

Consequently, if infants of poor minority teenage mothers are less vulnerable to infant mortality and other health risks than babies born to older mothers, as Geronimus suggests, it does not mean that funders should or will decrease support for special programs for teenage mothers. On the contrary, programs for teen mothers should be continued and additional resources should be allocated to increase access to health care for poor women during and after the teen years.

Let us now turn to the question posed by Furstenberg as to whether fewer teen pregnancies and births will improve the chances of poor youth. This question obviously has crucial policy implications. There is no evidence that efforts to reduce teen pregnancy and childbearing have been harmful. Data to prove that the returns on these programs are equal to the resources used by them are not available. I assume, however, that programs that reach poor pregnant and parenting teenagers—who often attend unsupportive schools and live in resource-poor neighborhoods— are a good investment in human capital. As stated above, comprehensive programs and special schools for pregnant and parenting teens have improved the lives of some teenagers. These programs usually reach teenagers after pregnancy and, at best, ameliorate the effects of early childbearing. If, however, our goal as a society is to provide children with opportunities to reach their full potential, then programs targeted to the reduction of pregnancy and childbearing deal with the symptoms, not the causes. Basic economic and social issues facing families in the lower third of the population should be addressed to deal with the underlying causes of early sexual involvement, pregnancy, and childbearing.

A full employment policy is fundamental to alleviating poverty. The majority of teen mothers come from poor families, and the majority of the partners of teen mothers are disadvantaged. Men who are unemployed and have no prospects of working do not marry. But employment policies that focus only on men will be misguided. Meaningful employment opportunities for poor young women may give them a compelling reason not to bear children early and provide an alternative to welfare. Black men who are the partners of teen mothers, even when employed, earn less than their White counterparts, in spite of having more education (Hardy and Zabin 1991). Thus the chances of Black teenage mothers and their children are not only determined by poverty but by race as well.

Further, policy and program initiatives have focused primarily on the teenage mother. Furstenberg (1991) reminds us that we know very little about the effects of teenage motherhood on the children, their fathers, and extended families. Until we can learn more about the impact of teenage childbearing on all affected parties, it will be difficult to fully know and assess the advantages and disadvantages associated with teenage childbearing.

It is much easier to seek changes by focusing on the behavior of the poor than to address the fundamental issues of poverty, unemployment, and poor schools. The behavioral changes being sought, such as abstinence and diligent contraceptive use, are radically at odds with the practices, if not the norms, of that segment of society providing the models for poor inner-city youth. Middle-class youth and women over twenty engage in many of the same behaviors as do poor teenagers without suffering the same consequences.

Over twenty years ago when teenage childbearing came to the attention of scholars, policy makers, and service providers, AIDS was unknown and cocaine use not widespread. Both of these serious, life-threatening problems disproportionately affect the populations at highest risk for early childbearing. Our inability to reach consensus about who should educate the young and what they should be taught about sexuality and contraception puts American youth at still greater risk for increased pregnancies, abortions, and births—and now, early death.

Government's abandonment of efforts to provide an effective safety net for all citizens, the abandonment of the cities, and a lack of support for public education affect all Americans, but disproportionately affect poor children most at risk for early sexual involvement and childbearing. In this climate, revisionist scholars have perhaps performed a service by reminding us that it is not age but economic and social factors that most influence outcomes for teen mothers and their children.

As scholars and citizens, we should emphasize economic and social change instead of attributing poor outcomes primarily to age. If we are committed to helping children delay sexual intercourse (a strategy approved of by liberals and conservatives) we shall find the dearth of age-appropriate activities supervised by adults unacceptable. *Instead, what would we offer as a reward for the postponement of parenthood?* This is a crucial question, since teenagers who do become parents have few compelling reasons not to do so.

Finally, we cannot expect teenagers to be wiser or behave better than do the adults in our society. Yet, we are alarmed when teenage girls follow their mothers and sisters in having unprotected sex or when teenage boys from female-headed families do not accept the responsibilities that accompany fatherhood. Whereas nonmarital births and teenage motherhood are disproportionately high among Blacks, the greatest growth in rate in nonmarital childbearing is among older White women. Racial attitudes have driven our presentation of teenage mothers, because the consequences of nonmarital childbearing are inextricably bound to AFDC, a program that is disproportionately Black. Here, too, revisionist scholars bring an important balance to the discussion of and debate over teenage motherhood by reminding us that teenage mothers have replaced the welfare mothers of the 1960s as objects of sexual and social control.

Summary and Recommendations

Recent research, including two longitudinal studies, confirms that there is no prototypical teen mother. However, early childbearing among poor teenagers should be viewed in context: namely, that sexual activity among teens from all classes is high; and the high rate of sexual activity among teenage girls is but one characteristic of numerous changes in the sexual and reproductive behavior of women. Further, sexual freedom is no longer considered the exclusive right of males. These changes have caused less attention to be focused on sexual behavior than on the consequences of the behavior.

Except for teenagers aged 15 or younger, childbearing does not lead to adverse health and educational outcomes. Poverty and a lack of prenatal care are more predictive of adverse outcomes for teen mothers and their children than is age. It is, perhaps, comforting to persons who view teenage pregnancy as a moral issue to believe that pregnancy and childbearing during adolescence lead to ruined lives. Such conventional wisdom, however, is not supported by research. Whereas there are sparse longitudinal data on the effects of teenage childbearing on children of teen mothers, and little is known about effects on their male partners and extended kin, two longitudinal studies on teens who became mothers in the 1960s indicate that the majority of those studied became economically self-sufficient in later life.

What policy directions might guide us through these issues? I suggest these: First, recognize that the major problem is not age but changes in societal norms and standards of sexual conduct among women. Second, seek to make teenagers aware of the difference in the consequences of sexual activity for them and for more economically secure and mature women and men. Third, improve programs for human development, for AIDS education, for the elimination and control of alcohol and other drugs, as well as programs that teach sexual abstinence and diligent contraceptive use. Fourth, create programs that deal with economic and social deprivation—conditions that contribute to early sexual activity and pregnancy—such as unemployment of males and females, with special attention to those groups disproportionately represented among the ranks of the jobless. Fifth, support the establishment of school-linked and school-based clinics. Sixth, target resource-poor neighborhoods and schools for after-school and recreation programs for children before they become at risk for pregnancy. Seventh, initiate studies to discover the effects of teenage motherhood on children, their fathers, and extended families.

These recommendations suggest that teenage sexual and reproductive behaviors are not anomalistic. Consequently, comprehensive policies and programs that take into account cultural, economic, and societal influences are more likely to succeed than those that focus on abstinence alone.

REFERENCES

Anderson, Elijah. 1990. *Streetwise: race, class, and change in an urban community.* Chicago: University of Chicago Press.

Bane, M. J.
   1986a. Household composition and poverty. In *Fighting poverty: what works and what doesn't,* ed. S. H. Danziger, pp. 209–31. Cambridge, Mass.: Harvard University Press.
   1986b. Welfare: is it part of the problem or solution? Paper presented at Prevention: Speakout '86, National Conference of the Children's Defense Fund, Washington, D.C., 26–28 February.

Bell, Winifred. 1987. *Contemporary social welfare.* 2d ed. New York: Macmillan.

Burton, L. M., and Bengtson, V. L. 1985. Black grandmothers: issues of timing and continuity of roles. In *Grandparenthood: research and policy perspectives,* ed. V. L. Bengtson and J. F. Robertson. Beverly Hills, Calif.: Sage.

Dryfoos, Joy G. 1990. *Adolescents at risk.* New York: Oxford University Press.

Franklin, D. L., and Smith, S. E. 1991. Adolescent mothers and persistent poverty: does delaying parenthood make a difference? Paper prepared for presentation at the Chicago Urban Poverty and Family Life Conference. October.

Frazier, E. Franklin. 1966. *The Negro family in the United States.* Chicago: University of Chicago Press.

Furstenberg, Frank F., Jr., 1991. As the pendulum swings: teenage childbearing and social concern. *Family Relations* 40 (April): 127–38.

Furstenberg, Frank F., Jr., Brooks-Gunn, J., and Morgan, S. P. 1987. *Adolescent mothers in later life.* Cambridge, England: Cambridge University Press.

Geronimus, Arline T. 1987. On teenage childbearing and neonatal mortality. *Population and Development Review* 13(2):245–79.

Geronimus, Arline T., and Korenman, Sanders. 1991. *The socioeconomic consequences of teen childbearing reconsidered.* Working Paper No. 3701. Cambridge, Mass.: National Bureau of Economic Research. May.

Hacker, Andrew. 1992. *Two nations: black and white, separate, hostile, unequal.* New York: Charles Scribner's Sons.

Hardy, J. B., and Zabin, L. S. 1991. *Adolescent pregnancy in an urban environment.* Washington, D.C.: Urban Institute Press, and Baltimore-Munich: Urban and Schwarzenberg.

Hayes, Cheryl D. 1987. *Risking the future: adolescent sexuality, pregnancy, and childbearing.* Vol. 1. Washington, D.C.: National Academy Press.

Horwitz, S. M., Klerman, L. V., Kuo, H. S., and Jekel, J. F. 1991. School-age mothers: predictors of long-term educational and economic outcomes. *Pediatrics* 87(6):862–68.

Jones, E. F., Forrest, J. D., Goldman, N., Henshaw, S., Lincoln, R., Rosoff, J. I., Westoff, C. F., and Wulf, D. 1986. *Teenage pregnancy in industrialized countries.* New Haven Conn.: Yale University Press.

Ladner, Joyce A. 1971. *Tomorrow's tomorrow: the Black woman.* New York: Doubleday.

McCrate, Elaine. 1989. *Discrimination, returns to education and teenage childbearing.* Research Seminar on Adolescent Issues. Wellesley College Center for Research on Women. October.

Makinson, Carolyn. 1985. The health consequences of teenage fertility. *Family Planning Perspectives* 17(3):132–39.

Moore, K. A., and Burt, M. R. 1982. *Private crisis public cost: policy perspectives on teenage childbearing.* Washington, D.C.: Urban Institute.

Moore, K. A., Snyder, N. O., and Daly, M. 1992. Facts at a glance. Washington, D.C.: Child Trends. January.

Moore, K. A., Snyder, N. O., and Halla, C. 1993. Facts at a glance. Washington, D.C.: *Child Trends.* March.

Moore, K. A., Wertheimer, R., and Holden, R. 1981. *Teenage childbearing: public costs.* Third Six-Month Report to the Center for Population Research, National Institutes of Health, Washington, D.C.

Nathanson, Constance A. 1991. *Dangerous passage: the social control of women's adolescence.* Philadelphia: Temple University Press.

National Center for Health Statistics. 1990. Advance Report of Final Natality Statistics. Monthly Vital Statistics Report. 39:4, suppl. Hyattsville, Md.: U.S. Public Health Service.

Stack, Carol. 1974. *All our kin.* New York: Harper and Row.

Vinovskis, Maris A. 1988. *An "epidemic" of adolescent pregnancy?* New York: Oxford University Press.

Williams, Constance Willard. 1991. *Black teenage mothers: pregnancy and child rearing from their perspective.* Lexington, Mass.: D. C. Heath.

Wilson, W. J. 1987. *The truly disadvantaged: the inner city, the underclass, and public policy.* Chicago: University of Chicago Press.

PART III

Social Problems and the Community

Inner-City Community Mental Health: The Interplay of Abuse and Race in Chronic Mentally Ill Women

Psychiatry in the Public Sector

THIS chapter describes some aspects of my work in a large inner-city community mental health center. It examines how sex and race shape identity, life experiences, and treatment options by focusing on two issues central to the lives of chronic mentally ill Black women—violence against women and AIDS risk. In mentally ill women of color, AIDS risk represents the lethal intersection of racism and sexism. Finally, the chapter offers some recommendations for treatment of chronic mentally ill women.

The Dr. Solomon Carter Fuller Mental Health Center, named after the first Black psychiatrist in the United States, is one of four public sector mental health centers for Boston and serves most of Boston's inner-city mentally ill Black and about half of its Latino population. About 68 percent of the Center's clients are Black, 18 percent White, 10 percent Latino, and the remainder Asian; about 55 percent are male and 45 percent female. The Center itself houses two twenty-bed inpatient units; two outpatient clinics; case management services; several day programs; and an intensive residential program for patients who can live on an unlocked unit, but who would be unable to manage in a residential program in the community. The Center shares a campus with Boston University Medical Center in the city's South End and is just blocks away from Boston City Hospital, whose patients come mostly from the same inner-city catchment area. Many of Boston's homeless shelters are within walking distance of the Center.

Center staff, also culturally diverse, includes psychiatrists, psychologists, social workers, nurses, mental health workers, case managers, and administrators. Although the issue of funding is not the primary focus of this chapter, it should be noted that the Center, the only minority mental health center in the state, has a history of chronic neglect and underfunding by the Massachusetts Department of Mental Health. Compounding these problems, the failing economy in Massachusetts has resulted in severe statewide funding cuts to mental health services. Clinician layoffs, programs' closing or decreasing services, and staff demoralization have all made it progressively harder to maintain an effective therapeutic presence (Dumont 1992).

The Center's catchment area, like other inner cities, is characterized by poverty, unemployment, homelessness, violent crime, drug abuse, and a high prevalence of HIV infection. The catchment area has been recognized by epidemiologists as an "excessive death zone," ranking first in the state in both excess mortality for 17 out of 34 independent causes of death and for total mortality (Jenkins et al. 1977). As Jenkins and colleagues comment, the number of excess deaths in the catchment area is larger than the number of deaths occurring in areas designated by the government as natural disaster areas. The Center treats more patients with AIDS and HIV infection than any other public mental health facility in Massachusetts and has a close working relationship with the immunodeficiency clinics at neighboring medical facilities.

The Center's clients are poor, and most receive some form of public assistance for their psychiatric disabilities. There is an active sex barter system—sex for money, cigarettes, coffee, food, drugs—within the client population, in which HIV risk is high. Some patients have been able to work with the support of vocational training programs or through their own resources. Many are parents who try to maintain some parental role, but most have been unable to care for their children, who are in the care of other family members or foster families. About one-third of the patients are homeless, and the remainder live with families or in residential programs either at the Center or in the community. Some of the homeless patients have rejected offers of supervised housing, because almost all of their monthly checks would go for room and board, leaving little for themselves.

The Department of Mental Health mandate to treat only the long-term mentally ill is reflected in the Center's population, most of whom are diagnosed with schizophrenic, schizoaffective, or severe bipolar and other affective disorders. Multiple hospitalizations are the norm for these patients, with decompensation usually the result of treatment noncompliance, drug abuse, and/or acute psychosocial stressors. Although most female patients and many males have significant histories of having been physically or sexually abused, post–traumatic stress disorders are rarely diagnosed but can be considered concurrent diagnoses for many. Chemical dependency is probably a concurrent diagnosis for a majority of males, and many females, with alcohol, crack cocaine, and marijuana representing the most common drugs of abuse.

The high crime rate in Boston's inner city leaves these patients extraordinarily vulnerable to victimization because of where they live or their homelessness and their inability to protect themselves due to their severe illness. Clinicians routinely hear about patients getting mugged, robbed, or raped. Most of the supervised residential programs are in unsafe areas, and patients are keenly aware of this; they hear gunshots outside their residences, they live down the street from crack houses, and they all know people who have been assaulted or murdered. This climate of poverty, violence, and continuing fears for their own safety serves as a severe chronic life stressor. This is what they talk to clinicians about.

The Role of Abuse in Chronic Mental Illness

In the last twenty years, the problems of violence in general, violence within families, and violence against women (Koss et al. 1994) have all been recognized as major public health issues. Indeed, violence can be considered the single greatest health risk factor for women. We owe much of this awareness to the successful efforts of the women's movement (through the anti-rape and shelter movements) to highlight the endemic nature of rape, wife-beating, and child sexual abuse in our culture. Violence against women occurs throughout the life cycle: physical and sexual abuse and rape in childhood; rape in adolescence and adulthood by strangers, acquaintances, dates, and husbands or partners; battering by marital and sexual partners; sexual harrassment in the workplace; and sexual abuse by some therapists and health care providers to whom they turn for help.

In a random sample of adult women, Russell (1984) found that more than one-third had been sexually abused by age 17. One woman in three and one man in ten are sexually molested in childhood (Finkelhor 1979). The prevalence of completed rape for adult women in the United States is reported as about 20 percent by a number of investigators (Russell 1982, 1984; Kilpatrick et al. 1987; Koss and Harvey 1991), with a range from 2 percent to 25 percent, depending on the data collection methods (Koss 1993). In a national sample of college students, 27 percent of women were found to be victims of rape or attempted rape that met the legal definitions, but only 5 percent had reported the assaults to law enforcement officials (Koss et al. 1987).

Family violence occurs in every social class and every racial, cultural, ethnic, religious, and educational group. Some of these families are highly disorganized; others appear to be in no way out of the ordinary or deviant. About 25 percent of adult women in the United States have been physically abused at least once by a male intimate, and domestic violence may be the single most common etiology for injuries presented by all women to health care providers. Estimates are that 20 percent of women seen in emergency rooms, 25 percent of obstetrical patients, and 50 percent of alcoholic women are in abusive relationships (Stark and Flitcraft 1985). An American Medical Association report on domestic violence (1992) estimates that 52 percent of female murder victims had been killed by a current or former partner. In a study of men in an inpatient alcohol rehabilitation program, 55 percent of those living with female partners reported that they had assaulted their partners in the last year (Gondolf and Foster 1991). In a subsample of their wives or partners, 82 percent of women compared with 52 percent of men reported an assault in the previous year. Families in which women are abused are also families in which children live at high risk for physical and sexual abuse.

Almost twenty years of investigation demonstrate the extent of physical and sexual violence in the lives of women. From these data, it seems clear that violence is a normative life experience for women (and a more reasonable explanation than masochism for why adolescent females begin to have more difficulty in school, become depressed or suicidal, or run away from home). As Rieker and I have written elsewhere (Rieker and Carmen 1984, 1986), it is in the body of work on victimization of women—rape, incest, and wife abuse—that the most extensive reformulation of traditional psychological theories of women's pain and suffering has occurred. In contrast to prevailing psychological explanations (such as masochism) that locate the problem within the victim, violence against women is more accurately conceptualized as one of the most destructive consequences of the sexual inequality in existing social institutions. What else besides inequality could explain why women and children are the most vulnerable targets of violence in families and of all forms of sexual abuse?

The Victim-to-Patient Process

In the last decade, we have learned about the extent of abuse experiences in the life histories of psychiatric patients and the link between chronic abuse and the development of psychiatric disorders. We know, for example, that up to 72 percent of psychiatric inpatients (depending on how the sample is defined) have histories of physical or sexual abuse experiences or both (Carmen et al. 1984; Mills et al. 1984; Bryer et al. 1987;

Craine et al. 1988). In an outpatient setting, Rose and colleagues (1991) studied the first 89 clients referred to an intensive case management program for chronic mentally ill clients and found that 41 percent of women and 9 percent of men were incest victims. Overall, 50 percent of women and 22 percent of men were sexually abused in childhood; the presence of alcoholic parents correlated highly with all forms of physical and sexual abuse in childhood.

The psychological legacy of chronic abuse is a disordered and fragmented identity or sense of self (Rieker and Carmen 1986; Carmen and Rieker 1989). This is observed clinically in the form of low self-esteem, self-hatred, affective instability, poor control of aggressive and sexual impulses, disturbed relationships with inability to trust and to behave in self-protective ways, and ongoing vulnerability to revictimization. Outcomes include depression (McGrath et al. 1990), suicidality, self-mutilation, substance abuse, violence toward others, sexual dysfunction, posttraumatic stress disorders (including transient psychosis), eating disorders, and borderline and multiple personality disorders. Not all victims, however, become mental patients. How can the processes that cause such enduring damage to self be understood?

All victims of physical or sexual violence are faced with a complex array of social, emotional, and cognitive tasks to make sense of experiences that threaten body integrity and life itself. Confrontations with violence challenge one's most basic assumptions about the self as invulnerable and worthy, and the world as orderly and fair. After victimization, the victim's view of self and world can never be the same again (Janoff-Bulman and Frieze 1983). The working-through process involves a reconstruction of self and world that incorporates the abuse experience.

The inevitability of the cognitive and affective processes set into motion by the abuse is well documented in the literature on psychic trauma and stress response syndromes. Such responses consist of involuntary recurrences of thoughts, feelings, and behavioral reenactments of the trauma alternating with periods of denial, psychic numbing, and behavioral constriction as a way of warding off the repetitive intrusions. At the heart of these processes is the necessity, at least temporarily, of dissociating or distancing oneself from affects and experiences that threaten to overwhelm an individual's adaptive capacities.

When victim and assailant are intimates, these processes are further complicated by the profound betrayal of trust and the ongoing vulnerability to physical and psychological danger when the abuser has continuing access to the victim (Hilberman 1980). Victim responses are also shaped by the chaotic and destructive psychological processes and relationship patterns that characterize many violent families. In these families, the child or adult victim's survival is often contingent on accommodating to a family system in which exploitation, invasiveness, and the betrayal of trust are normal and in which loyalty, secrecy, and self-sacrifice form the core of the family's value system. Thus, the victim's survival is dependent on adjusting to a psychotic world where abusive behavior is acceptable but telling the truth about it is sinful.

The victim's "adjustment" occurs by altering the reality of the victimization so that both the abuse experience and the victim's thoughts, feelings, and behaviors become congruent with family norms and expectations—namely, it didn't happen; it happened but it wasn't important and has no consequences; the victim provoked (and deserved) it; it wasn't abusive. The common features of the victim-to-patient process through which victims accommodate to the judgments that others make about the abuse include denying the abuse, altering the affective responses to abuse, and changing the meaning of abuse or, as Rieker and I have defined it, the disconfirmation and transformation of abuse (Rieker and Carmen 1986; Carmen and Rieker 1989). Victims thus repress and deny the trauma in order to survive. This isolation of victims is further reinforced by their helpless dependency and shame, offenders' threats of retaliatory violence, and the disbelieving responses of potential helpers outside the family.

AIDS Risk in Mentally Ill Women

All women are vulnerable to sexual assaults throughout their lives. Many mentally ill women have histories of sexual abuse in childhood. The sexually compulsive behaviors and failure of self-protection that represent the legacies of abuse combine with the poor judgment that derives from mental illness and chronic psychosis to further increase these women's risk for HIV infection. When these scenarios are enacted in inner cities where HIV, drug abuse, and violence are endemic, the risk for mentally ill women is extraordinary. This intersection of chronic mental illness, violence against women, and HIV risk in the inner city demonstrates how sexism and racism can come together with lethal consequences. For example, one of the first AIDS deaths at the Center was a battered woman who was repeatedly beaten and raped by her husband, an injection drug user. In our patient population, HIV infection and spectrum disorders are occurring at similar rates for men and women.

Some chronic mentally ill populations are at high risk for HIV infection (Brady and Carmen 1990; Carmen and Brady 1990). Their cognitive impairment, poor judgment, affective instability, and impulsivity often result in behaviors associated with HIV infection—namely, unsafe sexual practices and drug abuse. This is an urgent problem for mentally ill populations living in inner cities, communities with Black and Latino populations that, independent of mental illness, are at higher risk for AIDS. For example, a blind HIV seroprevalence survey of patients admitted to two psychiatric hospitals in New York City (Cournos et al. 1991) found a prevalence of 5.5 percent. Black patients accounted for 38 percent of the patients tested and 76 percent of seropositive results. Prevalence rates were similar for women and men.

In contrast to stereotypes of the mentally ill as asexual or neutered, many of the mentally ill are sexually active. Gender differences in sexual behavior are noteworthy. Test and Berlin (1981), reporting on a sample of young adult patients with a "revolving door" pattern of hospitalization, found that 54 percent of the women and 38 percent of the men had had sexual intercourse in the previous month. In a study of 80 chronic mentally ill women outpatients, Coverdale and Aruffo (1989) found that 73 percent had had at least one pregnancy; 31 percent had had at least one induced abortion, and 75 children had been born; 73 percent reported having sexual intercourse in the last year, 53 percent within the last three months.

Not only are the mentally ill sexually active, but they engage in very high risk sexual behaviors. In a preliminary report of HIV risk factors in 115 mentally ill patients, McKinnon et al. (1991) found that 55 percent of men and 66 percent of women had been sexually active in the previous six months. Women had an average of eight heterosexual partners and men three heterosexual partners in that six-month period; 17 percent of the men and 19 percent of the women sold sex as part of a barter economy (sex for drugs, cigarettes, rent, and so on). Almost one-third of both men and women used drugs during sex, and only 13 percent of patients used condoms. Our experiences at the Center are consistent with McKinnon's data. Sexual behaviors are often impulsive, anonymous, coerced, and divorced from relationship or health consequences.

Therapy with Chronic Mentally Ill Women

The new literature on victims has had little to say about the treatment of chronic mentally ill populations. At the Center, sexual abuse histories are the norm for most women and many men, and physical abuse experiences common among both. They are assaulted in families, on the street (especially the large numbers of homeless mentally ill patients), and sometimes in the psychiatric institutions that are supposed to protect them. Abused males are more likely to become sexual predators to both males and females, so that within the mental health center population we often have to protect female (and some male) patients from their male peers, as one of the following case examples demonstrates.

These case examples illustrate some common themes in the lives of mentally ill victims and in the responses of mental health professionals. All of these women tried to tell someone about the abuse when it was occurring, with inappropriate responses inside or outside the family. Some were told by family members that no one would believe them because they were mentally ill. These patients demonstrate the use of defenses that isolate and compartmentalize affects and experiences that would otherwise be overwhelming, through repression, dissociation, or altered states of consciousness. In this way, knowledge of the experience can be repressed or disconnected from the context: it is decontextualized (Rieker and Carmen 1986; Carmen and Rieker 1989). Decontextualization allows victims to report the abuse in such clinically bizarre ways as to be unbelievable or unrecognizable. For example, Ms. B tells the army recruiters that America is dangerous; Ms. C complains that she is hearing voices and needs hospitalization; and Ms. D calls the police emergency number and asks for help in finding an apartment. Decontextualization also allows victims to maintain their enmeshed attachments to family members and others who have abused them. For example, Ms. B, D, and E continually struggle with trying to separate from abusive families while at the same time fearing familial abandonment. These behaviors can be confusing to clinicians, who are left uncertain about the reality of abuse allegations.

Ms. A

Ms. A, a 30-year-old woman with a multiple personality disorder, spent the better part of two years in an inpatient unit under constant observation to keep her from killing or mutilating herself. She has a history of having been sexually abused by almost every adult in her family during childhood and adolescence. When she fled her family for the safety of an aunt and uncle during college, she was repeatedly raped by her uncle over a two-year period. The confusion she experienced as a consequence of her unrecognized dissociative disorder and amnesia resulted in a misdiagnosis of schizoaffective disorder for which she was treated with high doses of antipsychotic drugs. During her last hospitalization five years ago, she was sexually abused by a staff member. With an accurate diagnosis and a more direct focus on the abuse, she is recovering her memories and her identity, although she remains profoundly conflicted about the need to protect her family from her anger and to forgive them. Keeping secrets remains an important part of her identity. As she says, "if I have no secrets, then I've lost my whole personality." She takes no psychotropic medications and shows no evidence of a psychotic disorder.

Ms. B

Ms. B, a 40-year-old woman with a severe paranoid delusional disorder (possibly a variant of a post–traumatic stress disorder) was sexually abused in childhood by her father, with her mother's apparent knowledge and consent. She would often wander around the Center wearing dark sunglasses for protection and reminding me that everything about her life, sometimes including her name, must be kept "top secret" because America is a dangerous place. She thinks of herself as an alien; when she was acutely psychotic, she tried to join the army so that she would be sent to a country that would be safer than America. Her parents remain an intrusive force in her life and constantly tell her how awful, stupid, and crazy she is. She alternates between wanting to kill them and believing their assessment of her badness. When she obeys family loyalty oaths and denies the abuse, she becomes much more paranoid and psychotic. In the course of treatment, she has been able to move out of the parental home into a more nurturant residential setting. It was necessary to petition for a court-appointed guardian and a restraining order to stop her parents' continued intrusiveness and harrassment.

Ms. A and Ms. B demonstrate some of the dilemmas affecting diagnosis and treatment, and the relevance of diagnosis for treatment. Both women were functional, competent, and employed full-time until about ten years ago when intercurrent life crises occurred. Ms. A developed a disabling progressive medical illness that resulted in loss of employment and independence; Ms. B and her husband divorced and she moved back to her parents' home with her children. Ms. A has a psychiatric disorder that is a direct consequence of the child sexual abuse she sustained. Ms. B's psychiatric disorder may also be primarily of post–traumatic etiology; however, this is less clear because she appears so psychotic much of the time. Irrespective of diagnosis, these patients demonstrate how the experience of abuse remains, albeit disguised, the central organizing feature in their symptomatology.

Although both women had many hospitalizations in which the history of abuse was known to clinicians, one important difference seems to be that Ms. A's trauma history was incorporated into her psychiatric treatment, whereas for many years Ms. B's abuse was treated as irrelevant to her illness. Was Ms. A's initial misdiagnosis important? Early recognition of her dissociative episodes might have allowed some alternative treatment interventions; however, her clinicians were able to contain her life-threatening self-destructiveness and attend to the role of abuse in her illness. The later change in diagnosis, however, was a critical turning point in her treatment—in which many disconnected, out of control, and confusing experiences could finally be understood in a coherent way. Ms. B might have been given an accurate diagnosis, but she got the wrong treatment for many years. This is all the more remarkable given the centrality of abuse sequelae in her clinical presentation and clinicians' knowledge of her childhood sexual abuse.

Ms. C

Ms. C, a 33-year-old woman diagnosed with borderline mental retardation and schizoaffective and post–traumatic stress disorders, is the mother of two daughters. She and her children live with her mother who never believed her reports of sexual abuse in childhood during a time when she lived apart from her mother. Her mother and I are the only people she has told about the childhood sexual abuse. In her adult life, she has been sexually harrassed by her brother-in-law during his intermittent visits, but she was afraid to tell her mother for fear of disbelief or retribution. She is determined that her children will not have to suffer through such experiences and she remains ever vigilant when the abuser is visiting. One of the legacies of her childhood abuse is her sense that her only value is as a sex object, so that she engaged in high-risk sexual behavior with any male who approached her. Through discussions initiated about her HIV risk, she is learning to set limits about sexual encounters, and to decrease her risk behaviors.

During a recent crisis, she told one of my colleagues that she urgently needed to be hospitalized because she felt nervous and was hearing voices; initially, she could give no reason for her anxiety. Gentle inquiry revealed that an aggressive male patient has been making denigrating sexual remarks to her in the clinic waiting room and was pressuring her for a sexual contact. The male was confronted about his behavior and removed from the waiting area. (His harrassing behavior was addressed separately with him as a treatment issue.) Once she was assured about her safety and our willingness to hear her complaints, her symptoms abated. Subsequently, she has been able to tell her mother about her brother-in-law's harrassment in a way that elicited a supportive response. Her mother, who tends to infantilize her, has talked with her about having divorced the patient's stepfather because he had sexually abused the patient's sister, and has expressed her regrets about such victimization. Sadly, this sister has married an abuser, not an uncommon outcome.

Ms. D

Ms. D, a 28-year-old woman diagnosed with paranoid schizophrenia, frequently presented to the crisis service in a highly agitated state in which she was barely in control of homicidal impulses toward her step-father. At those times, she would request emergency shelter or hospital-ization because she would not return home. She lived at home with her mother, a violent alcoholic stepfather who had been in the home since she was two years old, an adolescent sister, and her 6-year-old son. She has an extensive history of sexual abuse beginning in childhood by multi-ple sexual partners of her mother and, starting at age 17, by her step-father. Her stepfather physically abused all household members and often terrorized her by playing with a gun in her presence. She described the onset of her stepfather's sexual assaults as the precipitant for the first of at least a dozen psychiatric hospitalizations, beginning at age 18. She reported the abuse during these hospitalizations, but the lack of response suggests that she was not believed. Similarly, she had made repeated emergency calls to the police, asking for assistance in finding an apart-ment for herself and her son but never mentioning the violence. It is not surprising that the police did not follow up these calls.

Because of her instability, custody of her son was awarded to her par-ents. She lived in terror of the abuse but was unable to leave home be-cause she was afraid of leaving her child and her sister in a vulnerable situation. The usual precipitant for these crises was her stepfather's sex-ual approach—repeatedly touching and grabbing her, and telling her he wanted to have a baby with her, and how he wished her mother would leave or die. Her mother responded to her allegations by telling her it didn't matter, while denying its occurrence to the outside world. She has coped with the lifelong assaults by pretending that she had a normal family and "blanking out" her mind so she can't feel anything that is taking place. These episodes of blanking out or dissociation were ob-served to occur at stressful moments in the interview and may account for an erroneous diagnosis of schizophrenia.

With severely damaged individuals, one cannot assume that domestic violence is a past occurrence, as exemplified by Ms. D., for whom the abuse continued into adulthood. She is one of a number of adult women who remained in the abusive parental home because parents have been given legal custody of the patient's children or guardianship of the pa-tient because of mental illness. For those who leave abusive families, vul-nerability to physical and sexual assault continues in mental hospitals and group homes, by other clients and staff members. For example, a young woman with a history of sexual abuse inside and outside the fam-ily was living in a supervised residence in which her boyfriend also lived. When they were alone, he would push and shove her and threaten further harm to her, but because he was a "model" client in his work program, she was accused of lying about the abuse. When her therapist insisted that he be evaluated, he was found to be using cocaine, and she then was blamed by staff for ruining his "model" record.

Ms. E

Ms. E, a 20-year-old homeless woman, has been intermittently hospitalized since age 18 for a psychotic disorder characterized by paranoid delusions, sexually inappropriate behavior, and threats to harm others, especially family members. She had lived apart from her family for much of her life until adolescence when she was reunited with them in Boston. At age 16, she became involved in a year-long relationship with a boyfriend who physically and sexually assaulted her, apparently with the knowledge of her family. She has intermittently claimed that family members have physically abused her, but these charges are usually retracted in the face of family pressure and her fears of abandonment. Although retracting the charges, she became homeless as the alternative to living with her family. In the shelter system, she was frequently noted to be only partially clothed, sexually aggressive, and engaging in prostitution.

When decompensated, she spends most of her disability check on bleaching and other skin creams because she wants to be White. As she asserted, "I'm sick of being Black, dirty, and ugly—don't I have the right to better myself?" She believed that were she White, any one of a number of prominent White male public figures whom she described as hating Blacks would love and marry her. She was outraged about her victimization and her life situation and believed that murdering her assailants would be within her legal rights. Because of her provocative sexual behavior and her multiple allegations of physical and sexual assault (many of which are clearly false), clinicians have tended to disbelieve her charges of family violence as well. (This is so, despite an observed episode in which a family member who was visiting her in the hospital became assaultive toward a staff member.) She has often been noncompliant with treatment because she doesn't believe she is mentally ill; she claimed that the hospital staff were part of a conspiracy to silence her and to prevent her becoming White by poisoning her food, which she refused to eat. She felt that were she White, she would be treated with the respect she deserves.

Ms. E has found an internal explanation for her experiences of abandonment and victimization. By blaming her Blackness, she protects her family and her connection to them, although at the expense of her own identity: it is not the abusive others who are bad, it is her Black self who must be transformed. Ms. E appears to be at the beginning of a pattern seen in many women who have made a chronic adaptation to homelessness. They alternate between homelessness and living with families who abused and scapegoated them in childhood. Inevitably, they become highly disturbed at home and either become homeless or have brief hospital admissions. They undermine attempts to help them find housing and, as a result, return to the streets or home. It may be that the homelessness itself is the repetition of the trauma—these patients are intensely preoccupied with finding a home but it never seems to work out even when adequate supports are provided.

Consistent with this dynamic, recent studies of homeless women reveal high lifetime rates of victimization. D'Ercole and Struening (1990) studied women in a single-adult shelter in New York and found that 63 percent had been battered, 58 percent raped, 51 percent attacked with a weapon, and 31 percent molested as children. In a study comparing homeless with housed female-headed families, researchers found that homeless mothers more often had been abused in childhood and adulthood (Bassuk and Rosenberg 1988). Although Goodman (1991) found no differences in abuse experiences in homeless and housed mothers, 89 percent of the total sample reported physical or sexual abuse, or both, in their lifetimes. The relationship between abuse and homelessness remains a topic of ongoing conceptual interest (Bassuk, this volume; Goodman et al. 1991).

Finally, within a chronic mentally ill population of survivors, the risk of HIV infection is high, as illustrated in the following example:

Ms. F

Ms. F, a 35-year-old woman with diagnoses of schizophrenia and cocaine dependency, was sexually abused by a family friend in adolescence, and this precipitated her first psychiatric hospitalization at age 18. She has continued to be physically and sexually victimized in adulthood and often presents with bruises acquired through either her sex trade for cocaine or her relationship with a variety of violent consorts. She has had multiple pregnancies, all but three aborted, and recurrent treatment for a spectrum of sexually transmitted diseases. Her three children are in foster care because of the severity of her illness. She has an intellectual awareness of HIV risk and prevention but continues to engage in unprotected sex with male partners, among them known seropositives and injection drug users. In response to recommendations that she insist her many sexual partners use condoms, she said, "I can't imagine telling someone to use a condom. I can't even tell anyone that I don't want to have sex with them. I just don't know how."

This may be an extreme example of the post-traumatic sequelae of childhood sexual abuse, but it underscores the promiscuous, impulsive, and sexually dangerous behaviors that may occur in adulthood. Ms. F and other mentally ill survivors remain at risk for HIV infection because of continued vulnerability to sexual exploitation. This heightened vulnerability is best understood as a behavioral legacy of the damaged self; it represents a confluence of many aspects of the survivor's identity disturbance. These include the survivor's definition of self as someone who is a legitimate object for sexual exploitation, whose own needs are irrelevant in the face of others' demands, and who is unable to think or act in self-protective ways, especially in sexual encounters. In countless ways, these survivors have learned through repeated trauma that they are powerless and worthless; they are devoid of any conception that they can (or should) have control over their bodies or their lives (Carmen and Rieker 1989; Carmen and Brady 1990).

Continuing Education for Clinicians

Despite the large numbers of victims found in psychiatric settings, mental health professionals remain generally unaware of the social and psychological consequences of abuse. There is still considerable confusion and resistance within psychiatry about how to conceptualize abuse and what its relevance and meaning is for understanding and treating psychiatric disorders. This confusion is reflected in a group of diagnoses that the American Psychiatric Association created (in preparation for the DSM-III-R and DSM-IV) in an ill-conceived attempt to acknowledge the role of real-life experiences such as victimization in psychiatric disorders. A proposed "masochistic personality disorder" was transformed into a "self-defeating personality disorder," leaving little doubt about who is to blame; in a later proposal, victims were viewed as suffering from a "victimization disorder," suggesting that to be victimized is itself a psychiatric disorder rather than a social problem. The lack of conceptual clarity is also reflected in treatment and research efforts. Although the physical and sexual abuse of children occurs in the same families in which their mothers are beaten and raped, most clinical research and treatment models still treat child and spouse abuse as separate and unrelated, with resources and research focused on abused children, whereas the victimization of adult women is not addressed.

Unfortunately, the new knowledge about trauma remains an elective rather than a required part of psychiatric training. Without adequate training, clinicians are less likely to ask about abuse experiences as part of psychiatric evaluations or to consider abuse-related diagnoses, such as post–traumatic stress and dissociative disorders. Consequently (as described in the case examples), victims are often misdiagnosed or inadequately diagnosed. Even a schizophrenic patient can have a post–traumatic stress disorder, a second diagnosis that might encourage some therapeutic interventions focused on the role of abuse in illness and symptomatology. In most of the case examples, the abuse histories were known to the clinicians and were well documented in the medical record. Nonetheless, the failure of clinicians to understand the relevance of abuse for psychological disorders results in disbelief, minimization, or inattention to patient complaints so that appropriate treatment is not offered.

A diagnosis of a major mental illness does not mean that one's other life experiences are no longer relevant; indeed, one could argue that a person diagnosed with schizophrenia or a major affective disorder might be more vulnerable to the effects of certain life stressors, among them physical or sexual abuse. Similarly, abuse experiences may be paramount to one's sense of self in the absence of a psychiatric diagnosis. As noted earlier, severe trauma histories transcend diagnosis and become, however disguised, a central organizing feature in symptom formation. Thus, a history of victimization should be considered a primary issue for exploration in an individual's treatment, regardless of diagnostic considerations.

The trauma literature rarely addresses the therapeutic needs of chronic mentally ill victims but tends to focus on treatment models developed for individuals with less disabling psychological impairments and more external resources. For example, recommendations for group therapy with adult incest survivors often include requirements that group participants be stable and not subject to frequent life crises. Few mentally ill survivors would meet such criteria for stability; further, many mentally ill victims may have neither the internal resources nor the external (social) supports needed to recover memories, grieve losses, and work through the trauma. The existing intervention models can be intimidating to clinicians who may question the value of asking about abuse in the absence of relevant treatment options. Nevertheless, repetition of the trauma continues and brings with it considerable risk for HIV infection. Given the large numbers of mentally ill victims, an urgent need exists to develop new treatment strategies tailored to meet their needs.

It is obvious that interventions must take into account the patient's vulnerabilities and ego strength and the severity of illness. In the earlier case examples, treatment efforts were modest in scope—acknowledging and affirming the patient's abuse experiences, recognizing the role of abuse in the patient's illness, supporting efforts to prevent revictimization, and helping victims to separate physically from their abusers. Such interventions increase the victim's feelings of safety and promote the gradual development of a therapeutic relationship with a clinician, which may allow these women to begin a process of emotional separation from abusive others. Alternatively, when clinicians fail to recognize the centrality of the victim-to-patient process, the therapist-patient relationship becomes another destructive repetition of the trauma, in which patients are again disconfirmed and left alone with their pain.

Stereotyping and prejudice have prevented aggressive interventions with mental patients at risk for AIDS. The largest proportionate increases in AIDS cases have occurred among women, Blacks and Hispanics, and persons exposed through heterosexual contact (*MMWR* 1991). One author asserts, "the heterosexual person most at risk for HIV disease in the U.S. is a Black woman whose social and economic conditions have led her to injection drug use or to having sex with an injection-drug-using man" (Myers 1992). Despite these trends, the stereotypes of AIDS as a White male homosexual disease persists, so that communities of color have been slow to intervene. To intervene, inner-city community leaders would have to acknowledge that HIV is endemic not only because of heterosexual and needle transmission, but because of homosexual and bisexual transmission as well. The public unfolding of the story of Earvin "Magic" Johnson's HIV infection has had more educational value among the Center's clients than any other single event, its homophobic aspects notwithstanding.

Stereotypes of the mentally ill as gender neutral also persist, preventing recognition that mentally ill women may have more sexual contacts, both voluntary and forced, than do men. Such stereotypes have had dangerous consequences: namely, the unavailability of sex education, contraception, and AIDS prevention programs for those at risk. Indeed, as we have developed intervention programs for Center patients, we have learned the extent to which mentally ill women and men are inadequately prepared to manage a wide range of health and lifestyle issues that confront them. Not only have mental health professionals not educated these vulnerable individuals about sex, health, and AIDS, but they often oppose such education (Test and Berlin 1981; Carmen and Brady 1990).

Recommendations for Treatment Programs

Clinicians at the Center have been providing clients with AIDS education for almost six years, with drop-in groups, condom distribution, and systematic HIV-risk assessment for patients (Carmen and Brady 1990; Brady and Carmen 1990). It was not so long ago that we learned how to ask about physical and sexual abuse experiences in the lives of our patients. The AIDS crisis demands that we ask new questions—the details of sexual and other risk behaviors such as number of partners, kinds of behaviors, sexual practices and gender of partners, injection and other drug abuse in self and partner, needle sharing, condom use, STDs, and concerns about AIDS. These data need to be integrated into the treatment process for all mentally ill patients so that we can actively engage them in changing risk behaviors. Although clinicians may feel uncomfortable discussing these details, patients' lives may depend on our active intervention.

Ironically, it is through the HIV risk assessment process that Center clinicians have learned about the extent and relevance of the abuse experiences of their patients and have begun to incorporate this information into diagnosis and treatment. As the case examples demonstrate, even with accurate diagnoses and formulations, these patients present complex treatment dilemmas. These examples, however, also demonstrate that it is possible to engage mentally ill survivors in treatment and to help them learn how to prevent revictimization and HIV infection. Many of these patients became ill in childhood and adolescence, thus disrupting the normal process of psychosexual development. As a result of this developmental deprivation, compounded by the abuse, they often have not learned the basic interpersonal skills required to negotiate the limits of a relationship or a sexual encounter. Thus, clinicians must also help them to learn what they need to know to live in the world—about health maintenance, sexuality, contraception, child care, social skills and relationships, and violence prevention.

I offer, finally, some recommendations (adapted from Brady and Carmen 1990). All patients should be asked about abuse experiences and about HIV-risk behaviors, and information about these issues should be incorporated into their treatment plans, as outlined below:

- All patients (inpatients and outpatients, adolescents and adults) should be educated about HIV transmission, risk reduction, and AIDS prevention as part of their treatment plans. These psychoeducational programs should be part of a comprehensive health, sex, and drug education curriculum and should include information about family violence and violence against women.
- All patients should have access to free condoms and basic instruction about how to use them.
- Same-sex groups should be offered to help men and women deal with such issues as sexuality, physical and sexual violence, and AIDS risk and prevention. Groups should be designed for mentally ill subpopulations at particular risk, such as adolescents, men who engage in homosexual behavior, adult survivors of child sexual abuse, and women in abusive relationships.
- All mental health centers should have close liaisons promoting access to community programs that offer treatment to rape victims

and battered women. Interventions should be developed that focus on the special needs of mentally ill victims. Ideally, all mental health centers should have on-site treatment programs for mentally ill victims.

- Similarly, mentally ill substance abusers should have easy access to drug and alcohol treatment programs geared toward the special needs of dually diagnosed patients. Given the high prevalence of substance abuse in mentally ill populations, substance abuse programs should be available on-site at mental health centers. Such programs should integrate information about AIDS prevention (including needle sharing and needle cleaning) and violence prevention.

Chronic mentally ill women are not a homogeneous group. Within this population, there are important differences in culture, ethnicity, family roles, sexual orientation, alcohol and drug use, diagnosis, intellectual and functional capacity, abuse experiences, and life circumstances such as poverty and homelessness. Since mentally ill women don't speak the language of clinicians, researchers, or policy makers, they have remained an invisible population of underserved and inappropriately served women. Like all women, they have been underrepresented as subjects for research on women's health and mental health. Mentally ill women, in all of their variety, must be included in the new research initiatives on women's health, in such areas as psychopharmacological effects in women (Hamilton, this volume); the physical and mental health sequelae of abuse as these relate to stress and severe mental disorders; the development of effective interventions for mentally ill victims of physical and sexual violence; strategies for AIDS prevention in mentally ill women at risk; and the development of effective psychological and social supports for HIV-infected women.

REFERENCES

American Medical Association. 1992. *Diagnostic and treatment guidelines on domestic violence.* Chicago: American Medical Association.

Bassuk, E. 1994. Lives in jeopardy: women and homelessness. In *Mental health, racism, and sexism,* ed. Charles Willie, Patricia Rieker, Bernard Kramer, and Bertram Brown. Pittsburgh: University of Pittsburgh Press.

Bassuk, E., and Rosenberg, L. 1988. Why does family homelessness occur? A case-control study. *American Journal of Public Health* 78(7):783–88.

Brady, S. M., and Carmen, E. 1990. AIDS risk in the chronically mentally ill: strategies for prevention. In *Psychiatric aspects of AIDS and HIV infection*, ed. S. M. Goldfinger. New Directions for Mental Health Services No. 48. San Francisco: Jossey Bass.

Bryer, J. B., Nelson, B. A., Miller, J. B., and Krol, P. A. 1987. Childhood sexual and physical abuse as factors in adult psychiatric illness. *American Journal of Psychiatry* 144(11):1426–30.

Carmen, E. (H.), and Brady, S. M. 1990. AIDS risk and prevention for the chronic mentally ill. *Hospital and Community Psychiatry* 41(6):652–57.

Carmen, E. (H.), and Rieker, P. P. 1989. A psychosocial model of the victim-to-patient process. *Psychiatric Clinics of North America* 12(2):431–43.

Carmen, E. (H.), Rieker, P. P., and Mills, T. 1984. Victims of violence and psychiatric disorders. *American Journal of Psychiatry* 141(3):378–83.

Cournos, F., Empfield, M., Horwath, E., McKinnon, K., Meyer, I., Schrage, H., Currie, C., and Agosin, B. 1991. HIV seroprevalence among patients admitted to two psychiatric hospitals. *American Journal of Psychiatry* 148(9):1225–30.

Coverdale, J. H., and Aruffo, J. A. 1989. Family planning needs in female chronic psychiatric patients. *American Journal of Psychiatry* 146(11):1489–91.

Craine, L. S., Henson, C. E., Colliver, J. A., and MacLean, D. G. 1988. Prevalence of a history of sexual abuse among female psychiatric patients in a state hospital system. *Hospital and Community Psychiatry* 39(3):300–304.

D'Ercole, A., and Struening, E. 1990. Victimization among homeless women: implications for service delivery. *Journal of Community Psychology* 18:141–52.

Dumont, M. T. 1992. *Treating the poor*. Belmont, Mass.: Dymphna Press.

Finkelhor, D. 1979. *Sexually victimized children*. New York: Free Press.

Gondolf, E. W., and Foster, R. A. 1991. Wife assault among VA alcohol rehabilitation patients. *Hospital and Community Psychiatry* 42(1):74–79.

Goodman, L. 1991. The prevalence of abuse among homeless and housed poor mothers: a comparison study. *American Journal of Orthopsychiatry* 61:489–500.

Goodman, L., Saxe, L., and Harvey, M. 1991. Homelessness as psychological trauma: broadening perspectives. *American Psychologist* 46(11):1219–25.

Hamilton, J. 1994. Gender as a critical variable in psychotropic drug research. In *Mental health, racism, and sexism*, ed. Charles Willie, Patricia Rieker, Bernard Kramer, and Bertram Brown. Pittsburgh: University of Pittsburgh Press.

Hilberman, E. 1980. Overview: the "wife-beater's wife" reconsidered. *American Journal of Pschiatry* 137(11):1336–47.

Janoff-Bulman, R., and Frieze, I. H. 1983. A theoretical perspective for understanding reactions to victimization. *Journal of Social Issues* 39(2):1–17.

Jenkins, C. D., Tuthill, R. W., Tannenbaum, S. I., and Kirby, C. R. 1977. Zones of excess mortality in Massachusetts. *New England Journal of Medicine* 296(23):1354–56.

Kilpatrick, D. G., Saunders, B. E., Veronen, L. J., Best, C. L., and Von, J. M. 1987. Criminal victimization: lifetime prevalence, reporting to police, and psychological impact. *Crime and Delinquency* 33:479–89.

Koss, M. P. 1993. Detecting the scope of rape: a review of prevalence research methods. *Journal of Interpersonal Violence* 8(2):198–222.

Koss, M. P., Gidycz, C. A., and Wisniewski, N. 1987. The scope of rape: incidence and prevalence of sexual aggression and victimization in a national sample of higher education students. *Journal of Consulting and Clinical Psychology* 55:162–70.

Koss, M. P., Goodman, L., Fitzgerald, L., Russo, N. F., Keita, G. P., and Browne, A. 1994. *No safe haven: male violence against women at home, at work, and in the community*. Washington, D.C.: American Psychological Association.

Koss, M. P., and Harvey, M. R. 1991. *The rape victim: clinical and community interventions.* Newbury Park, Calif.: Sage.

McGrath, E., Keita, G. P., Strickland, B. R., and Russo, N. F., eds. 1990. *Women and depression: risk factors and treatment issues.* Washington, D.C.: American Psychological Association.

McKinnon, K., Cournos, F., Horwath, E., Margoshes, E., Caraballo, L., and Currie, C. M. 1991. HIV risk behaviors among the severely mentally ill. Paper presented at the 144th annual meeting of the American Psychiatric Association, New Orleans, May 13.

Mills, T., Rieker, P. P., and Carmen, E. (H.), 1984. Hospitalization experiences of victims of abuse. *Victimology: An International Journal* 9(3–4):436–49.

Morbidity and Mortality Weekly Report (MMRW). 1991. Update: Acquired Immunodeficiency Syndrome, 1981–1990. 40(22):358–63, 369. June 7.

Myers, M. T. 1992. The African-American experience with HIV disease. *Focus: A Guide to AIDS Research and Counseling* 7(4):2. March.

Rieker, P. P., and Carmen, E. (H.), eds. 1984. *The gender gap in psychotherapy: social realities and psychological processes.* New York: Plenum Press.

Rieker, P. P., and Carmen, E. (H.). 1986. The victim-to-patient process: the disconfirmation and transformation of abuse. *American Journal of Orthopsychiatry* 56(3):360–70.

Rose, S. M., Peabody, C. G. and Stratigeas, B. 1991. Undetected abuse among intensive case management clients. *Hospital and Community Psychiatry* 42(5):499–502.

Russell, D. E. H.

1982. The prevalence and incidence of forcible rape and attempted rape of females. *Victimology: An International Journal* 7:81–93.

1984. *Sexual exploitation, rape, child sexual abuse, and workplace harrassment.* Beverly Hills, Calif.: Sage.

Stark, E., and Flitcraft, A. H. 1985. Spouse abuse. In *Source book for Surgeon General's Workshop on Violence and Public Health.* Leesburg, Virginia, October 27–29.

Test, M. A., and Berlin, S. B. 1981. Issues of special concern to chronically mentally ill women. *Professional Psychology* 12(1):136–45.

Lives in Jeopardy: Women and Homelessness

OMEN have changed the face of homelessness and now comprise at least one-quarter of the overall homeless population in
the United States (Slavinsky and Cousins 1982; Rossi 1990). Just
as poverty has become feminized, so has homelessness (Bassuk 1987).
Experts have identified a variety of marco and micro level factors that
may lead to homelessness, including economic hardships and individual
vulnerabilities (Bassuk and Cohen 1991). Researchers have paid little attention, however, to how these economic and personal variables are
linked.

Many poor women have limited earning power and little education
and are overwhelmed by child-care responsibilities. Women heading
households—an ever-increasing population—have sole childrearing and
homemaker responsibilities. Yet they have no place in the current labor
market, which is designed to serve an outmoded fantasy world of nuclear
families and staunch male breadwinners. As a society, we have not yet
acknowledged that women must support families; if they are to do so,
they must have jobs and ancillary supports that meet their needs.

We are now witnessing the devastating results of our negligence. The
gap between women's and men's income remains wide. Women are further limited by occupational segregation and gender-related discrimination. Service sector jobs and AFDC are too low paying to help a woman
out of poverty. And more recently, the crisis in the availability of decent
affordable housing has added another ugly feature to women's poverty:
homelessness.

Many women have survived these struggles with the help of other
women and sometimes men. Unfortunately, many other national factors,

237

such as the housing crisis, the explosion in violence and drug abuse, and the collapse of institutional supports in many inner-city neighborhoods have eroded and even destroyed these life-saving networks. Poor women with children are now frequently in desperate circumstances. As a result, many women suffer from emotional disorders and addictions; others try to take their own lives.

This chapter considers the relationship of gender to homelessness. I argue that economic and personal factors are bound together in a constellation of difficulties that can only be understood as a synthetic whole. Homeless women suffer disproportionately from every catastrophe specific to their gender and race. The problems they experience mirror those of low-income women and are further compounded for women of color. These problems obstruct all women, but not with the same intensity or frequency.

Despite the gains of the last decades, women and children are poorer than ever before. If we expect to halt the growing number of women and children living below the poverty level and on the streets, we must first acknowledge the deeply rooted structural causes of poverty. Family homelessness dramatically demonstrates how gender-related inequalities in large measure determine women's experiences. Until we address this problem, we cannot hope to effect long-lasting change.

Gender-Related Problems Associated with Homelessness

Economic Inequity

Compared to men, women are more likely to be poor and to remain poor (McLanahan 1986; Wilson 1988). The incomes of women aged between 30 and 64 years are less than half that of men (Smith and Ward 1984; Zopf 1989). The income gap is even greater for women who are working part-time. Given these economic constraints it is more difficult for poor women to pull themselves out of poverty. According to Zopf (1989), the disparity in income may in fact be "the primary direct cause of women's higher poverty rates" (132). Although increasing numbers of women have joined the workforce over the past two decades, they still face severe discrimination. Nearly half of all poor women aged 18 to 64 years go to work, but they are frequently underemployed and have fewer unemployment benefits. Those who can find year-round, full-time employment often work in service or retail jobs or in government positions, occupations characterized by low wages and meager opportunities for advancement (Sidel 1986; Zopf 1989).

In part, this wage differential has been explained by the fact that women generally have less education and work experience than men. Recent studies have shown, however, that even when men's and women's educational levels and employment experiences are equivalent, men are still likely to be paid more than women. Education and experience may narrow the wage disparity, but they do not eliminate it entirely. According to Zopf (1989), there is a substantial residue of structural and attitudinal flaws, such as sexism, racism, the 'old-boy network,' persistent job segregation and gender-typing, and socialization for certain careers over others" (138). Scott (1984) emphasizes how occupational segregation and gender-based discrimination and harassment in the workplace contribute to the income gap.

Economic discrimination virtually ensures that women do not have the material resources to raise families unaided. However, in recent years, the numbers of households headed by women have increased dramatically. In 1970, one in ten families was headed by women; Moynihan (1985) has projected that by the year 2000 one in five families will be female headed. The disintegration of the traditional two-parent family has been ascribed to an increase in out-of-wedlock births, an increase in divorce, a decrease in remarriage, and by the growing numbers of women who choose to remain single (Jencks and Peterson 1991).

Families headed by women are among the poorest in our society; more than one-third live below the poverty level (McLanahan 1986; Bassuk 1991). Members of female-headed families are significantly poorer than members of intact families; they are also poorer than disabled and aged individuals (McLanahan 1986). And they are likely to stay poorer longer. In contrast to the majority of poor individuals and families who receive public assistance for less than two years, many single mothers are or will become what sociologists term the "persistent poor," those who live below the poverty level or remain on welfare for at least eight years (Gelpi 1986). For minority women, this problem is amplified. According to Belle (1990), "Black women heading families face a risk of poverty that is more than 10 times that of White men heading families, and Puerto Rican female family heads face a poverty rate that is almost 15 times that found among White male family heads" (385).

Many women heading households have limited education, few job skills, and insufficient child-care resources. They frequently turn to welfare for help. Yet, AFDC is well below the federally established poverty level in most states. Although social welfare spending increased over the past decade, both in real dollars and in percentage of GNP, most of this outlay has been for social security benefits for the elderly, not for the poor (Bassuk 1991). More than 85 percent of homeless families in Massachusetts, for example, are not currently in the workforce and have been receiving cash assistance instead (Bassuk, Rubin, and Lauriat 1986).

The economic plight of homeless women is even graver than the plight of low-income women in the workforce and of housed women on AFDC. In general, homeless women are alone and have limited educational backgrounds, inconsistent work experience, and several children. Some have worked sporadically at low-paying service jobs, such as sales clerks, waitresses, cashiers, and babysitters, but generally not in the year before becoming homeless (Bassuk, Rubin, and Lauriat 1986; Bassuk, Carman, and Weinreb 1990; Russell 1991). Crystal (1984) found that, compared to homeless men, homeless women were three times more likely to have never worked. More than 85 percent of homeless families in Massachusetts are not currently working and have been receiving AFDC (Bassuk, Rubin, and Lauriat 1986). Given the limitations imposed by extreme poverty, it is difficult to imagine how women in these circumstances can ever hope to become self-sufficient.

Low-Income Housing Crisis

The severity of the low-income housing crisis poses an immediate threat to low-income women. The gap between income and housing costs has widened, leaving more poor families precariously housed. Not only have the numbers of poor renters increased substantially between 1974 (4.5 million) and 1987 (7 million), but they are poorer, in part because their AFDC benefits have relatively less purchasing power. At the same time, median rents of unsubsidized low-income units climbed 41 percent nationally. Condominium conversion and neighborhood gentrification have diminished the supply of decent affordable housing, and the federal government has virtually ceased to support new construction or rehabilitation programs for low- and moderate-income housing. These combined factors have caused a critical shortage of housing (Bassuk 1984, 1991).

Families headed by women, because they are poorer than other families, are particularly at risk in this housing market. If a family loses its home, it must find an affordable apartment. Because of the marked discrepancy between median rents in many locales and income or benefit levels, many families spend far more on rent and utilities than the 30 percent allotment that is considered feasible, and hence have little left for other essential expenditures. For example, in 1987 more than two-thirds of families living below the poverty level spent at least 50 percent of their income on rent and utilities and/or lived in substandard housing (Bassuk 1991).

Even if a woman is working full-time and has arranged free child care, her housing expenses still comprise an inordinate percentage of her income. Any unexpected negative change in either her income or her expenses may force her onto the streets. Low-income housing in most cities is largely unavailable and public housing waiting lists are years long. Even if a family is lucky enough to obtain a housing voucher, in some cities less than half of the families with vouchers are able to find permanent housing. Thus, families who are able to survive with even minimal after-rent income are in an extremely precarious situation, in some cases only one crisis away from homelessness.

Motherhood and Homelessness

The weight of the economic evidence explains why more than one-third of women in the United States eke out a bare existence on the margins of society. Yet poverty alone does not fully account for women's homelessness. Rather, poverty chips away at women's buffers, enabling the events of their lives to become catastrophes. Against a backdrop of minimum subsistence, motherhood (and single parenting in particular) may jeopardize a woman's ability to maintain her home. Women must combine their role as worker with that of single parent and homemaker, a challenging position even for women with adequate financial resources and social supports.

Given conditions of extreme poverty and deprivation, as well as the insufficiency of federal child support legislation and the virtual lack of government-sponsored child care, it is not difficult to understand why single motherhood is a risk factor for homelessness (Lerman 1989). Children are a financial burden, and the demands of mothering further constrain many women's job possibilities and already limited earning power. Mothers on the streets are, in the vast majority of cases, women who are alone. When families split up, the economic burden is largely carried by the women. Few women receive adequate support, whether material or emotional, from their male partners. In addition, federal and state governments offer homeless women very little.

Pregnant women living below the poverty level are in a particularly vulnerable position. An estimated 12–35 percent of women on the streets are pregnant—far higher than the pregnancy rate of 10.8 percent reported among the general population (Bassuk 1991). Data from a study of poor women requesting shelter in New York City's Emergency Assistance Units (Knickman and Weitzman 1989) suggested that pregnancy or the recent birth of a child may be a significant risk factor for homelessness. Although housing policies were more favorable for homeless mothers during the time of this study, its authors suggested that pregnant women or those who had newborns were more likely to be extremely stressed and living in unstable housing situations.

Family Violence

In the story of women's homelessness, the role of sexual and physical abuse may well be the great unknown. Abuse is prevalent and is perhaps the rule rather than the exception for most homeless women. Abuse is the salient feature of their childhoods, as well as of their adult lives. Women suffer the debilitating consequences of abuse for the rest of their lives.

Homeless women, like the general female population, are more frequently assaulted by partners, relatives, or friends (Anderson, Boe, and Smith 1988; Bassuk, Rubin, and Lauriat 1986; Bassuk and Rosenberg 1988; D'Ercole and Struening 1990). According to Angela Browne (1990), "even when compared with poor housed female-headed families or with black women in urban populations, groups in which violent victimization rates are known to be high, a larger percentage of homeless women have experienced child physical or sexual abuse, rape or battering by an adult partner" (119). In a recent Boston University study, Lisa Goodman (1991) reported shockingly high rates of victimization: more than two-thirds of homeless mothers had been abused as children, and 90 percent overall had been sexually or physically abused at some time in their lives.

The risk of victimization is heightened in neighborhoods plagued by extreme poverty and violence, in situations where women are alone and lack adequate protection, and in relationships with men who suffer from addictions. In our Massachusetts study (Bassuk, Rubin, and Lauriat 1986; Bassuk and Rosenberg 1988), homeless mothers characterized their relationships with men as unstable, chaotic, and often violent. Approximately 40 percent described at least one major relationship in which they had been battered. More recent studies suggest that these figures may be underestimates.

We know that violent victimization is commonly a precipitant of homelessness among women. Although eviction and housing-related problems are generally the most immediate cause of homelessness, serious interpersonal conflict is frequently a significant factor.

Relationships

Women's self-esteem is largely defined by their affiliations with others. Carol Gilligan (1982) and Jean Baker Miller and Irene Stiver (1991), for example, have posited that women's sense of self derives from their connection to, and sense of responsibility for other people. Homeless women are no exception; the homeless women in Russell's (1991) ethnographic study of Baltimore's shelters, soup kitchens, and daytime missions identified themselves in terms of their dual role as wife and mother. Similarly, Rowe and Wolch's (1990) ethnographic study of homeless women living in Skid Row, Los Angeles, documented that the formation of "social networks were particularly vital to the restoration of a positive and valued personal identity" (191).

Solid relationships contribute to more than women's psychological well-being. Partly as a consequence of the economic and social exigencies of their lives, women in many classes and cultures work especially hard to develop and maintain hardy and extensive support networks. During times of crises, poor families headed by women rely on interconnected kin and non-kin domestic networks comprised primarily of women. As Stack (1974) and Susser (1982) have described in their studies of inner-city ghetto neighborhoods, close relations with female friends and family serve both to ease members' daily existence and to protect them in times of economic and social stress. Not only do supports ameliorate stress once crises have occurred, but they also can prevent crises. Support networks are women's capital, a resource on which poor women and women in crisis must often draw very heavily. However, although supports may be hardy, they are not invincible. When supports are sufficiently depleted, especially in this housing market, poor women are at high risk of becoming homeless.

Many homeless women have exhausted their supports after months and sometimes years of doubling up in overcrowded and often substandard apartments. In fact, almost 85 percent of the homeless mothers in our Massachusetts study had lived with friends or relatives immediately before they came to the shelter; more than 50 percent of these women had also been in other shelters (Bassuk, Rubin and Lauriat 1986). It is even more devastating when entire communities face the problem of disintegrating supports. Poverty, violence, and the housing shortage sometimes combine to disrupt relationships and dislocate longtime residents, destroying networks that have been years in the making (Bassuk and Rosenberg 1988).

Unfortunately, as homeless women themselves recognize, their actual experiences of family and community life fall far short of their ideals. Homeless women have fewer and more fragmented support networks than poor housed women. When a 1986 Massachusetts study asked homeless women "who were the three people most important to you that you could depend on during difficult times?" Twenty-six percent of the respondents were unable to name anyone, 18 percent could name only one person, and 20 percent named only two. Approximately 25 percent claimed that their child—often a preschooler, in all cases a minor—was their only support (Bassuk, Rubin, and Lauriat 1986). Although recent studies suggest that some mothers may have adequate numbers of supports, researchers did not learn about the nature and quality of these supports, especially the availability of material resources such as cash, transportation, and child care (Knickman and Weitzman 1989).

A significant proportion of homeless women may never have had the robust social support networks that enable many poor women to make ends meet. Traumatic childhood experiences such as sexual or physical abuse may rob women of their capacity to form and maintain supports. Women who do not have anchoring, non-contingent relationships during critical development years may have difficulty later sustaining relationships. Without this valuable capital, they have fewer defenses against the onslaught of poverty and homelessness (Bassuk and Rosenberg 1988).

How Women Experience Homelessness

Once homeless, the terrors of a woman's life are grotesguely magnified. Homeless women are more regularly raped, assaulted, and robbed than the average woman. A San Francisco study documented that homeless women are more frequently raped and assaulted (Kelly 1985). D'Ercole and Struening (1990) calculated that their sample of 141 sheltered women in New York City were 106 times more likely to be raped, 41 times more likely to be robbed, and 15 times more likely to be assaulted than a housed African American female.

The stresses of living on the streets or in shelters are overwhelming for most people, and especially for women with young children. Daily life is unpredictable and is focused largely on survival needs. In some cities, shelters are only open at night and families must walk the streets during the day. Many shelters are overcrowded and unsafe. Families have little privacy and generally live in cramped quarters, sometimes with the entire family sleeping in one bed. In accord with some shelters' policies, parents must relinquish responsibility for setting rules for their own children.

The lack of daily routine, structure, and rules in some shelters and most welfare hotels increase the stress and chaos within the family. Because of the lack of child care, mothers have little respite from their children's constant demands. If one child awakens in the middle of the night, the entire family doesn't sleep. Similarly, if one child must see a doctor, the entire family has to go for the visit. Homeless women, like most women, define themselves in terms of their relationships and connectedness to others, especially their children. Despite the creativity and adaptability of many homeless mothers, their desperate situations often cause them to be anxious and depressed about their role as parents. Because they are extremely stressed by the condition of homelessness itself, they often have little energy left to meet the demands of young children who are also chronically stressed. Understandably, raising children on the streets leads to feelings of shame and failure.

Other Factors: Causes and Consequences of Homelessness

Poverty, discrimination, and disappointment do not leave poor and homeless women unscathed. Partly as a result of the constricted realities of their lives as well as their orientation as caregivers, low-income and homeless women suffer disproportionately from emotional disorders and substance abuse problems (Belle 1990). Researchers have not been able to determine with certainty whether these problems are a cause or an effect of poverty and homelessness. It is clear, however, that homelessness is an extremely stressful situation that may exacerbate existing disorders. Researchers also concur that the stresses of homelessness frequently precipitate emotional crises, and that the condition of homelessness impairs a person's sense of well-being and ability to cope. For some, homelessness contributes to the emergence of psychiatric or substance abuse disorders requiring treatment. In others, preexisting problems contribute to the loss of a home. Most importantly, it is virtually impossible to provide adequate care on the streets for those women who suffer from emotional or substance abuse disorders.

Mental Illness

Homeless women are "quintessentially stressed women" (Hammen 1991, 47–48). They not only suffer from the stresses of extreme poverty, including disproportionate rates of violent victimization, but also from the condition of homelessness itself. Similar to low-income women, they "experience more frequent, more threatening, and more uncontrollable life events than does the general population" (Belle 1990, 386). Because their supports are frequently limited, they are more likely to develop emotional problems. In fact, persons suffering from major psychopathology are two-and-a-half times more likely to come from the lowest social class (Belle 1990, 385).

Despite the methodologic shortcomings of existing studies, most researchers agree that, overall, approximately 25–50 percent of homeless adult individuals (including both homeless men and homeless women, but not women in families) suffer from chronic mental illness, particularly schizophrenia (Koegel, Burnam, and Farr 1988). Most studies indicate that the rates of severe mental illness among homeless women are far higher than among homeless men (Burt and Cohen 1989b; Crystal 1984; Hagen 1987; Fischer 1989). However, researchers who study the prevalence of all DSM-III Axis I disorders (that is, chronic mental illness and less serious non-psychotic disorders such as anxiety states) have discovered even greater disparities. For example, in a recent study of adult individual homeless men and homeless women in Baltimore, Breakey et al. (1989) documented that 91 percent of men and 80 percent of women had Axis I diagnoses. They found that "among conditions that are less severe, but nonetheless impairing, 28% of men and 44% of women had phobic, panic, or anxiety disorders" (1989, 1355).

The high percentage of Axis I diagnoses, particularly schizophrenia, is explained in part by the shoddy implementation of deinstitutionalization. Some adult individuals were discharged without adequate follow-up to non-existent supports in the community, while others were discharged to fragmented supports and tenuous placements. Although the closing of state hospital beds peaked in the early 1970s, some deinstitutionalized patients managed to stay housed from many years before they exhausted their resources and lost their homes. In addition, many patients today who might have been hospitalized years ago are now treated as outpatients (Bassuk 1984).

Few studies have explored the prevalence of psychiatric disorders among homeless women who have children with them (that is, families). To date, the data indicate that psychoses are not overrepresented among homeless mothers and that, unlike individual adult homeless women, very few had been deinstitutionalized from state hospitals. However, the Massachusetts study of sheltered homeless mothers (Bassuk, Rubin, and Lauriat 1986) found that approximately 25 percent suffered from some kind of Axis I psychiatric clinical syndrome (this figure includes substance abuse disorders), but these diagnoses did not cluster into a single category.

These data may be confounded by the somewhat arbitrary construction of the categories of homeless adult individuals versus homeless families. Many women who are on the streets alone or are residing in shelters for so-called "singles" are also mothers, but their children have been placed in foster care or are with relatives. Recent literature suggests that many women alone on the streets have lost their children because of severe mental illness, and that these two groups represent a continuum.

The use of Axis II disorders within the context of poverty and homelessness has stirred additional debate. These disorders are largely responses to serious deprivation and "problems in living" and are therefore more subject to class, gender, and race biases. Criteria for making these diagnoses are no more than descriptions of long-term social dysfunction, which predates the homelessness episode. Since these diagnoses do not consider context, they may exaggerate the degree of psychopathology. For example, preliminary data from the Massachusetts study of homeless mothers found that 71 percent suffered from "personality disorders" (Bassuk and Rosenberg 1988).

Moreover, with the exception of work by Browne (1990) and D'Ercole and Struening (1990), the relationship between so-called "personality disorders" and past–traumatic stress disorders in homeless women has been largely ignored. The high rates of violent victimization experienced by homeless women certainly suggest that many of their symptoms could be accounted for by their experience of victimization.

Given the oppressive systemic and personal circumstances that engulf many homeless women, it is not surprising they have astonishingly high rates of attempted suicide. Burt and Cohen (1989a, 1989b) studied 1,704 homeless users of soup kitchens and shelters nationwide in twenty cities with populations of 100,000 or more. They reported that 26 percent of homeless single women reported at least one suicide attempt (compared to 21 percent of homeless single men); and 14 percent of homeless women with children reported such behavior, a figure five times as high as the general population. Researchers have not yet correlated suicidal behavior among homeless women with victimization, substance abuse, or DSM-III diagnoses. However, one can surmise that their feelings of helplessness, hopelessness, and despair can partly be accounted for by the extreme stresses they have experienced throughout their lives, the ineffectiveness of their supports, and their disconnectedness from family and community. It is hard to imagine how women can experience such pervasive stress and misfortune and still feel optimistic about their lives. Furthermore, the real barriers to self-sufficiency are so great that some women's hopeless assessment of their circumstances may be accurate.

Substance Abuse

Although alcohol problems are common among all socioeconomic groups, races, and genders, they are disproportionately represented among persons living in poverty, especially those who are poorly educated (Shuckit 1990). Given these facts, it is not surprising that alcoholism is the most prevalent disorder among the homeless (Breakey et al. 1989). The estimated lifetime prevalence of alcohol disorders is 25–40 percent among homeless men (Institute of Medicine 1988) and 30 percent among homeless adult individual women (Smith and North 1991). Although greatly overrepresented among both homeless men and homeless women, as compared to housed persons, the gap between the genders is far less than among the housed (Smith and North 1991). Similarly, the rates of other drug abuse problems are high (Benda and Dattalo, 1990).

In contrast to homeless adult individual women, mothers with children on the streets have lower lifetime prevalence rates of substance abuse. However, no systematic epidemiologic studies have explored this question. Rates of substance abuse among homeless female heads of families are estimated at 10–30 percent (Weinreb and Bassuk 1990; Smith and North 1991). Anecdotal reports from shelter providers suggest that these may be underestimates.

Women with substance abuse disorders experience a unique set of gender-related problems. First, they are more likely to develop pregnancy complications and to place their newborns at significant risk of developing congenital and neurobehavioral problems, such as fetal alcohol syndrome. Second, women with addictions suffer from more severe medical sequelae (such as neurologic deficits) than men. Finally, detoxification and rehabilitation beds are relatively unavailable for women, especially for those with children.

Discussion

Family homelessness dramatically demonstrates the virulence of societal inequity, disregard, and discrimination along lines of gender. Only when we acknowledge the specific economic and relational needs of women, and we differentiate the unique character of women's poverty from womens' dependence on men (Scott 1984), can we develop effective policies and programs. The catastrophes peculiar to women's lives should not be viewed as unrelated events but should rather, be understood within a gender-related context. Policy makers must keep in mind that womens' self-worth is based on their interconnectedness and affiliations.

A critical step in ameliorating some of the problems of poor and homeless women is to increase public awareness of the relationship among poverty, homelessness, and "the invidious effects of the socialization of women and the limited opportunities for women" (Benda and Dattalo 1990, 77). Until we understand how gender-related inequalities in large measure determine women's experiences, we cannot hope to effect any long-lasting changes. Advocates must make public education about these issues a primary part of their agenda. Although it is hard to be optimistic about changing society's prejudices about women, extreme poverty, and persons with disabilities, small changes are certainly within our reach.

Programs designed to serve homeless women must account for their specific pathways into homelessness, their experiences on the streets, and gender-related needs such as child care. First and foremost, homeless women must have their survival needs met. They require decent, affordable permanent housing, job training and opportunities, comprehensive services coordinated by case management, sustaining supports, and adequate child care. Some women also need help to cope with feelings of hopelessness, desolation, and anger arising from life-long oppression and victimization (Benda and Dattalo 1990). These feelings often become obstacles for women struggling to get off the streets and back into mainstream society. Through encouragement, personal support, empowerment, and advocacy, "deeply rooted, enslaving, self-deprecatory feelings and attitudes" can be worked through and resolved (Benda and Dattalo 1990, 78).

The homeless population includes those groups in our society who have been discarded, denigrated, and abandoned on the basis of extreme poverty, and sometimes on the basis of disability and individual difference. With the feminization of homelessness, we can now add gender-based discrimination to the picture. Reflecting our priorities as a nation, homelessness tells a story about whom we value. It also mirrors the gaps in our service system and the holes in our "safety nets." Sadly, women and children have become a growing proportion of our country's casualties.

Appendix

Homeless persons can generally be subdivided into the following three discrete but overlapping categories, which correspond to divisions in the shelter network and differences in service requirements. These categories include:

(1) *Adult Individuals.* They comprise the majority of the homeless population and include the unemployed, the elderly and veterans, as well as chronically mentally ill persons and substance abusers. With the increase in numbers of women, the ratio of men to women now approaches 3:2. Their average age (early thirties) is younger than a decade ago (Institute of Medicine 1988). In contrast to homeless men who tend to have never married, many homeless women have married and have children who are now in foster care, with relatives, or alone. Contrary to popular belief, these women are actively involved (Crystal 1984) with their children and have hopes of being reunited with them (Hagen 1987; Maurin et al. 1989).

Although many adult individual men and women are homeless because of economic hardships, particularly unemployment, some suffer from serious disabilities. Approximately 25–50 percent are chronically mentally ill and are casualties of the deinstitutionalization policy. At least one-fourth suffer from alcoholism, have more "severe patterns of drinking," and many have dual diagnoses as well (Koegel and Burnam 1988). In addition, the prevalence of both acute and chronic medical problems is higher than in the general population (Institute of Medicine 1988).

(2) *Families with Children.* These consist of a parent or parents with a child in tow. The fastest-growing segment of the homeless population, families account for more than 40 percent of the overall numbers. Recent conservative government estimates indicate that on any given night at least 68,000 to 100,000 children in families are homeless and an additional 186,000 may be precariously housed in overcrowded living arrangements. Families are predominantly headed by women in their late twenties with approximately two or three children, most of whom are preschoolers (Johnson 1989; Bassuk 1991).

(3) *Homeless and Runaway Youths.* This subgroup generally consists of teens who are on

the street alone. Many have been extruded from dysfunctional and abusive families or are dropouts from foster care placements.

This chapter focuses primarily on homeless adult individual women and mothers in families. Although the relationships among these subgroups have not been systematically studied, they probably represent a continuum. Overall, women residing on the streets alone (that is, without children) tend to be more disabled than women in homeless families. A large percentage of homeless adult individual women suffer from chronic mental illness (far more than the overall estimate of one-third) and substance abuse, and some have lost their children because of their disability. In contrast, chronic mental illness (for example, schizophrenia) is not overrepresented among homeless female heads of families.

NOTE

I would like to thank Rebecca Carman, Deborah Cohen, and Jody Dushay for their comments and suggestions.

REFERENCES

Anderson, S., Boe, T., and Smith, S. 1988. Homeless women. *Affilia* 3:62–70.
Bassuk, E. L.
   1984. The homeless problem. *Scientific American* 251:40–45.
   1987. The feminization of homelessness: families in Boston shelters. *American Journal of Social Psychiatry* 7(1):19–23.
   1991. Homeless families. *Scientific American* 265:66–74.
Bassuk, E. L., and Cohen, D. A. 1991. *Homeless families with children: research perspectives.* Washington D.C.: NIAAA and NIMH.
Bassuk, E. L., and Rosenberg, L. 1988. Why does family homelessness occur? a case-control study. *American Journal of Public Health* 78(7):783–88.
Bassuk, E. L., Carman, R., and Weinreb, L., eds. 1990. *Community care for homeless families: a program design manual.* Washington D.C.: Interagency Council for the Homeless.
Bassuk, E. L., Rubin, L., and Lauriat, A. 1986. Characteristics of sheltered homeless families. *American Journal of Public Health* 76:1097–1101.
Belle, D. 1990. Poverty and women's mental health. *American Psychologist* 45:385–89.
Benda, B. B., and Dattalo, P. 1990. Homeless women and men: their problems and use of services. *Affilia* 5:50–82.
Breakey, W., Fischer, P., Kramer M., et al. 1989. Health and mental health problems of homeless men and women in Baltimore. *JAMA* 262:1352–57.
Browne, A. 1990. Family violence and homelessness. In *Community care for homeless families: a program design manual,* ed. E. Bassuk, E. (H.) Carmen, and L. Weinreb, pp. 119–28. Washington D.C.: The Interagency Council for the Homeless.
Burt, M., and Cohen, B. E.
   1989a. *America's homeless: numbers, characteristics, and programs that serve them.* Washington D.C.: The Urban Institute Press. July.
   1989b. Differences among homeless single women, women with children, and single men. *Social Problems* 6:508–24.

Crystal, S. 1984. Homeless men and homeless women: the gender gap. *Urban and Social Change Review* 17:2–6.

D'Ercole, A., and Struening, E. 1990. Victimization among homeless women: implications for service delivery. *Journal of Community Psychology* 18:141–52.

Fischer, P. J. 1989. Estimating the prevalence of alcohol, drug, and mental health problems in the contemporary homeless population: a review of the literature. *Contemporary Drug Problems* 16:333–89. Fall.

Gelpi, B. 1986. *Women and poverty.* Chicago: University of Chicago Press.

Gilligan, C. 1982. *In a different voice: psychological theory and women's development.* Cambridge: Harvard University Press.

Goodman, L. 1991. The prevalence of abuse among homeless and housed poor mothers: a comparison study. *American Journal of Orthopsychiatry* 61:489–500.

Hagen, J. L. 1987. Gender and homelessness. *Social Work* 32:312–16.

Hammen, C. 1991. Parenting. In *Homeless families with children: research perspectives,* ed. E. L. Bassuk and D. A. Cohen. Washington D.C.: NIAAA and NIMH.

Institute of Medicine. 1988. *Homelessness, health, and human needs.* Washington D.C.: National Academy Press.

Jencks, C., and Peterson, P., eds. 1991. *The urban underclass.* Washington D.C.: The Brookings Institution.

Johnson, A. 1989. Female-headed homeless families: a comparative profile. *Affilia* 4:23–29.

Kelly, J. T. 1985. Trauma: with the example of San Francisco's shelter program. In *Health care of homeless people,* ed. P. W. Brickner, L. K. Scharer, B. Conanan, et al. New York: Springer-Verlag.

Knickman, J. R., and Weitzman, B. C. 1989. *A study of homeless families in New York City: risk assessment models and strategies for prevention.* Final report. Vol. 1. New York: NYU Health Research Program.

Koegel, P., and Burnam, A. 1988. Alcoholism among homeless adults in the inner city of Los Angeles. *Arch Gen Psych* 45:1011–101.

Koegel, P., Burnam, A., and Farr, R. 1988. The prevalence of specific psychiatric disorders among homeless individuals in the inner city of Los Angeles. *Arch Gen Psych* 45:1085–92.

Lerman, R. 1989. Child support policies. In *Welfare Policy for the 1990s,* ed. P. Cottingham and D. Ellwood, pp. 219–46. Cambridge: Harvard University Press.

McLanahan, S. 1986. Problems of mother-only families. In *Single mothers and their children: a new American dilemma,* ed. I. Garfinkel and S. McLanahan, pp. 11–43. Washington D.C.: The Urban Institute.

Maurin, J., Russell, L., Memmott, R. J. 1989. An exploration of gender differences among the homeless. *Res. Nursing and Health* 12:315–21.

Miller, J. B., and Stiver, I. 1991. *A relational reframing of therapy.* Wellesley College: Stone Center, No. 52.

Moynihan, D. P. 1985. *Family and nation.* The Godkin lectures. Harvard University. April 8–9.

Rossi, P. 1990. The old homeless and the new homeless in historical perspective. *American Psychologist* 45:954–59.

Rowe, S., and Wolch, J. 1990. Social networks in time and space: homeless women in Skid Row, Los Angeles. *Annals Assoc. Amer. Geographers* 80:184–204.

Russell, B. G. 1991. *Silent sisters: a study of homeless women.* New York: Hemisphere.

Scott, H. 1984. *Working your way to the bottom: the feminization of poverty.* London: Pandora.

Shuckit, M. 1990. *Drug and alcohol abuse.* New York: Plenum Press.

Sidel, R. 1986. *Women and children last: the plight of poor women in affluent America.* New York: Viking.

Slavinsky, A., and Cousins, A. 1982. Homeless women. *Nursing Outlook* 30:358–62.

Smith, E., and North C. 1991. Impact of substance abuse on homeless families. In *Homeless families with children: research perspectives*, ed. E. L. Bassuk and D. A. Cohen. Washington D.C.: NIAAA and NIMH.

Smith, J. P., and Ward, M. P. 1984. *Women's wages and work in the twentieth century.* Washington D.C.: R-3119-NICHD. October.

Stack, C. 1974. *All our kin: strategies for survival in a Black community.* New York: Harper and Row.

Susser, I. 1982. *Norman Street.* New York: Oxford University Press.

Weinreb, L., and Bassuk, E. L. 1990. Substance abuse: a growing problem among homeless families. *Family and Comm. Health* 13:55–64.

Wilson, J. B. 1988. Women and poverty: a demographic overview. In *Too little, too late: dealing with the health needs of women in poverty*, ed. C. A. Perales and L. S. Young, pp. 21–40. New York: Harrington Park Press.

Zopf, P. 1989. *American women in poverty.* New York: Greenwood Press.

Turbulence on the College Campus and the Frustration-Aggression Hypothesis

OVER two decades ago, Thomas Pettigrew, in his book *Racially Separate or Together* (1971), reminded us that the American racial scene has always been "highly complex, . . . defying facile generalizations" (264). This is an apt description of race relations on college campuses today—complex and confusing.

We have not understood the association between pluralism and racial turbulence probably because the focus of our analysis has often been too limited. We have focused on ways of recruiting diverse student bodies without examining the social structures and processes that have excluded certain groups in the past. We have not adequately examined how majority-group students adapt to campuses that are more reflective of the diversity in society and the world at large. The literature on African American students at predominantly White colleges is growing, but there are few studies of the range of responses of White students to their new personal experiences of campus pluralism and, in some cases, of minority status.

Studies conducted by social scientists such as Willie and McCord (1972), Thomas (1981), Astin (1982), Fleming (1984), Allen (1986), Blackwell (1987), Nettles (1988), and others examine the increasing enrollment of Blacks in predominantly White institutions. They concluded that Black students on predominantly White college campuses do not fare as well as they should.

It is time now to examine turbulence on the American college campus. Institutions that are undergoing intensified experiences of pluralism could, because of their diverse and multicultural populations, become laboratories of conflict resolution, thereby leading to a new social reality in our nation. A goal of this chapter is to diagnose what contributes to campus turbulence and to analyze possibilities for overcoming it.

Pluralism on the Campus: A Historical Overview

The termination of the twenty-year-old *Adams* case mandating the federal government's active responsibility for insuring pluralism in publicly supported colleges and universities in eighteen states was evidence that in the 1980s the U.S. government had stopped vigorously pursuing student body integration on college campuses. Eileen O'Brien notes,

> The lawsuit's termination indicates that the Federal Government—as well as the courts—will no longer serve as the "guardian" for rights for Blacks and minorities, and that minority advocates will have to fight at the state level to ensure access and equity for minorities in higher education. . . . One affirmative action officer said, "with the [federal] government backing off, I don't think they will keep up the efforts. The states were headed in the right direction, but I don't think they're going to comply unless there is some kind of pressure to comply. Already, I'm seeing some retrenchment." (O'Brien 1990, 7, 11)

The association, if any, between turbulence on the college campus and the function of formal institutions such as state and federal governments will be examined.

Since passage of the Civil Rights Act of 1964, an increasing number of African Americans, other people of color, and women have enrolled in predominantly White schools. Most Black students now enroll in such schools. Although the student bodies of their schools are experiencing increased diversity, White students—the majority population in these schools—have not shown a corresponding increase in interracial understanding. An annual survey of freshmen in U.S. colleges revealed that only 35 percent believed that "helping to promote racial understanding" is an essential or even very important objective of college education. The fulfillment of personal goals such as "being well off financially" or "being able to make more money" were the more salient objectives of higher education for these students. Two-thirds of the female first-year students and three-fourths of the male first-year students said that "the chief benefit of college is that it increases one's earning power" (Astin 1989).

Maintaining enrollment, according to administrators, is an important way of achieving institutional financial stability. This was the chief concern of senior administrators of colleges and universities as reported in a survey conducted by the American Council on Education in 1989. When asked to indicate their perceptions of the challenges facing institutions of higher education during the next five years, only 13 percent indicated that diversity would be a major issue. Another way of ascertaining the level of concern about diversity is to ask if serving new populations might be a major challenge in the next half-decade. When diversity was put in these terms, 18 percent of the college and university officers identified it as a major issue that would challenge their institutions in the near future (*Chronicle of Higher Education* 1989, 56).

Race relations, diversity, and serving new populations of students appeared to be of limited concern among most White administrators and White students in colleges and universities in the United States. Despite this limited concern, diversity in colleges and universities is increasing. In 1964, when the Civil Rights Act was passed, 93 percent of all students enrolled in institutions of higher education were White (U.S. Census Bureau 1965, 109). Approximately one generation later, the proportion of Whites among the total student population had decreased to 85 percent (U.S. Census Bureau 1990, 131). White students' proportion of the total higher education population is closer now to Whites' actual proportion in the total U.S. population. The U.S. Department of Education also reports that another source of diversity for institutions of higher education is "older students who enroll to prepare for career changes" (U.S. Department of Education 1989, 2:46). Whether students and administrators acknowledge it, the general characteristics of students in colleges and universities are changing.

Examining Racism and Prejudice on the Campus

In the early 1990s, with the increase in pluralism on college campuses there has been much debate about a concept called "political correctness." The term *political correctness* was first developed by Marxists and progressives as an expression of self-criticism in situations in which opinions were formed without the benefit of careful, independent thought (Stimpson 1991, A40). Recently, the term has been used by some conservatives to describe challenges that they face because their attitudes and actions may not embrace multiculturalism or sanction the validity and worth of various styles of living. Thus, the concept of political correctness is being used pejoratively by dominant people of power to ridicule those who demand sensitivity to and consideration for subdominant people of power. Some who sneer at political correctness contend that their right to free speech is compromised when their cruel, insensitive, and abusive remarks to others are challenged.

In a more positive vein, political correctness has been described as a way of building community in a pluralistic population consisting of diverse racial, ethnic, and gender groups. The boundaries of the debate have extended over into curriculum development, language, and public use of signs and symbols. It is no longer a debate limited to professional academics about appropriate discourse. *Newsweek* magazine featured the political correctness issue as a cover story and asked if it is "the New Enlightenment or the New McCarthyism?" (*Newsweek* Dec. 24, 1990). Despite the widespread attention that it has attracted, the political correctness debate has made its greatest impact on college campus communities.

Duke University has a chapter of the National Association of Scholars, a predominantly White organization. The association, founded in 1987, has chapters on more than twenty campuses. The *New York Times* described the group as one "devoted to preserving the traditional Western curriculum in colleges and universities. The group is troubled by the introduction of women's and ethnic studies into the curriculum" (*New York Times* Oct. 21, 1990:45). One professor, opposed to the formation of the Duke chapter, said that the association is "widely known to be racist, sexist and homophobic." He said that the Western curriculum that the association was organized to protect reflects a White European male political bias. The professor and ninety-three others were so concerned about the possible harm that could result from the activities of the National Association of Scholars that they named themselves the Duke Association of Scholars who "applaud all efforts to acknowledge the rich diversity of our society in the curriculum of [the] university" (*New York Times* Oct. 21, 1990:45).

As the final decade of the twentieth century commenced, *Newsweek* reported that on college campuses "almost everyone, it seems, is mad about something: racial slurs, affirmative action, separatism, multiculturalism or . . . the PC [political correctness] movement." *Newsweek* continues, "the lofty notion of the college campuses as havens of tolerance . . . seems . . . archaic" (Newsweek 1991, 26).

The Organization of American Historians, whose members are affiliated largely with colleges and universities, joined the political correctness debate with regard to the issue of curriculum. Its statement maintained that "history courses should be based on sound historical scholarship." They rejected "history that asserts or implies the inherent superiority of one race, gender, class or region of the world over another" (*Chronicle of Higher Education* 1991:A5). Other mass media reports indicate that some academicians view expressions like the one mentioned above and other changes as "a new wave of repression" (*Boston Globe* July 8, 1991:7). They are unhappy with schools like the University of Arizona, which has initiated a new series of humanities courses in which students "study Dante and Pope, but also Kiowan Indian mythology" (Stimpson 1991).

In the early 1970s, while Vice President for Student Affairs at Syracuse University, Charles Willie joined Ruth Burton, a psychiatrist in Student Health Services, to co-teach a seminar on racism and prejudice. The seminar consisted of campus student leaders (who were invited to participate) and students that had been involved in interracial altercations (who were required to participate). Students earned course credit. Professional staff of the Office of Student Affairs also participated as seminar members. In the seminar, students discussed parental and societal responses to interracial dating and marriage. They discussed the feelings evoked when minority-group students prefer to sit together at dining hall tables and chose segregated housing arrangements. They discussed whether the negative feelings people experience when members of their race date members of another race is the same for Whites and Blacks and whether these feelings are based on jealousy, prejudice, pity, resentment, pride, stereotyping, ethnocentricity, fear of genetic annihilation, or other factors. They questioned Black males who missed several sessions of the seminar and asked if their absences were due to discomfort with the class and/or with the discussions. They asked Puerto Rican students why they did not speak up in class and give voice to their concerns. They talked about a variety of intergroup encounters both on and off campus.

Three months into the seminar, the teachers realized that most of the discussion had focused on minority-group class members—their feelings, attitudes, and behaviors. One member of the seminar—a student— hypothesized that the class had not dealt with the feelings, attitudes, and behaviors of majority-group class members—particularly White males— because they were not ready to discuss themselves within the context of racism and prejudice. One seminar leader—the psychiatrist—hypothesized that groups such as White Anglo-Saxon Protestants probably did not feel threatened and/or felt that they did not have to defend anything, and could therefore view these issues as someone else's problem. Thus, they were not inclined to discuss their circumstances as issues of concern in the seminar on prejudice and racism. Also, other motivations could have been responsible for their silence.

Samuel Osherson observes that the "classic male chauvinistic patronizing perspective" of many college-educated White men derives from their "feeling of clear superiority" over others (Osherson 1986, 88). This theory could explain the diminished participation of White males in the seminar discussions. Another explanation suggested by Osherson's work is that of fear and anxiety. Osherson states that those "who equate maturity with being in control" may have fears and anxieties when others become self-determining and less dependent on their controlling authority. Osherson believes that such individuals, when they are not fully in control, "may feel embarrassment over not living up to the strong male image in which they believe" (Osherson 1986, 90). Thus, feelings of superiority on the one hand, or fear and anxiety on the other, could be associated with the level of participation by White males in the seminar on racism and prejudice.

Similarly, Jayminn Sanford—a student of higher education for nine years in three predominantly White institutions—has experienced the same phenomenon from a different perspective. Syllabi outlining the course content for the semester will often devote only one class discussion to issues that are of special concern to minorities. When racism and prejudice become issues of discussion in courses, the "majority perspective" is often presented by the instructor and discussed by the class as a whole. The "minority perspective" is then sought as an adjunct idea, a different way of seeing things as opposed to the way things "really are." When themes of racism and prejudice are discussed, African Americans and people of color are clearly expected to assume leadership. At the end of the appointed time, the course content reverts to the majority viewpoint and Whites reenter the conversation as if the previous discussion had been a digression from the major purpose of the course.

The various complementary and contradictory perspectives that students of different racial and ethnic backgrounds bring to the classroom are rarely grappled with and tackled head on. There is little substantive debate. Often there is uncomfortable silence or hurried discussion to get back to the main material of the course. The minority perspective is presented and received in isolation, separated from the whole—not understood as a reality without which there is no whole.

The *Chronicle of Higher Education* reports that many White students are forming racially homogeneous groups to protect personal interests that they believe are being eroded by increasing pluralism in higher education. These students have formed "White Students' Unions" as organizations through which to press their claims. White students are "angered by admissions and financial-aid policies that they say unfairly favor minority students." They are described as feeling "squeezed out of opportunities," because of special arrangements made by colleges to recruit equitable numbers of minority students. The *Chronicle of Higher Education* attributes these issues to the policies that began during the Reagan administration. "These students have grown up with a national leadership that hasn't accentuated the need for an atmosphere which is inclusive of all citizens," says an associate dean of students at Temple University. A senior at the University of Florida says White males are frightened that women and members of minority groups are now competing with them for jobs.

"There is a growing realization by White males that they may not long have their privileged advantage" (*Chronicle of Higher Education* 1990a).

Newsweek acknowledges that tension between the races is nothing new. What is new, according to the magazine's investigation, "is the apparent rise in racial incidents of all sorts . . . namecalling, scapegoating, accusations and recriminations" (*Newsweek* May 6, 1991:27). Findings of the National Institute Against Prejudice and Violence at the University of Maryland's Baltimore campus indicates that "one in five Black students reports some form of racial harassment and that racist episodes have been reported at more than 300 colleges and universities [during a five-year period]." Schools hit by race-related incidents in recent years, according to *Newsweek*, are located in all regions of the nation (*Newsweek* May 6, 1991:27). Examples of racist incidents on college campuses include:

- At Olivet College in Michigan, thirty-five of the college's fifty Black students decided to leave after a brawl involving the students and a White fraternity. Other campus groups such as the basketball team have been accused of making racial slurs against Black teammates (*Wichita Eagle* April 9, 1992:79).
- At the University of Delaware, an unidentified caller to the Center for Black Culture threatened to bomb "every Black Center in the world" if a demonstration planned against the campus newspaper was carried out the next day (*Newsweek* p. 23).
- At the University of Illinois in Chicago, the university refused to discontinue its war dancing and use of a mascot known as Chief Illiniwek during sports events despite protests from Native American students (*Newsweek* p. 27).
- At the University of Florida in Gainesville an article in the campus newspaper read: "To put it bluntly, many Black students gained entrance into universities they were neither qualified nor prepared to attend" (*Group Tensions in American Colleges* 1989, National Institute Against Prejudice and Violence.)
- Sharon Parker, director of multicultural development at Stanford University, said "There is not a university in the country that hasn't had some [bias incident] . . . it goes with the territory; it goes with life" (*Black Issues in Higher Education*, July 16, 1992, p. 50).

The Frustration-Aggression Hypothesis

The discussion thus far indicates that frustration may be prevalent and increasing among White faculty members and students on college campuses. Several decades ago, John Dollard explained intergroup hostility as resulting from frustration that leads to aggression. His hypothesis, published in 1939, provides a social science perspective on intergroup relations on college campuses. Based on the belief that aggression is frequently a function of frustration, Dollard explains:

the occurrence of aggressive behavior always presupposes the existence of frustration and, contrariwise, that the existence always leads to some form of aggression. . . . [P]eace with the "we group" and hostility against the "others group" seems to be [a] correlated factor. Aggressive responses are often merely displaced from in group members and find substitute target in the out group. This is a clear case of a displacement of an original in group aggressive response[:] . . . Out groupers are, as it were, blamed for the frustrations which are actually incident to in group life; and a host of aggressive responses are displaced to them. . . . For the out group to be a good scapegoat it must be so far removed from the in group by differences in custom or feature that it [the scapegoat] will not be included effectively within the scope of in group taboos on aggression. Out groupers may then be thought of merely as perennial frustrators, as traditional enemies and threats to the integrity of in group life. Often, of course, they are not such in reality; but they are invariably so represented in order to seem to justify the displacement of aggression to them. Opportunities for displacement and limited expressions are available and are utilized, such as maintenance of order within the group or attacking some of the sources of frustration as by scientific research (Dollard 1939, 89, 90).

While we invoke Dollard's hypothesis in the analysis of frustration and aggression in the White population of the United States, we believe that it also helps to explain behavior among subdominant people of power. Our hypothesis is that aggression among dominant people of power is usually displaced or expressed outwardly, whereas aggression among subdominant people of power is often expressed inwardly or against members of their own group. Moreover, we believe that the frustration-aggression hypothesis is applicable nationally and internationally. Following this analysis, we will consider alternative ways of overcoming frustration and aggression.

Frustration Aggression among Dominant People of Power

Lois Mark Stanley has described an unfortunate experience in the 1980s, in community organization for race relations, that may be a direct consequence of the frustration-aggression hypothesis. She was involved in an effort to integrate her predominantly White neighborhood, attempting to enrich her community with a modest experience of racial diversity. Community members threatened her if she persisted in her efforts to secure a home for her Black friends. Already, there had been a cross-burning on the lawn of one Black property owner who had purchased an undeveloped lot in the neighborhood.

We agree with Stanley's assertion that these forms of aggression are products of unrelenting frustration of Whites, particularly of White males, who considered their previously all-White world natural and normal (Stanley 1989, 28). Stanley's experience indicates that middle-class Whites who feel threatened may respond with aggression. Such activity is not limited to the working class and poor, as the following examples indicate: The occurrence of racial violence in the Mobile, Alabama, public schools a quarter of a century ago is similar to some problems taking place on college and university campuses today. The governor of Alabama tried to prevent the desegregation of Mobile public schools, particularly Murphy High School, the largest and one of the finest all-White schools in the community. Then, as now, Whites used violence to hold on to what they believed were their prerogatives and entitlements. The governor mobilized the National Guard to prevent Black children from entering the high school. When the National Guard was federalized so that it could not be used in this way, the local White Citizens' Council went into action. It urged Whites "to instruct their children to make things unpleasant for Black students who were legally admitted to Murphy. . . . [A]lmost 300 White students participated in a noisy demonstration" (Foley 1981, 180). The affluent Whites in Murphy High School used violence to resist their eroding power—a predictable response.

Our discussion has thus far focused on racial violence, but we hypothesize similar outcomes for gender as well. There now is increasing evidence that violence against women on college campuses may also represent a manifestation of the frustration-aggression hypothesis. "A fraternity sent its pledges out on a 'scavenger hunt' in which they were to return with photos of themselves with [Asian] girls" (National Institute against Prejudice and Violence 1992). "Access to women for sexual gratification is a presumed benefit of fraternity membership [in some organizations. It is] promised . . . through brothers' conversations with new recruits" (Martin and Hummer 1989, 466). Joseph Weinberg at the 1990 annual meeting of the American Psychological Association indicated that "All-male groups that foster admiration for macho behavior are more likely to engage in inappropriate sexual aggression" (*Boston Globe* 1990). This is the shared conclusion of several studies on date rape and other forms of violence against women on college campuses.

The *Uniform Crime Reports* of the Federal Bureau of Investigation indicate that forcible rape had increased from 76,000 cases in 1979 to 93,500 cases in 1988—a 21.5 percent increase during the 1980s. However, the rate for murder—typically a male-against-male crime—decreased during the same ten-year period. Forcible rape is typically a male-against-female crime (*The World Almanac and Book of Facts* 1988). It is difficult to obtain data on violent crimes by race. The FBI's *Uniform Crime Reports* give data on arrests by race, however. These data may be used by law enforcement officials as an indication of assumed criminal activity. A minority of the individuals arrested for robbery and murder (36 percent and 46 percent, respectively) were White males. However, 50.2 percent of the people arrested for forcible rape during a single year were White males (*Information Please Almanac* 1989). These findings pertaining to White males and rape are particularly significant because they are at variance with "a widening of the racial gap in arrests" for other offenses (Jaynes and Williams, 1989 458). We hypothesize that forcible rape is an example of an outwardly directed or displaced aggression on women by White males who are frustrated by their diminished power. It probably is no coincidence that the increase in this violent crime comes at a time when women represent a growing proportion of successful, independent individuals.

According to Senator Daniel Patrick Moynihan, "Ours is a society which presumes male leadership" (U.S. Department of Labor 1965). A similar observation was made by Dairl Gillespie, who said that "Once upon a time, the function of culture was to rationalize the predominance of the male sex" (Gillespie 1979). When Moynihan made his observation in 1965, only four of every ten college students were female. "[I]n 1988–89, women earned the majority of associate, bachelor's and master's degrees . . . and by [the year] 2000, women are expected to have earned 50 percent or more of the associate, bachelor's, master's, and doctorate degrees" (U.S. Department of Education 1989). There has been a "substantial rise in the number of degrees awarded to women. The majority of students in colleges are female" (National Center for Educational Statistics 1988). Since the society to which Moynihan referred includes college and university campuses, White males are clearly losing ground as reflected in the number of college degrees conferred upon women.

Not only have White males fallen behind in numbers in higher education, they also are falling behind in standardized aptitude test scores as well. On the mathematics portion of the Standardized Aptitude Test, the mean score for Asian Americans exceeds that of Whites. The composite average score of Asian Americans on English, mathematics, social studies, and natural sciences tests of the American Council on Education is higher than that of Whites or other racial and ethnic groups in the United States (*Chronicle of Higher Education* 1990b). Our society, including our schools, no longer can presume White male leadership. In the light of Moynihan's assertion, one could characterize the diminishing power of White males as one of their grievances, a source of frustration possibly resulting in displaced aggression. (Historical examples of this contemporary manifestation of aggression are discussed below.)

The Dred Scott case—formally known as *Scott v. Sandford* (1857)—resulted in an opinion by the Supreme Court that prohibited Congress from forbidding slavery in the territories. According to that opinion, Dred Scott remained a slave despite his previous residence in a free territory. Moreover, the opinion concluded that one whose ancestors were sold as slaves was not entitled to the rights of a federal citizen and, therefore, had no standing in court. Later, Supreme Court Chief Justice Roger B. Taney would say that a Negro had no rights that White men were bound to respect (*New Columbia Encyclopedia* 1975, 795). Despite endorsement of their dominant power by the highest court in the nation, Whites would experience its erosion just six years later.

The Emancipation Proclamation, issued in 1862, became effective on January 1, 1863. The Proclamation was issued by President Abraham Lincoln as Commander in Chief of the armed forces. It freed all enslaved persons in states that were in rebellion against the federal government. With passage of the Thirteenth Amendment to the Constitution in 1865, less than a decade after the Dred Scott decision, slavery in the United States was abolished. (The Fourteenth Amendment gave citizenship to all people born in the United States, including people whose ancestors were enslaved persons, and prohibited states from enacting laws that abridged the privileges of citizenship. The Fifteenth Amendment guaranteed all citizens the right to participate in the democratic electoral process regardless of race or previous status of servitude or enslavement.)

Two civil rights bills were enacted following the Civil War, one in 1866 and another in 1875. In 1883, however, an all-male and all-White Supreme Court outlawed the Civil Rights Act of 1875. As a result, Southern states were able to return to racial segregation as a lawful practice. The requirement to accept integration after the Civil War frustrated Whites' belief in their supremacy. The action of the Supreme Court in 1883 was an aggressive way of reasserting White supremacy, as was the practice of lynching African Americans. "The long and bloody chapter of the lynching of Blacks in America had social gain and psychic need [for Whites] as powerful moving forces behind it" (Comer 1972, 133). Records held at Tuskegee University indicate that "more than 4,700 Blacks died from the mob action between 1882 and 1956 . . . [there were] more than 150 lynchings in an average year" (Comer 1972, 166). Psychiatrist James Comer concluded that "the role of the black as a convenient target for the discharge of white aggression is deeply embedded in American folkways" (Comer 1972, 134). The linkage between frustration and aggression was revealed in the reflections of a 41-year-old White worker employed in an

African American community development project during the 1960s. His Black co-workers expressed anger toward him and constantly found fault in his work. He felt unappreciated and beaten up. Increasingly, he said he got "fed up with the whole damn business." One day, after a particularly frustrating series of conversations with Black co-workers, he exclaimed, "G-ddam it, I'd like to hang everyone of those Black sons-of-b-tches by their necks; they are destroying me; I'd like to string them all up!" The White worker had had dreams that revealed murderous impulses. At first, he did not understand the dreams until he blurted out his feelings after the frustrating and revealing conversation. He acknowledged at least at night in his dreams that he actively did away with all the Blacks in his life. Close association with Blacks constituted the difficult, upsetting life circumstances that challenged his authority and professionalism and stimulated his "previously dormant or little noticed sadistic attitudes and wishes" (Ordway 1973).

Frustration Aggression among Subdominant People of Power

As stated earlier, we believe the frustration-aggression hypothesis is applicable to subdominants as well as dominants. The difference, however, is that the aggression associated with frustration tends to be inwardly rather than outwardly directed among subdominants. The higher homicide rate among African Americans is probably an accurate indicator of the inward direction of aggression toward members of this in group. The National Research Council's Committee on the Status of Black Americans found that "most Black criminal offenders victimize other Blacks." This pattern is particularly true for most crimes of violence (Jaynes and William, 1989). Black-against-Black violence probably is a manifestation of intense frustration.

Because the homicide rates among Blacks in 1941 and in 1983 were similar, one might conjecture that frustration which materializes in this kind of aggression has existed over the years in this population. An excellent example of the frustration-aggression hypothesis in operation is the high rate of homicide in the Black community, which climbed rapidly in 1968, the year Martin Luther King, Jr., was assassinated; the homicide rate remained high for the next decade or so. As many may recall, these were years of great frustration for African Americans. In Martin Luther King, Jr., African Americans had offered their best and he was murdered.

Richard Wright poignantly describes the internalization of aggression within the African American community in *Twelve Million Black Voices:*

We watch strange moods fill our children, and our hearts swell with pain. The streets, with their noise and flaring lights, the taverns, the automobiles, and the poolhall claim them, and no voice of ours can call them back. They spend their nights away from home; they forget our ways of life, our language, our God. Their swift speech and impatient eyes make us feel weak and foolish. We cannot keep them in school . . . we fall on our knees and pray for them; but in vain. The city has beaten us, evaded us; . . . young bodies filled with warm blood, feel bitter and frustrated at the sight of the alluring hopes and prizes denied them. It is not their eagerness to fight that makes us afraid, but that they go to death on the city pavements faster than even disease and starvation can take them. As the courts and the morgues become crowded with our lost children, the hearts of the officials of the city grow cold toward us. As our jobs begin to fail in another depression, our lives and the lives of our children grow so frightful that even some of our educated Black leaders are afraid to make known to the nation how we exist. They become ashamed of us and tell us to hide our wounds. (Wright 1941, 136)

This observation, published in 1941, is an appropriate description of the experiences of many young African Americans in urban settings.

Aggression associated with frustration, however, is not always violent. Sometimes the outcome is estrangement. This is another form in which the frustration-aggression hypothesis manifests itself among subdominant populations. A study of Black students at White colleges revealed estrangement from the out group and estrangement from the in group as consequences of the small numbers of Blacks on campus. When the number in their group or a combination of minority groups is less than one-fifth, an insufficient critical mass is present to make a meaningful impact on the total campus community. Unable to have their legitimate interests appropriately considered, small Black student populations tend to feel estranged from the campus community (Willie and McCord 1972). This was expected.

The unexpected finding, however, is that members of racial-minority populations also are estranged from each other when their number in the campus community is small. This is the explanation offered by Willie and McCord: When Blacks believe that they are more or less totally dependent on each other for social life, and their number is small, there may be an insufficient range of personality and social types present within the minority population to fulfill the companionship needs of all. Under these conditions, one member of a dyad of mutually attracted individuals may move prematurely for the formation of an exclusive relationship. Such a move may be prompted by fear that others of similar characteristics are not available in the small population. To resist entrapment in an exclusive relationship that is premature, many of the members of a small minority community on campus tend to "hang loose in their relationships with each other, exhibiting standoffish and indifferent attitudes." (Willie and McCord 1972, 17). Also, in a campus community where the number of individuals in a particular group is small, many social relations take on the character of an extended family. The almost unlimited access that the students in a minority group have to each other in such a setting is socially stifling and suffocating for some. Their way of handling these feelings of frustration over the absence of privacy and autonomy is to distance themselves or become estranged from the in group (Willie and McCord 1972).

James Comer tells the story of another source of frustration. A young Black college student, a football player at a college on the West Coast, was frustrated because he feared the consequences of aggression. Having grown up in the South, the student athlete grew up knowing that aggression by Black men could result in death. The Black football lineman's fears were of course solidly grounded in the racial realities of the South. For example, an alleged aggressive action by fourteen-year-old Emmett Till—whistling at a White woman—cost him his life in 1955.

The football player was being pushed around the field by his White teammates in an early scrimmage session. He was unable to be physical because in the part of America he came from, Black males are taught from early childhood that Black aggression will not be tolerated. . . . His insightful coach was eventually able to convince him that aggression toward Whites—at least on the football field— would not bring retribution, and the [football player] went on to become an outstanding athlete. (Comer 1972, 143)

One might classify this story as an example of inwardly directed aggression, since the individual at first denied himself the privilege of expressing his extraordinary athletic ability because of fear. Such denial surely must be an experience of immense frustration and unexpressed anger.

The frustration-aggression hypothesis is documented in the history of other populations of subdominants. In 1890, for example, the Oklahoma territory was formed out of the western half of the "unorganized" Indian territory. This was the year in which Chief Sitting Bull was assassinated. At least twenty-two Sioux were slaughtered by U.S. troops. This was the year of the "last major Indian out-break," a year of great frustration for Native Americans (Linton 1985). Adolph Bandelier's study of Pueblo Indians offers a dynamic description of an Indian Council meeting of clan representatives. Bandelier describes the outbursts of one of its participants in the council meeting as aggression anchored in frustration. They were clearly a response to the frustration of the Native Americans having had their land taken and the lives of their kin destroyed. Bandelier said "weak individuals . . . when they see themselves driven to the wall become frenzied . . . [and may] explode like a loaded weapon" (Bandelier

1971). However, the aggression was expressed inwardly toward other Native Americans, not outwardly.

Testimony offered to the President's Commission on Mental Health revealed that in Alaska, suicide and alcoholism are reaching epidemic proportions among Native peoples (Willie 1983). One might characterize these as the ultimate forms of inward aggression and self-destructiveness: abuse and annihilation of one's own personhood.

Likewise, Alexander Leighton's (1946) study of the social life of Japanese people in relocation camps in the United States during World War II revealed that "the situation most likely to lead to aggression is that in which frustration predominates." He added, "Attacks on persons who had little or nothing to do with the causes of stress appeared when evacuees suspected of being 'dogs' (informers) became targets for hate. Because it was not safe to express anger directly against Whites in the Administration and the other agents who cause much suffering, gangs broke into barrack rooms in the night and beat supposed 'dogs' [other Japanese] after the usual fashion of the Ku Kux Klan and other vigilante organizations." Leighton discovered that "when aggression cannot spend itself on the forces directly responsible for the stress from which the individuals are suffering, then there is a tendency to attack substitutes." Leighton concluded that "hating and beating these 'dogs' gave the people a feeling of doing something, of 'making somebody suffer for this,' [since] they were unable to control the outside world which had oppressed them" (Leighton 1946, 272).

Frustration Aggression: A Global Perspective

The frustration-aggression hypothesis is not exclusively a U.S. phenomenon. There is general agreement among scholars that the seeds of Nazi Germany's aggression, which resulted in World War II, were planted by the treaty that terminated World War I. Winston Churchill called the economic clauses of the treaty that required reparations "silly" requirements that "no defeated nation . . . [could] ever pay." The triumphant allies tried to squeeze Germany "until the pips squeaked." Churchill described post–World War I Germany as "impoverished" and "loaded with measureless indemnities" (Churchill 1959, 3). If it was unreasonable for Germany to pay the reparations, the requirement to do so must have resulted in great frustration. According to Arthur Solemssen, poverty and frustration left the German people vulnerable to the aggressive proposals of Hitler, which were laid before them as one way out of their misery. Hitler promised to return Germany to some kind of order (Solemssen 1980). The frustration that made the German people vulnerable to the aggressive proposals of Hitler was not limited to lower-status people. The middle-class and dominant people of power facilitated his rise. Churchill said it was "indispensable" that Hitler should make "an alliance with the governing elite." By 1932, he had "gained the allegiance of the controlling forces in Germany" (Churchill 1959, 13). The outcome of Hitler's rise to power in a frustrated Germany is the tragedy of unlimited social aggression operating on a tremendous scale.

Dealing with Frustration Personally and Socially

Beyond diagnosis of conditions under which the frustration-aggression hypothesis is applicable, this analysis seeks to understand how to adapt to and transcend frustration in an effective way. Several years ago, psychiatrist James Comer stated that adversity has the possibility of "turning one on" as well as "turning one off" (Comer 1972, 23). The goal of this section is to examine how to transcend frustration by successfully managing adversity. Frustration need not always lead to aggression.

A brief clarification of the definition of successful adaptation is needed: "It does not refer to adjustment to and acceptance of a racist [or sexist] environment in a fatalistic way. Indeed, a success response could be the attempt to transform a racist [or sexist] society or transcend it if transformation is impossible" (Willie 1977, 214). René DuBos makes a similar statement: "A successful life is not one without ordeal, failure and tragedies, but one during which the person has made an adequate number of effective responses to the constant challenges of his physical and social environment" (DuBos 1968, 162).

The responses of Black students to three situations at Syracuse University a few decades ago indicate the beneficial effects of dominants' and subdominants' embracing alternative forms of adaptation. The Blacks in that campus community were assertive, cooperative, and withdrawing. The multiple adaptive strategies that Blacks pursued proved to have survival value for their group and reformed the campus community in a positive fashion. Leighton points out that cooperation, or withdrawal, or assertiveness may be either a successful strategy or a failure, depending upon the person, the circumstances, and the interaction among these (Leighton 1946). No single approach can always be effective. Thus, flexibility in response to adversity is essential in making a successful adaptation.

Eight Black athletes were suspended from the Syracuse University football team because they boycotted spring training sessions. They boycotted spring practice as a way of registering their discontent over the all-White coaching staff. As a result of the boycott and the report of a trustee, faculty, and student committee appointed to investigate the controversy, the Black football players were reinstated and a Black assistant coach was hired. The investigating committee labeled the suspension of the Black athletes, "a form of institutional racism unworthy of a great university because the university had not taken into consideration the racist condition of an all White coaching staff that gave rise to the boycott" (Willie 1977, 215). Here, then, was a racist episode at a predominantly White university to which the Black students responded by withdrawing. This adaptive response was successful in that it achieved the students' intended goal.

A couple of years after the effective boycott, a fight broke out between Black and White students in a meeting of the Student Assembly of Syracuse University. The assembly had responsibility for allocating the student activity fee to student organizations. Black students said that they needed more funds to support their expanding programs, which an enlarged Black student group required. In rejecting the request for more funds, some White student representatives in the assembly made remarks that some of the Black students considered insulting. Beyond the fight, which probably was unnecessary, the assertiveness of the Blacks was manifested through continuous demonstration in front of a campus movie theater each evening while the final decision on their request was pending. The assertiveness of the Black students was intended to demonstrate that their request be treated equitably and seriously. While these demonstrations were in progress, the Student Assembly met, rescinded its earlier action of rejection, and voted to allocate the student Afro American Society a sum of money that was about four-fifths of the increased amount requested. The Syracuse University administration made up the difference so that there was full funding of the society's budget; peace and calm then returned to the campus. This was an adaptive, effective, and assertive response.

Shortly after this event, student body elections were held at Syracuse University for the leadership positions of the Student Association for undergraduates and the Graduate Student Organization. Black students were elected as the heads of each organization. These Black students were part of the student establishment and, therefore, represented the interests of all students at the University. A cooperative relationship between these student leaders and others was necessary to fulfill the functions of their offices. For these leaders, cooperation was an effective strategy that enabled them to gain a measure of control over campus decision making.

The African American students at Syracuse University were able to successfully adapt to their environment because they used a variety of strategies. They probably would not have been as successful if only one form of adaptation had been used in each of the three situations. It seems that flexibility and ingenuity are all useful in making successful adaptations to varying situations and their particular requirements. The activities of the Black students at Syracuse University were flexible; they were also successful because these students refused to cooperate in their own oppression. These flexible strategies are appropriate behavior for both dominants and subdominants.

The activities of the Black students at Syracuse University were effective, also, because they were rewarded by the establishment for their efforts. Rather than permanently suspending the Black athletes who brought to the university the bad news that its discriminatory employment practice for football coaches was racist, the university hired a Black assistant football coach and, after sufficient pressure was brought to bear on the Athletic Department, reinstated the student athletes who had boycotted spring practice. The students who demonstrated and peacefully disrupted an orderly campus community in the long run were rewarded with more funds to support expanded services for Blacks. Finally, the Black undergraduate and graduate student officers were rewarded with all the rights, privileges, and responsibilities pertaining to the new posts to which they were elected. This case study of minority-majority student interaction at one university is illustrative of the efficacy of using flexible strategies in community organization.

Likewise, the actions of a group of female graduate students at the Harvard Graduate School of Education is a second illustration of the benefits of a flexible approach to problem solving that includes assertiveness and cooperation. A small group of women enrolled in a professional degree program called Administration, Planning, and Social Policy (APSP) began meeting informally to share their campus experiences. A concern that arose during their discussions was the lack of attention paid to issues in education that are of particular interest to women. Also, group members had a common concern about the disproportionate use of male-oriented materials in courses and the absence of inclusive language in class lectures. The group met for several months and formulated an action plan.

After extensive research and preparation, the group presented its concerns to the APSP Department of the Harvard Graduate School of Education at a regularly scheduled faculty meeting. The women's group indicated the changes it wanted. Further, the group offered its members as change agents, if appropriately compensated. The members would help professors review syllabi for the purpose of eliminating non-inclusive language and adding readings that focus on issues of concern to women as well as men. The women's group was sufficiently assertive to persuade a predominantly male faculty to take effective action. Half of the membership of the women's group was hired the semester following the peaceful confrontation to review the course syllabi of several professors.

The women's group neglected to include people of color in its membership. The faculty might have questioned how serious the women's group was in attempting to achieve justice for all. Accordingly, the group invited women of a variety of racial and ethnic backgrounds to join. African American women, Latina, and women from other countries were asked to join the women's group and to embrace the agenda that had already been developed. This effort was unsuccessful, however. Women of color refused to participate because the mission and the focus of the group had been established without their input. By refusing to participate, the women of color forced the White women's group to come to terms with its own racially exclusive composition. Obviously, the racial exclusiveness of the women's group diminished its credibility as a potential promoter of diversity. Having had little success convincing women of color to join the group and adopt their already formulated agenda, the women's group realized that it had to find a way to become representative of all women on campus.

Another group consisting of male and female African American, Asian, Latino, Latina, and Native American students had been meeting regularly with faculty and administrators appointed by the dean of the Graduate School of Education to address issues of concern to all people of color at the school. The group had been successful in helping the school to recruit a multicultural student body, to recruit a faculty member of Latino background, and to retain two institutional programs that offered services to campus minorities and to the community.

The women's group asked for one of its issues to be placed on the agenda of the first spring monthly meeting of the coalition of people of color. During this meeting, the groups decided that they could be supportive of each other and that they could work on common issues together. Consequently, representatives from both groups met with the chair of the APSP department to press for action on their common concerns. By compromising and embracing a broader population and agenda, the women's group was able to continue and thrive as a vital force in the Harvard Graduate School of Education. These examples show how subdominant groups establish coalitions that are mutually beneficial to all participants.

We also examine how groups of the dominant people of power control behavior contraindicated for community living. The best way to control abusive behavior by individuals who believe they are entitled to do whatever they wish whenever they wish to do it because they are dominant is to punish them for violating the norms of fairness and the personhood of others. Reward has been recognized as a way of inducing people to behave in a prescribed way, but punishment should be recognized as equally important. Punishment is particularly appropriate for dominant people of power who aggress against others as a way of fulfilling the entitlement that they have self-righteously arrogated to themselves. Beyond controlling such behavior with punishment, we also explore ways to prevent it. To prevent dominant people of power from harming subdominants, the dominants should be informed by community authorities that all who violate mutually agreed upon customs of community living will experience immediate application of community sanctions in a firm and fair way. This message must become a community norm. The declaration that socially irresponsible behavior is unacceptable and will not be tolerated, among the high and mighty or among the meek and lowly, has a good chance of contributing to the achievement of community on the college campus and elsewhere. Our communities, including campus communities, have been reluctant to punish in a swift and decisive way dominant people of power who violate community norms.

Summary and Conclusion

This analysis demonstrates that the frustration-aggression hypothesis is applicable to a range of individuals and groups, including dominant people of power and subdominant people of power. It has also argued that dominants tend to adapt to frustration by outward aggression toward others, especially toward those who are members of the out group and who are usually subdominant. The pattern of adaptation to frustration among subdominants tends to be the opposite. Subdominants tend to adapt by way of inward aggression toward either themselves or toward other members of their own group.

Subdominants have demonstrated that the most effective way to adapt to frustration is to be flexible in action strategies. According to the requirements of the situation, such flexibility may dictate assertiveness, cooperation, or withdrawal as the most appropriate action to take. This discussion has pointed out how subdominant people of power can make an appropriate adaptation to a pluralistic learning environment and cope effectively with prejudice and discrimination if they are rewarded for their actions.

Aggression, particularly by dominant people of power against subdominant people of power, often is the outcome of the dominants' sense of entitlement. We call this attitude a pathological adaptation. It is found among some men who believe that "force is an acceptable means of acquiring . . . favors" (*Boston Globe* July 25, 1991). When Supreme Court Justice Roger Tanney, midway through the nineteenth century, said that Blacks have no rights that Whites were bound to respect, he was giving voice to a certainty of absolute entitlement that existed among some Whites. Robert Coles has described smug, self-satisfied, and self-centered people as manifesting narcissistic entitlement (Coles 1977). Such individuals tend to act out their anger when they are frustrated, targeting others unlike themselves as scapegoats. People who manifest such behavior should be punished if it harms others.

Thus, reward and punishment are ways of inducing people in a community to behave in prescribed and appropriate ways. However, punishment is a particularly effective way of controlling aggression resulting from frustration among dominants who exhibit the entitlement syndrome. And reward is an effective way of controlling aggression resulting from frustration among subdominants who suffer from self-preservation anxiety. By emphasizing the community sanctions of punishment as well as reward, intergroup hostility is recognized as arising from institutional factors as well as from interpersonal ones.

The prevention and control of attitudes of prejudice are of value; but these approaches also must be linked with methods that prevent and control actions of discrimination. No one has the right to hoard privileges for a special population without offering compensating opportunities to others.

REFERENCES

Allen, W. R. 1986. *Gender and campus race differences in black student academic performance, racial attitude, and college satisfaction.* Atlanta, Ga.: Southern Education Foundation.

Alves, Michael, and Willie, Charles V. 1990. Choice, decentralization, and desegregation. In *Choice and control in American education,* ed. William Clune and John Witte. New York: Palmer.

American Council on Education. 1989. *Eighth annual status report: minorities in higher education.* Washington, D.C.

Astin, Alexander W.
    1982. *Minorities in higher education.* San Francisco: Jossey-Bass.
    1989. *The American freshman, norms for fall 1989.* Los Angeles: American Council on Education and University of California at Los Angeles.

Bandelier, Adolf F. 1971. *The delight makers.* New York: Harcourt Brace Jovanovich.

Black Issues in Higher Education. 1990. Adams dismissal marks end of an era. Vol. 7, no. 11. August.

Black Issues in Higher Education. 1992. Vol. 9, no. 10. July 16.

Blackwell, James E. 1987. *Minorities in higher education.* San Francisco: Jossey-Bass.

Boston Globe.

1990. Macho stereotypes linked to sex abuse rate. August 15.

1991. Putting "PC" in its place. July 8.

1991. Why do some men think it's OK to commit rape? July 25.

Chronicle of Higher Education.

1989. *The Almanac of Higher Education 1990.* Chicago: University of Chicago Press.

1990a. New white students on some campuses are sparking outrage and worry. April 18.

1990b. Almanac. Washington, D.C. September 5.

1991. Organization of American Historians backs teaching of non-Western culture and diversity in schools. February 6.

Churchill, Winston, and the editors of *Life.* 1959. The Second World War. Vol. 1. New York: Time Inc.

Coles, Robert. 1977. *The privileged ones.* Boston: Little, Brown.

Comer, James. 1972. *Beyond Black and White.* New York: Quadrangle Books.

Dollard, John.

1938. Hostility and fear in social life. In *Readings in social psychology,* ed. Theodore M. Newcomb and Eugene L. Hartley. New York: Henry Holt.

1939. *Frustration or aggression.* New Haven: York University Press.

DuBos, René. 1968. *So human an animal.* New York: Scribner's.

Farrell, Walter, Jr., and Cloyzelle, James. 1988. Recent racial incidents in higher education: a preliminary perspective. *Urban Review* 20. Fall.

Fleming, John E. 1984. Blacks in higher education to 1954: a historical overview. In *Black students in higher education,* ed. Gail Thomas. Westport: Greenwood Press.

Foley, Albert S. 1981. Mobile, Alabama: the demise of state-sanctioned resistance. In *Community politics and educational change,* ed. Charles V. Willie and Susan L. Greenblatt, pp. 174–207. New York: Longman.

Franklin, J. H. 1967. *From slavery to freedom.* 3d ed. New York: Knopf.

Gillespie, Dairl. 1979. Who has the power? the marital struggle. In *Socialization and the Life Cycle,* ed. Peter Rose. New York: St. Martin's Press.

Information Please Almanac. 1989. Boston: Houghton Mifflin.

Jaynes, Gerald, and Williams, Robin, eds. 1989. *A common destiny: Blacks in American society.* Washington, D.C.: National Academy Press.

Kardiner, Abraham, and Ovesey, Lionel. 1962. *The mark of oppression.* Ohio: Meridan.

Leighton, Alexander H. 1946. *The governing of men.* Princeton: Princeton University Press.

Linton, Calvin D. 1985. *American headlines year by year.* New York: Thomas Nelson.

Martin, Patricia Yancy, and Hummer, Robert A. 1989. Fraternities and rape on campus. *Gender and Society* 3:457–73.

National Institute Against Prejudice and Violence. 1992. *Forum* 6:1–12. March.

National Center for Educational Statistics. 1988. *Digest of educational statistics.* Washington, D.C.: U.S. Government Printing Office.

Nettles, Michael T. 1988. *Toward black undergraduate student equality in higher education.* Westport, Conn.: Greenwood Press.

New Columbia Encyclopedia. 1975. New York: Columbia University Press.

Newsweek.

1990. December 24.

1991. The new politics of race. May 6.

New York Times. 1990. Duke scholar's group accused of bias, divides faculty. October 21.

O'Brien, Eileen. 1990. Adams dismissal marks end of an era. *Black issues in higher education.* August, no. 11.

Ordway, John A. 1973. Some emotional consequences of racism for Whites. In *Racism and mental health*, ed. C. V. Willie, B. M. Kramer, and B. S. Brown. Pittsburgh: University of Pittsburgh Press.

Osherson, Samuel. 1986. *Finding our fathers*. New York: Fawcett.

Pettigrew, Thomas. 1971. *Racially separate or together*. New York: McGraw-Hill.

Solemssen, Arthur. 1980. *A princess in Berlin*. New York: Ballantine Books.

Stanley, Manfred. 1978. *The technological conscience*. New York: Free Press.

Stimpson, Catharine R. 1991. New "politically correct" metaphors insult history and our campuses. *Chronicle of Higher Education*. May 29.

Thomas, Gail, ed. 1981. *Black students in higher education*. Westport, Conn.: Greenwood Press.

U.S. Census Bureau.

    1965. *Statistical abstract of the United States*. Washington, D.C.: U.S. Government Printing Office.

    1990. *Statistical abstract of the United States*. Washington, D.C.: U.S. Government Printing Office.

U.S. Department of Education. 1989. The condition of education. *Postsecondary education*. Vol. 2. Washington, D.C.: U.S. Government Printing Office.

U.S. Department of Labor. 1965. *The negro family*. Washington, D.C.: U.S. Government Printing Office.

Willie, Charles V.

    1977. *Black/Brown/White relations*. New Brunswick: Transaction Books.

    1983. *Race, ethnicity and socioeconomic status*. Dix Hills, N.Y.: General Hall.

Willie, Charles V., and Greenblatt, Susan L., eds. 1981. *Community politics and educational change*. New York: Longman.

Willie, Charles V., and McCord, Arline. 1972. *Black students at White colleges*. Westport, Conn.: Praeger.

World Almanac Book of Facts. 1988. New York: Pharus.

Wright, Richard. 1941. *Twelve million Black voices*. New York: Viking.

Stress Analogs of Racism and Sexism: Terrorism, Torture, and Disaster

THE victims of racism and sexism are stressed by unrelenting oppression and discrimination. The oppression and discrimination is distributed on an individual and group basis. It may be overt or covert, acute or chronic, mental or physical. It varies in intended seriousness from lethal hatred to subclinical amusement. For the victim, depending on perceptions and circumstances, the stress may seem omnipresent and ubiquitous. It is therefore common for many, if not most, victims of racism and sexism to believe at some time that their lives are in danger, because of actual or threatened terrorizing and torture from the oppressor.

Much of the conscious activity of any victim of racism and sexism is devoted toward elaborating and applying adaptive techniques. These techniques dilute, postpone, or deflect stress about anxieties of disaster, terror, and torture that could be brought about by an oppressive individual or collective. Yet the dread usually is unformulated, perhaps because people need certainty, security, and stability in their lives. Powerful active and passive denial mechanisms allow victims to coexist with oppressors, even at the cost of participating in and permitting much of their own catastrophe. On the other hand, most Whites and males are largely oblivious to the stress they create merely by their potential for exerting power. Almost all oppressors are unmindful of the withering effects of cumulative, individual, and collective microaggressions toward victims, even honestly believing that they themselves have inflicted no damage upon socially devalued persons.

An important need is to reveal and illuminate the origins and structure of the blind spots and the taken-for-granted but less examined mundane features of victimization and oppression in racism and sexism. Even in obvious, gross, and extreme instances of terrorism, torture, and disaster, these features often are found to be critical and persuasive in how any individual or group performs and survives. This essay is intentionally theoretical and discursive. It proposes to highlight analogues between the stress of disaster, terrorism, and torture and the dynamics of racism and sexism. It will be based upon study of the literature on stress, torture, terrorism, and disaster. In addition, it will draw largely on personal experience of a Black clinician and consultant who has done research on animals and humans. The personal experiences pertinent to this essay include: professional concerns related to space travel; cultural translocations of sojourners; adjustment of submariners and persons in the Arctic and the Antarctic; military and civilian incarcerations during war and peace; media analysis; observations on drilling rigs and in refugee camps; observations of sufferers in mass disasters; problems in elite athletic performance; studies in police-community relations; experiments in racial psychodynamics; and the subjugation of animals.

Stress in Racism and Sexism

Inherent Problems

The academic study of racism and sexism in the United States is hampered by inherent operational prejudices that are institutionalized and widely applied and that produce and sustain stress in the victim. Especially in the investigation of racism, three of the most pernicious are these variations:

- Almost always in academic studies the dominating agent uses the submissive agent as the target to be understood, helped, analyzed, categorized, altered, and controlled. Hardly ever is the dominator the subject of study by the dominated.
- Almost never in academic studies is the viewpoint of the submissive agent sought. If it is sought or considered, there is frequently a conscious or unconscious presumption that it is trivial, irrelevant, marginal, or even immature, miniature, and worthless.
- Almost exclusively the dominant agent serves as gatekeeper and arbiter of what is published or taught, as well as when, where, and how it is published or taught.

It cannot be argued that theories and studies created by minorities or females would be superior to those created by Whites and males. It can be argued, however, that such work might be different and could lead to new perspectives and resolutions. Further, the elimination of these operational prejudices would relieve stress in the academic community and perhaps ultimately in the community at large.

Another set of inherent difficulties that must be acknowledged in considering the stress of racism and sexism exhibits more obvious parallels with individuals in classic situations of terror, torture, and disaster. These difficulties are as indifferent to tides and wind as they are to political ideology or philosophical assumptions. They are found commonly in any dominant-submission pattern, whether it be a coach-player, parent-child, teacher-student, White-Black, male-female, employer-employee relationship, or any situation rife with terror and grief. These fundamental questions must be addressed in any submission-dominance engagement: (1) Can both the oppressed and the oppressor be happy and content at the same time? (2) When, how, where, and how much does the oppressed resist victimization, versus when, how, where, and how much does the oppressed accommodate oppression? (3) How does the oppressed differentiate when a dominant agent's actions and/or words represent an individual viewpoint versus when they represent a collective viewpoint? (4) When there seems to be some degree of acceptance or validation, how does the oppressed recognize when this acceptance indicates being wanted or welcomed, versus when it indicates being merely tolerated or needed?

The need to resolve this set of problems is daily, regular, and ceaseless in many submission-dominance dyads including those involving race or sex. The manner and thoroughness of their resolutions generate the quality and quantity of stress produced and sustained in these interactions.

Common Traits in Racism and Sexism

Besides the need to handle these inherent problems, there are other common traits in racism and sexism that also are seen in those who are captive to terrorists or torturers, or who suffer from disastrous conditions. In all these situations, there are forces compelling people to do what they might not otherwise do. In all these situations the victim is challenged, often beyond available resources, to maintain hope, options, self-esteem, and group esteem. Complete subjugation in any of the analogous conditions is attained when one individual or group is so compliant to another individual or group that the defeated are bereft of hope, option, self- and group esteem.

The oppressive agent or situation promotes an unrelenting devaluation, manifested by controlling the victim's space, time, energy, and motion (STEM). The more rigid and unyielding this control, the more victimized the individual or group. All blind spots and mundane features of stress are aggravated in this control by factors that increase unpredictability and unexpectedness in the victims' lives. These factors are intensified also by control or disruption of vegetative functions including eating, sleeping, urinating, and defecating. This cluster of traits tends to make any victim feel diminished and tyrannized, whether observed in a prisoner of war being brainwashed, an upper-middle-class mother of a newborn child, or a homeless man in an inner city. The negative end result of oppression is a shattered self-image, a failure in adaptation, a hatred and dissatisfaction about one's own group and self. There is also a tendency to dwell on what cannot be done, rather than a devising of what can be done to alleviate the duress. By the time this result is reached, the victim feels and believes that on every tomorrow no new support will appear.

A working definition of stress: When one lacks support, one is stressed. Hypothetically, if one had perfect support, biologically, sociologically, and psychologically, stress would not exist. For victims of racism and sexism, the relative lack of support defines the degree of stress. Therefore, clarifying and reinforcing the types and sites of needed support offers preventive, intervening, and curative possibilities. In both racism and sexism there is a never-ending struggle by a designated, demeaned group to obtain sufficient support, so that offenders can no longer abuse, exploit, injure, and humiliate solely because of an individual's skin color or gender. This submission-dominance struggle describes racism and sexism.

Many participants on every ideological side agree that what is essential about this struggle is the presumption of inferiority in a target group, which allows the "superiors" to enjoy prerogatives with the "inferiors" that they would never exercise among themselves. Even when abundant evidence is presented to invalidate these claims of inferiority, they are not abandoned. The persistence of a false belief in the face of contrary evidence constitutes delusional thinking.

By this definition probably everyone indulges in some "delusional thinking." This makes racism and sexism intrinsic variables in almost all social, political, and economic interactions. Americans have continued for decades to be held hostage to this delusional thinking. Many would agree that the ramifications of delusional thinking have led to tragic consequences both in the United States and in the rest of the world. Perhaps more would agree that such a delusion, at minimum, has retarded and abbreviated overall development of the potential of humankind.

Consequences of Submission-Dominance

In racism and sexism, as in all submission-dominance relationships, the chief consequences follow from the curbing of space, time, energy, and freedom of mobility of the victim. A major consequence is that the victim becomes "defensive" in thought. Defensive thinking then becomes increasingly necessary as the victim must anticipate assaults and offensive strategies from the dominator. These assaults may come from any direction, at any time or place. Any person required to manage more uncertainty and unpredictability becomes increasingly wary and hypervigilant. In essence, the victim's thinking becomes more focused on general monitoring and surveillance tasks needed to thwart expected and unexpected offenses.

The thinking process is defensive in that it is tentative, apologetic, deferential, and impressionistic. It is rapid, since decision making incorporates the anticipation of incessant racial and sexual assaults. It perhaps makes the victim more sensitive to appraising end-result or summative aspects of situations rather than to processing concerns and formative aspects of situations. It stresses the victim even more because often one's plight is to possess defensive responsibility without commensurate authority, liberty, or power.

Probably the most grievous of offensive mechanisms spewed at victims in racism and sexism are microaggressions. These are subtle, innocuous, preconscious, or unconscious degradations, and putdowns, often kinetic but capable of being verbal and/or kinetic. In and of itself a microaggression may seem harmless, but the cumulative burden of a lifetime of microaggressions can theoretically contribute to diminished mortality, augmented morbidity, and flattened confidence. An example of a microaggression: the lone Black among a group of seventy full professors is asked to move the chairs so a meeting can commence. Another: a White female passenger joins two male seat companions who occupy a middle and window seat on an airplane. By chance, she is on the aisle, seated next to a Black man. Immediately she turns on a light, although no one else in the plane has done so because it is broad daylight. Wordlessly, she shows she is agitated, perhaps fearful. Across the aisle from her are seated three White men. The man nearest her, sensing her distress, gallantly says, "Perhaps you'd be more comfortable sitting here." With almost palpable relief, she sighs gratefully, "Oh yes, yes, thank you!" They exchange seats. She is now still seated on an aisle next to two men—White men. Most astonishing and galling from the viewpoint of the offended Black: as soon as the gallant White man sits down next to him, he attempts to initiate friendly small talk, probably to make the White feel good about himself and for the Black to indicate happy acceptance of the insult. The Black passenger, afflicted by another set of microaggressions by Whites, suffers additional stress. For him these racially inspired microaggressions represent simultaneously a microterror, a microdisaster, and a microtorture.

The most baffling task for victims of racism and sexism is to defend against microaggressions. Knowing how and when to defend requires time and energy that oppressors cannot appreciate. Gauging, titrating, regulating, expressing appropriate, safe outrage is never an easy task, even though one may handle thousands of microaggressions in a lifetime. However, in a real sense, one's adaptation to the stress of a dominator depends on how well one defends self-image, how carefully one selects which microaggressions to defend against, to deflect, or to allow to pass. Most microaggressions have to be allowed to pass, to protect one's time, energy, sanity, or bodily integrity. Racism and sexism then are stress-related public health illnesses. They can be approached in terms of questions about segregation, quarantine, and immunization. Answers must be found relative to who is afflicted, who afflicts, and why they afflict.

Similarities Among Analogs

Terrorism, torture, disaster, racism, and sexism are all stressful and may be viewed in terms of submission-dominance patterns. In addition, sometimes they are simultaneously congruent, complimentary, and supplementary. A medical model could classify all of them as public health illnesses manifested by stress to *all* participants. Therefore, these represent public health illnesses such as smallpox since they affect masses of people, are unresponsive to treatment on a one-by-one basis; would require large sums of money to eradicate; and would leave biological, social, and psychological sequelae when eliminated.

As customarily defined, terrorism is actual or threatened violence to gain attention for non-criminal political purposes, which in turn cause people to exaggerate the strength of the terrorists and the importance of their cause. Often the methods are deliberately shocking. In the submission-dominance engagement between races and sexes, the oppressor frequently meets the definition of a terrorist. The aim of the terrorist is to inspire fear. For example, the victim of a wife-batterer may fear for her life. She makes constant and deliberate accommodation to her husband's wrath. She realizes that swift and hearty acknowledgment of her husband's "cause," no matter what it is, may be lifesaving.

Similarly, a definition of torture may be conceptualized as being congruent with racism or sexism, especially at the micro as opposed to the macro end of a continuum of definition. The World Medical Association (1975) definition of torture is "deliberate, systematic infliction of physical and mental suffering to induce confessions or to obtain information for any reason." In this general sense, majority people and males are torturers. The oppressor extracts and uses information to control space, time, energy, and movement (STEM). Probably there are few Blacks who have not heard of chilling sabotage to a fellow Black employee by a Black informant. The Black informant is motivated by a perceived or actual need to act, or else lose his or her own job. In such instances, the White employer's institutionalized expectations meet the definition of torture. The aim of the torturer is to strengthen control. As will be discussed later, torture terrorizes victims and others into conforming. In this sense, torture and terror both function to shape victims and victimizers into accepting an etiquette based on supreme advantage for the oppressor. For the oppressed such acceptance can be disastrous—again on a micro-to-macro continuum of definition.

Disaster is a sudden departure from the expected that is of sufficient magnitude to require relief and assistance; it is associated with physical and/or mental trauma and/or environmental loss. Tragic end results of oppression such as unemployment and wife-battering are disasters for the victims. Incidentally, it may be that environmental loss is particularly underemphasized even though it is commonplace. For example, the "Not in My Backyard" syndrome almost always implies or suggests that environmental degradation is more acceptable in Black neighborhoods or Black countries, that is, wherever the oppressor deems it best suits the purposes and convenience of STEM.

Disaster, torture, and terror—like racism and sexism—are public health illnesses, which often overlap in their structure, function, and definition. Therefore, they can be studied together to see how each informs the other in approaches to research, education, or service. In this way, perhaps we can find new methods for prevention, intervention, and rehabilitation.

Public Health and Violence

Besides an inherent relationship to stress, these public health illnesses all have an inherent relationship to violence. For the victims both stress and violence speak to noxious stimuli, situations, or persons. Surcease for victims arrives only by diluting these conditions, being removed from the conditions, or having the conditions removed from the victims. For victims of these public health illnesses, violence and stress are oppressive, dehumanizing, and offensive. These illnesses place the victims on the defensive by life-threatening infringement of STEM. Often the inciter of the action displays demonstrable physical and/or mental disdain, disrespect, or indifference for the victim.

In the history of science it has proved valuable to congregate similar phenomena as a method of expediting progress. For example, the design of the periodic table in chemistry enabled accurate predictions to be made about the behavior of closely related elements. Nosological categorizations helped advance prognosis, treatment, and prevention of illness. Perhaps some benefit may result from studying racism and sexism by speculating that they are part of a group of public health illnesses characterized by stress and violence, which includes terrorism, torture, and many features found in persons in the midst of natural or artificial disaster.

As in many illnesses there is a range of manifestations and complications that can be generated. In any population, as well, there are people who are variously affected or spared, or who are subjected to exacerbated difficulties on an episodic, cyclic, or phasic basis. The public health questions of "Who gets sick? when? how? and why do they get sick?" are as pertinent to offenders and offended in racism and sexism as they are to participants in conditions of disaster, torture, or terror. The variability in vulnerability demands more investigation of both so-called normal and abnormal responses in all these conditions. The practical problem is to define who does well and discover why they do so, despite exposure to situations that tend to make one a victim or a victimizer. Perhaps the crucial psychodynamics are how resolutions are managed in an ongoing submission-dominance contest involving conflicts about entitlement, depreciation, and capitulation.

Crucial Psychodynamics

The most harrowing management problem in these analogs is how to recognize and eliminate entitlement dysfunctions in all the relevant participants. Clashes of entitlement arise from either the aggressor, the aggrieved, or both. The participants may be designated or potential dominator versus designated or potential subordinate. Entitlement dysfunctions are real or imagined conflicts, microscopic or macroscopic. Interpersonal confrontations about prestige and status are more expressed, more salient, and more important than frustrations and obstacles resulting from problems concerning sex, dependency, and aggression.

Basically, in entitlement dysfunctions, perceptual differences exist among communicants regarding rights, duties, obligations, and privileges. These dysfunctions concern which, if any, person, agency, collective, or institution has coercive and regulatory hegemony over the issue being considered. Typically, as in racism and sexism, the issue involves a perception of disrespectful, undignified use, misuse, or abuse of someone's time, space, energy, or freedom of movement. Thus an important ingredient in the consideration of these illnesses speaks to the zeal and priority by which an individual or group seeks or maintains pride, as well as the sensitivity and quality of respect one person or group must—or should—show to another individual or group.

Closely related to the psychodynamics of entitlement dysfunction are feelings of depreciation. These feelings come about from guilt, shame, and impotent rage over allowing some person, group, or inanimate force to impress its will on an individual or group. The bottom line for the successful victimizer is to gain power to impress one's will on another. This is seen readily in everyday interactions in the United States between races and sexes. What is less obvious but increasingly well documented from the other analogs is that the victimizers and other observers might also suffer from identical feelings, often at a later time. For example, a torturer, seemingly content to do his terrible deeds, may later develop serious symptomatology, understood to be a direct or indirect result of the grisly performances. Perhaps, often, victimizers feel obliged to be oppressive for reasons that they feel they do not understand or that are beyond their control.

Similarly, for the designated disfranchised in situations of racism, sexism, torture, terror, or disaster, there is a need to focus on if, when, and how one should capitulate. Too ready and too easy capitulation often aggravates depreciation and verifies one's submission in terms of entitlement for respect. This amounts to a self-validation of one's inferiority. Yet too slow and too difficult a capitulation could be fatal. On the other hand, failure to exact capitulation may be unpardonable for the would-be victimizing terrorist or torturer. So the victimizer also is enthralled by conflicts about capitulation. And, of course, there is no solace for the victim that these conflicts of capitulation and depreciation may—at the time or later—cause even slight discomfort and problems for the tormentor.

The submission-dominance psychodynamic considerations stemming from the triad of conflicts of entitlement, self-depreciation, and capitulation are germane to the public health because they are intrinsically stressful and potentially dangerous for all participants. When this triad is too overwhelming for any person or group, hopelessness is born. Hopelessness and its mirror image, foreclosure of options, are the chief enemies of any who roam in climates of threat and danger, such as those occurring in situations of disaster, torture, or terror, as well as those curbed by racism and sexism.

The literature on torture, terrorism, and disaster—unlike the literature on racism and sexism—its more devoted to understanding and helping victims by studying successful adaptation. If analogs hold, then perhaps a search for common strengths exhibited or required for successful adaptation in situations of terrorism, torture, and disaster would be particularly useful in providing insights into overcoming racism and sexism.

Before seeking some of these distillates, some minimal important background considerations about torture, terrorism, and disaster must be understood. These considerations also emphasize the public health role in disorders of violence or stress.

Torture and Terrorism

From the viewpoint of the sufferer, existential questions are prominent. Sufferers stay preoccupied with questions such as "Why me?" "Can I survive?" and "How do I minimize the brutality and callous disregard?" Terror and torture both aim at producing physiological and psychological distress. Preferably this distress must be accomplished in such a way that if there are survivors, none can be elevated to martyrdom in the eyes of other victims, victimizers, or other relevant audiences. Similarly, it is preferable that no survivor should leave the encounter in such a way that he or she can be unequivocal and copious in self-congratulation about his or her performance during the event. An example: A newly graduated Black MBA arrived at an investment firm. His superiors gave him a portfolio that they knew would generate noticeably less income than those given to White peers who entered the firm at the same time. To the enormous surprise of his superiors, by a combination of creativity, daring, and chance, the Black employee made one of the largest profits the company had ever enjoyed. While making this profit, the Black felt tortured by threats, hypersurveillance, and isolation in terms of performance evaluations. Traditionally, in the firm, a major success such as he had achieved was rewarded by a generous bonus, a large salary increase, and a promotion to a vice-presidency. In this instance, he was offered only a modest salary increase. Shocked and discouraged by these events, this man entered an entirely different profession.

As in the torture and terror of racism and sexism, much of the success of these aims, from the viewpoint of the aggressor, depends on deliberate or inadvertent cooperation and/or control of a variety of media, especially over an indefinite period of time. The tighter the control, the greater the array of channels of media involved and the longer the time available about a message, the more likely the aggressor is to convince victims, victimizers, and any other relevant audiences that certain actions and behavior are in everyone's best interest. Thus if every textbook, statue, billboard, magazine and newspaper ad, television program, radio newscast, and civic ritual reinforces a message, it will be seen as typical, desirable, and probable. There will be little tendency to resist it, and everyone might be persuaded and indoctrinated to its reasonableness and appropriateness. The aggrieved may be particularly compliant to the message, even as they suffer progressive stress, violence, and loss of freedom. The victims become isolated, unable to organize effective action against the message.

An example: A tardy arrival at a soirée of privileged middle-class Blacks mentioned that his plane had been late. Then he joked that the plane had a Black pilot. After a round of guffaws, he quipped that when he spied the Black pilot he didn't know whether or not to get on the plane. These victims, by their own acceptance of stereotypes about Black abilities and competence, demonstrated pro-racism, a principle basis for perpetuating the etiquette for submission-dominance. Yet, too, the important and well-known role of humor in overcoming adversity must not be discounted. But humor can also be based on rejecting stereotypes, glorifying the oppressed, and empowering the victim. It need not perpetuate only dangerous messages.

Meanwhile, terrorists and torturers find it easier to increase anxiety in the victims, often by resorting to blatant theatrics. With the aggrieved in disarray, the aggressors find it easier to work and train together, and to support each other, thereby gaining more sympathizers. It is known now that what binds the terrorist or torturer is loyalty to a cause and the repetition of aggressive acts. To obtain such boundless, often mindless loyalty, one selects "normal" people and makes them believe they are elite and superior to a designated dehumanized group. With the provision of special privileges and indulgences, particularly in comparison to a despised or weak "them," the process of loyalty binding is complete and sustaining. To break or modify this cycle is the task of all champions of sufferers from racism, sexism, terrorism, and torture. In all instances what seems monumental, if not implacable, is how to persuade "normals" that it is in their best interest to relinquish advantages that not only seem natural to them but often have been granted to them formally by church and state and informally by family and society.

It may require dedicated craftiness, courage, and systematic enterprise to select the kind and amount of defense the sufferer should launch against such entrenchment. The weight of history shows, however, that some combination of consciousness raising, informing public opinion, and confrontation can alter power relationships. Unfortunately, history may bear witness, too, to the fact that it is insufficient to change the aggregate behavior of victimizers merely by getting them to become aware or even outraged. Some members of the group of aggrieved victims must be able and willing to sacrifice themselves at great cost, in order to demonstrate to their oppressors that it is no longer in the interests of the oppressors to continue their exploitation.

Social scientists and mental health workers need to contribute whatever they can toward understanding what creates entitlement in torturers and terrorists. "Normal" Whites and "normal" males continue to enjoy advantages in spite of turbulent struggle in recent decades. Yet there seems to be little academic understanding of how these attitudes develop in White children and in males of all races. Especially lacking is the understanding of how and why females in their undoubtedly enormous socializing roles as mothers and grade school teachers continue to shape "normal" Whites and "normal" males to expect as unremarkable that they should have privileges and prerogatives that minorities and females do not have.

Like torturers and terrorists, sexists and racists believe what they do is good and significant. Similarly, the results of this "good and significant" behavior damage individuals, families, and communities. The damaged people develop a gamut of acute or chronic symptoms including fear, tension, somatic complaints, withdrawal, phobias, guilt, and sleep disturbances. The imposed psychosocial burdens put them at risk of becoming pathogenetic to others, including their victimizers.

Disaster

For victims of terrorism, torture, sexism, or racism, life can be disastrous. At any given time, this disaster may be conceived of as being mundane or exotic for the individual. It may be more or less intense, and its scope may range from a gross disaster to a mini- or a microdisaster. However it is conceptualized in the person's life, the disaster is associated with some degree of danger and a corresponding abbreviation of spatial and temporal fields in consequence of the unusual situation.

The result of any endured disaster is unpredictable because it is modified in many ways by the specific circumstances. For instance, one may be better prepared or more knowledgeable about the circumstances. The magnitude of disruption to crucial systems—including communications systems—will vary. The duress may vary according to distance and affect the individual's perception of its significance. Help of some sort may prove more abundant or more adequate. The individual's defense system may be stronger or weaker depending on factors such as one's hope, one's ability to gather vital information, one's religious or spiritual resistance, and one's repertoire of psychological mechanisms such as numbing, denial, or projection. Finally, the victim's physical and mental state before and after the disaster is a governing factor in vulnerability for morbidity of any sort as well as the risk for death.

What may be more predictable is that however one responds to a disaster, including disastrous racist and sexist events, a smoother resolution, is achieved when the person quickly mobilizes short- and long-term defenses and has some means to quickly desensitize the event. This usually includes being able to give a rigorous, honest, but appreciative evaluation of one's negotiation of the event. Formative and summative assessment is necessary in managing any disaster. What elements of one's environment should be included in such an assessment depends on one's judgment and accuracy regarding the extent of the disaster, how it has or might touch oneself, other victims, victimizers, caretakers, and other family and community members.

A target for racism or sexism can feel as if his or her life is in a disaster, characterized by features of terrorism and torture. Frequently one seems to be dislocated and held captive in an extreme situation. What can be distilled from the experiences of survivors of disasters, terrorism, and torture that might be helpful for research in the prevention or treatment of racism and sexism?

Selected Distillates

Captivity

A person in a disaster is captive to an unwanted, unpleasant situation. Everything is focused on and revolves about the captivity. Those who do best in captivity demonstrate the importance of having strong convictions. Also an ability for effective group cooperation probably enhances both the likelihood of survival and its quality. Important components for prisoner-of-war survival include prior knowledge regarding the conditions of imprisonment; staying active; keeping one's personal integrity; one's desire to live. Following the disaster of captivity with reentry into the general society, there is a need to consolidate and integrate. This requires some ability to "forgive and forget."

Perhaps the importance of a cause has most relevance for racism and sexism. A cause can keep integrity robust. Those prisoners who did well had a strong belief in God, country, family, and companions. They were proud of their identity as military personnel and maintained it. They had faith that their families would survive.

Prisoners' own knowledge of what to expect also was critical. It was important to know that one might become fearful of fellow inmates or that one would have to develop some tolerance for others' human foibles, such as crime, theft, drug use, graft, sexual behaviors, and collaboration. Being prepared realistically for appropriate followership or leadership, as well as for having to undergo grief for fellow companions was also helpful.

Those who did well had an admirable situational plasticity. They could make obligatory modifications and adjustments, while staying busy, occupied, and structured over an indefinite time.

Keeping alive included having patience and recalling the good past, while expecting a good future. Of lifesaving importance was to know how to obtain the truth from the captor; or how to obfuscate the truth, and knowing when and how much truth you should yield to the captor. Many may find it surprising or instructive to learn that keeping alive included preserving a modicum of hatred for the captor.

These articles of faith, tenacity, captor-interaction, and group cohesion might translate into areas to pursue in the study of racism or sexism. Similarly, there are lessons from those in disasters that might be useful for those caught in the disasters of racism and sexism.

Extremity

In disaster a victim feels daunted and diminished by the unusual and extraordinary. Almost routinely one can predict in extreme situations that the habitués will feel intense ambivalence and anger toward those who are not in their plight. The outside others will be seen as uncaring, insensitive, selfish, uninterested, and uninformed. Yet, almost always, any person in this plight recognizes at some level that relief from stress and even survival may depend on these outside others.

Those who are caught in extreme situations must cherish hope and do for themselves, while expecting support from outside others. Even when the support is safely and reasonably assured, compounding issues concern the quality, willingness, abundance, appropriateness, and timeliness of support. Those who do well in extreme situations generally have fewer doubts and conflicts about support. At the same time, those who do well can believe they are capable of helping themselves. Furthermore, they are clear, strong, and satisfied about the importance and urgency of what they must achieve. Abundant feedback from relevant sources frequently has engendered and sustained these positive valuations.

To do well in situations of racism and sexism the oppressed must take decisive actions while striving toward goals that are understood, applauded, and approved. At the same time they must do all they can to feel confident and secure about the existence of outside support. All this helps reduce feelings of captivity and dislocation.

Dislocation

In disaster, a victim is dislocated and forced uncomfortably from customary behavior, thoughts, and goals. Fire drills and life-boat drills give testimony that there is value in individuals being prepared in advance for the unforeseen. This amounts to anticipatory guidance for a potential victim. Theoretically, the more the potential victim knows about a disaster, the more effectively will he or she respond in an emergency.

Related to anticipatory guidance is vulnerability awareness. This concept assumes that the more an individual knows about what might occur in a strange situation, the better that person can prevent disaster. Racism and sexism may well require dedicated educative anticipatory guidance and vulnerability awareness for everyone. As with persons dislocated by disaster, sufferers of racism and sexism may have to mobilize themselves to contend with fear, distrust, ignorance, or ineptitude when seeking available help. Overcoming these barriers while realizing that one is exploited by discriminatory or whimsical disadvantages can engender exquisite grief.

Just as in the case of disaster, the ability to function after the impact of a racist or sexist event or circumstance varies from individual to individual. Usually, most will be able to continue to function at some level. Predictably, some will have an emotional and cognitive disruption that leaves them defeated, dependent, and resigned. A scientific objective in disaster, as well as in racism and sexism, is to sharpen the ability to detect what conditions influence which persons toward effective adjustment.

Conclusion

The possibility seems quite remote that racism or sexism can be eliminated in the next quarter of a century. The goal of total elimination should remain the standard, but the immediate steps should be to dilute and diminish these negative forces.

This chapter has presented theoretical similarities among racism, sexism, torture, terrorism, and disaster. It is postulated that knowledge from any one of these public health menaces is useful in understanding the others. Since all relate to submission-dominance dynamics, they represent struggles for control on a matrix of gross to microscopic stress and violence.

Mathematically, victimization is defined by the degree of control an oppressor has over the space, time, energy, and freedom of movement of the oppressed. The more the oppressed can regain command or control over space, time, energy, and freedom of movement, the less he or she is oppressed. Such mathematical postulates allow oppression to be measured and objectified. Such measurements might lead to newer, more effective methods of cure and prevention of victimization.

Functionally, victimization has developed because of legal, economic, social, and even religious factors. There is also a long history of an etiquette among victims of racism and sexism, in which they themselves have given over gratuitously and unbidden much of their own space, time, energy, and freedom of movement. To dilute victimization and to work toward its elimination, the oppressed must attend simultaneously to both these developmental and etiquette obstacles. In an ideal world, at least some oppressors would join in the search for discovering why it is not in their own best interests to continue insisting upon domination.

The academic world reflects society at large. It must somehow rectify its own extensive institutional involvement in racism and sexism. In the instance of racism, the ripe areas of academic concern for social scientists and mental health specialists include propaganda analysis, group dynamics, and child development. Knowledge in all these areas might be advanced by scrutinizing what is known about torture, terrorism, and disaster. It may be true that those who do best against the horrors and inequity of racism are similar to those who do best against the awfulness of torture, terrorism, and disaster. In all cases decided benefits accrue if one has extensive cognitive awareness and if one retains unshakable hope. To decrease racism, the awareness and hope of both potential victim and potential victimizer must be guided and shaped so that both see it as not advantageous to engage in draining submission-dominance contests based on skin color.

For many decades persons who have endured duress have developed symptoms given such labels as "post–traumatic stress syndrome," "shell shock," and "traumatic neurosis." Some persons who endure racism and sexism—like those who have suffered terrorism, torture, and disaster— also must develop these symptoms. Yet there is a more challenging and immense chore to address in the future. We must classify and understand which perpetrators and victims of racism and sexism develop continuing and perhaps cumulative symptoms. We must learn why some may be relatively immune to or more easily cured of perpetrating or suffering from racism and sexism.

From a Black perspective at the close of the twentieth century, racism and sexism continue to be public health menaces. They feature receiving or delivering violence at both gross and microscopic levels. Racism and sexism can result in post–traumatic stress syndrome, with possibilities of compounding "continuing traumatic stress syndrome."

Since the writing of this essay, the "Rodney King Riots" have occurred in Los Angeles. It is not a mere academic exercise to study and treat torture, terrorism, and racism together. Many American people, minority and White, when viewing the tape of Rodney King being beaten with disgusting brutality by Los Angeles policemen, have no trouble believing racism, torture, and terrorism exist together very comfortably. The astonishing verdict in this case, not surprisingly, precipitated grievous, costly, and disastrous counterviolence against the maldistribution of entitlements in the United States. It turns out that the three barbaric, stress-violent human rights abuse illnesses (racism, torture, terrorism), are all entitlement dysfunctions, which significantly disrupt the public health and the very fabric of the society.

REFERENCES

Gibson, Janice T., and Haritos-Fatouros, Mika. 1986. The education of a torturer. *Psychology Today* (November): 50–58.

Goldstein, R. H., and Breslin, P. 1986. Technicians of torture. *The Sciences* (April): 14–19.

Green, B. L., Lindy, J. D., Grace, M. C., Gleser, G. C., Leonard, A. C., Korol, M., and Winget, C. 1990. Buffalo Creek survivors in the second decade: stability of stress symptoms. *Am J Orthopsychiatry* 60:43–54. January.

Jones, D. R. 1985. Secondary disaster victims: the emotional effects of recovering and identifying human remains. *Am J Psychiat* 142:303–7. March.

Mollica, R. F. 1988. The trauma story: the psychiatric care of refugee survivors of violence and torture. In *Post-traumatic therapy and victims of violence,* ed. F. M. Ochberg. New York: Brunner/Mazel.

Pierce, C. M. 1992. Public health and human rights: racism, torture, and terrorism. Paper presented at the annual meeting of the Presidential Seminar at the American Psychiatric Association, 4 May. Washington, D.C.

Segal, Julius. 1974. *Long term psychological and physical effects of the POW experience: a review of the literature.* Report no. 74-2. Naval Health Research Center, San Diego.

Segal, J., Hunter, E. J., and Segal, Z. 1976. Universal consequences of captivity: stress reactions among divergent populations of prisoners of war and their families. *International Social Science Journal* 28:593–609.

Studies and Analysis Service. 1980. *Veterans Administration: study of former prisoners of war.* Superintendent of Documents. Washington, D.C.: U.S. Government Printing Office.

Terr, Lenore. 1979. Children of Chowchilla. *The Psychoanalytic Study of the Child* 34:547–623.

Wilkinson, C. B. 1983. Aftermath of a disaster: the collapse of the Hyatt Regency Hotel skywalks. *Am J Psychiat* 140:1134–39. September.

PART IV

*Teaching, Learning, Research,
and Training Issues*

Sex and Gender as Critical Variables in Psychotropic Drug Research

Overview and Introduction

I N 1985 the U.S. Public Health Service Task Force *Report on Women's Health Issues* documented that women were disadvantaged in health care and research (Hamilton 1992a,b). As one example of bias in research, there had been a preference, historically, for using males as study subjects. In view of such problems, the newly reemerging field of women's health (Zimmerman 1987) has sought to achieve equity in health care research and clinical practice for both sexes. Since pharmacotherapy is a critical treatment modality in modern medicine, it is important to ensure its efficacy and safety in demographically diverse populations. Women use drugs at least as often as men (Moeller and Mathiowetz 1989), and some studies suggest an excess of prescription drug use by women (Rossiter 1983), especially in older populations (Braude 1986).

In clinical pharmacology overall, there has been increasing concern about generalizing to females from predominantly or exclusively male samples (Brett 1989; Leaf 1989; Cotton 1990; Levey 1991). In recognition of these problems, important changes in federal policy concerning drug testing occurred in the United States in March 1993. The Food and Drug Administration (FDA) announced that it would "end its ban on women's participation in most drug safety tests and require companies to carry out analysis by sex in virtually all applications for new drugs" (Hilts 1993). The FDA announcement followed a report issued in October 1992 by the General Accounting Office (GAO) (a congressional investigative group), entitled *FDA Needs to Ensure More Study of Gender Differences in Prescription Drug Testing*. Federally funded clinical treatment trials will also largely

297

require the inclusion of women and the analysis of data by sex (Merkatz et al. 1993; Bennett 1993).

One subspecialty in clinical pharmacology—psychopharmacology—relates to drugs that have predominately mental effects (known as psychotropics). The medical specialty most concerned with studying psychotropics is psychiatry. Psychotropics are used frequently for a wide variety of mental conditions and disorders. This chapter examines implications of sex or gender bias for the study of psychopharmacology and the use of psychotropic drugs. As part of an overall critique, I shall examine research practices and reasons for the development of psychopharmacology, considered and interpreted in terms of an implicit theory guiding biomedical research. Distinctions between sex- and gender-related effects will be explored, although I shall generally refer to sex/gender differences. Findings suggesting sex differences in response to drugs will be summarized and gaps in knowledge identified. I shall propose a contextualized approach to research, offering an ideal methodology for gender-sensitive evaluation, treatment, and research. Reasons for the neglect of sex/gender will be reevaluated and a method for targeting drugs requiring intensive sex/gender study identified. Finally, I shall explore some implications of an improved, sex/gender-sensitive methodology in psychopharmacology for women's mental health.

Clinical depression has been identified as a key mental health issue for women (McGrath et al. 1990). There are numerous subtypes of clinical depression, and many occur more commonly in women than in men. The most widely recognized sex difference is in rates of unipolar depression (as opposed to bipolar disorder—previously referred to as manic-depressive illness), which is observed twice as commonly in women as in men.

As one class of psychotropic drug, antidepressants represent an instructive illustration because of the clear excess of depression among females and the resulting higher use of antidepressants by women. Survey data from 1984 show that about two-thirds of prescriptions in the United States for heterocyclic antidepressants (tricyclics and newer cyclic products) were given to women (Baum et al. 1988; note that the rate of antidepressant use in this study appears to be consistent with the 2:1 ratio of depression in females compared with males). The first antidepressant used in the United States was imipramine (IMI), and it continues to be considered the "gold standard" for evaluating treatments for non-bipolar depressions. For these reasons, IMI will be the subject here of a case study of possible sex/gender biases in psychopharmacology research.

Policy decisions regarding the study of sex/gender differences in psychopharmacology were made in the United States at the National Institute of Mental Health (NIMH) in the early 1980s. The NIMH oversees both psychiatric and other research related to mental illness and its various treatments. In terms of psychopharmacology research, NIMH has been charged with primary responsibility for investigating psychotropics. It has both intramural and extramural research programs, but here the attention focuses on the intramural research program. What happened at NIMH is important, because NIMH has served as the premier training ground for biomedical research in the United States. Data from clinical trials of IMI available to NIMH decision makers in the early 1980s will be carefully evaluated, although the literature on IMI and other antidepressants through 1991 will also be considered.

Critique of Psychopharmacology Research Practices

The relative neglect of sex/gender as a critical variable in modern pharmacology research has been documented in a series of articles that have appeared over the past decade (Hamilton and Parry 1983; Hamilton et al. 1984; Hamilton 1986; Hamilton and Conrad 1987; Hamilton et al. 1991). Many leaders in psychiatry are proponents of current research practices, however, and do not believe that a problem exists. These experts assume that sex- or gender-related effects generally are negligible. For example, a draft of the American Psychiatric Association's (APA) *Practice Guidelines for the Treatment of Major Depression* asserted that "the factor of the patient's sex plays only a minor role in the treatment of depression" (Karasu and Work Group, personal communication 1992, 21). This position was only slightly revised by the APA, which sponsored and endorsed the Karasu guidelines (1993, 18–19; that is, the APA acknowledged just one of the many sex/gender-related pharmacotherapy findings to be discussed here). Findings are suggestive, however limited, because of the lack of systematic research attention given to the issue.

Recent Research Practices

Until 1993 (Hilts), women in the United States had been explicitly excluded from the earliest phases of drug testing as a matter of federal policy since at least the late 1970s. The FDA (1977) had defined the four phases of drug testing:

- *Phase I.* Drugs are screened for toxicity and safety, and early dose ranging and pharmacokinetic studies are performed.
- *Phase II.* Relative safety is further established and efficacy is more systematically demonstrated; expensive teratology studies of animals are required (before including women).
- *Phase III.* Expanded trials are aimed at further demonstrating effec-

tiveness for specific indications and more precisely defining adverse drug reactions (ADRs) or side-effects.

- *Phase IV.* The drug is marketed and post-marketing surveillance follows—for example, there may be large-scale studies of drug effects on morbidity and mortality, and side effects are further reported, however voluntarily.

In summary, women typically were excluded from the first two stages of testing, at least until animal teratology results became available.

Several authors have documented that women also had been "under-represented" in at least some clinical pharmacology trials even in the later phases of testing (Kinney et al., 1981; Reitman 1990). However, the standard for determining appropriate representation remains controversial even now: for example, should representation in research be proportional to representation in the general population [51 percent female], or should it rather be proportional to representation among those having the target illness? Even when women have been included in the later phases of testing, studies typically have not been designed to assess sex/gender differences, and frequently findings have not been reported by age or sex (Hamilton 1991; Levey 1991; GAO 1992).

More specifically, these practices have been documented in psychopharmacology research. Consistent with the FDA guidelines, one of the first papers on IMI that explicitly excluded women appeared in 1980, when Feighner wrote that "[f]emales at risk of conception were not permitted to enter the study" (p. 250). In an earlier (non-comprehensive) review of a different type of antidepressant, MAO-enzyme inhibitors (MAOIs), only 3 out of 25 (12 percent) studies of the MAOI phenelzine tabulated data by either the sex or age of subjects (Hamilton et al. 1984). In recognition of widespread problems in the field, officials at the Center for Studies of Affective Disorders at NIMH recommended that voluntary guidelines for depression research include the reporting of data by age and sex (Hamilton and Hirschfeld 1984).

A Preliminary Survey: Theoretical Development of the Field

The development of the field is illustrated by the policy of excluding women from the early phases of drug testing, although I will demonstrate that such practices actually preceded that policy. The official policy arose in part from experiences in the United States with the drug thalidomide, in the 1960s. Thalidomide is now known to be a potent source of developmental defects (see Zimmerman 1987). The Belmont Report (1979), commissioned in 1974, summarized ethical issues regarding informed consent in the United States. It specifically addressed the need for extra protection for infants (or the fetus) and young children to avoid harmful exposure to drugs. As we shall see later, however, there has been a great deal of ambivalence about protection and extra-protection for women.

In 1980–1981, while serving in a three-year post-residency fellowship in clinical neuropharmacology at NIMH (at the NIH Clinical Center in Bethesda), I first asked whether there might be sex differences in psychopharmacology. The question, asked innocently enough, was greeted with derision (Hamilton 1992a). My lab chief informed me that there could not possibly be an important clinical effect of sex, "because if there were, we'd already know about it." He said this despite the fact that our group did not examine clinical treatment responses to antidepressants by age or sex. Although this may have been statistically the norm for clinical pharmacology research in the United States at the time (Levey 1991), we engaged in these practices even when we studied antidepressants associated with sizable sex differences in animals studies (that is, clomipramine [CMI] and pargyline, an MAOI). As a friend and colleague in another part of NIMH said later, "Some people are so expert they don't even need data." This example illustrates the likelihood that just the asking of a question in itself challenges implicitly held beliefs. Only gradually did I come to understand why the question had provoked such a reaction.

Biological primacy is an error in thinking. The biomedical model traditionally supports studies aimed at discovering laws of physiology or biological invariants. The implicit theoretical orientation is this: Whereas multiple factors may contribute to a particular effect, biological factors are assumed to be causal. Hence biology is assumed to subsume psychosocial or situational co-contributors to variance (Fausto-Sterling 1992; Hamilton 1993).

The primacy of the biomedical model is consistent with an error in thinking that is well known to social psychologists: a tendency to underestimate the role of context as determinant of a person's behavior and to overestimate the significance of internal (in this version, biological) factors. This value-laden bias is so well documented in Western cultures that it has been labeled the "fundamental attribution error" (see Jones and Harris 1967; Ross 1977; Travis and Moore 1988).

I maintain that the fundamental attribution error has shaped the way that modern, biomedically based pharmacology research developed. According to Fingl and Woodbury, writing in Goodman and Gilman's (1975) text *The Pharmacological Basis of Therapeutics*, "[t]he net effect of drug therapy is the sum of the *pharmacological effects* of the drug and the nonspecific placebo effects associated with the therapeutic effort" (34; emphasis added). This conceptualization presupposes the existence of situationally neutral (that is, "real" or purely pharmacological drug effects) that can be studied without reference to the context of the studies (Hamilton 1987).

From this perspective, demographic variables such as sex, age, and race may be considered secondary concerns when it comes to "real science," such as biomedical research. The existence of possible contextual effects is trivialized by assuming, without proof, that they will be negligible if compared with the essential pharmacological effects (Hamilton 1986; Hamilton and Alagna 1988; Hamilton and Jensvold, in press). The feminist critique of science also addresses the need for contextualized research (Fausto-Sterling 1992; Tuana 1989). Hence, I believe the derision I encountered was triggered, in part, because my question had challenged implicit theoretical assumptions about the conduct of science.

Concerning sex and gender, the study of "sex differences" in pharmacology, as in any field, is inherently complex because differences observed between males and females may have various explanations. For example, differences or similarities between men and women could be due to:

- one's sex (that is, sex as a demographic or descriptive variable);
- sexual anatomy, which might be imperfectly linked to genetic sex (defined as the presence of xx or xy chromosomes, and further, these concepts must be differentiated from the sex act or sexual behaviors);
- sex-related prenatal hormone exposure (organizational effects);
- sex-related natural hormonal fluctuations during the menstrual cycle or menopause, or treatment with synthetic hormones, or both (known as activational effects);
- social roles such as gender (Deaux, 1993);
- some other confounding variables (for example, males and females might vary on some other dimension independently affecting outcome measures, thereby complicating interpretation of results).

Even if seemingly "pure pharmacological" effects could be measured and "sex" differences were found to be unimportant (Karasu and Work Group 1992), the possibility remains that "gender" differences in treatment might prove to be profoundly important. By the term *gender,* I refer to a socially constructed, contextual variable (Deaux, 1993) related here specifically to women's unequal, devalued social role. Contextual variables represent a special case of those factors often called confounding. For example, gender roles are expected to differentially affect responses to weight gain as a drug side effect because the societal preference for being thin is greater in females than in males. Gender-role pressures may make more females unwilling to tolerate weight gain.

Even if one's initial purpose is not to sort out the relative contributions of diverse factors such as these to the observation and analysis of sex differences, what is judged a meaningful *pharmacological* difference may hinge on what is thought to be a "true drug effect" as opposed to an artifact. It is crucial here to understand that what we objectively determine in most drug studies is the role of sex as a demographic or descriptive variable. Investigators in pharmacology almost never assess gender-role orientation or attitudes toward women (as one exception, see Marinier et al. 1985). Therefore, it is imprecise and ill advised to write about "gender" differences in psychopharmacology (Yonkers et al. 1992), even though the role of gender may ultimately account for some observed differences between males and females.

Findings in Clinical Studies of Antidepressants

Despite objections to studying women, could it possibly be true that there are statistically significant and clinically meaningful sex differences in psychopharmacology? The two broad divisions in pharmacology research are (1) pharmacokinetics, which deals with getting drugs to and away from the site of action (that is, absorption and bioavailability, distribution, metabolism, and elimination); and (2) pharmacodynamics, which involves mechanisms of action (that is, receptor functioning). Sex differences in animals and humans for each area have been reviewed in greater detail elsewhere (Hamilton and Conrad 1987; Hamilton et al. 1991). The following discussion, however, emphasizes data in humans, especially those concerning clinical antidepressant outcome studies.

In keeping with current research practices, I shall present data on sex differences for antidepressants as if the effects were purely "pharmacological" in origin. Subsequent discussion, however, will challenge this assumption and argue for a more complex, more accurate perspective regarding the origins of sex differences in psychopharmacological research. If a sex/gender difference were observed in clinical outcome studies, the next logical steps would be to examine possible confounding factors and pharmacokinetics, and lastly, to analyze possible pharmacodynamic explanations.

Pharmacokinetic studies reveal sex differences in multiple variables affecting drug absorption and bioavailability, distribution, metabolism, and elimination. As examples, sex-related effects on physiological processes underlying pharmacokinetics include: gastric emptying, basal gastric acid secretion, gastric oxidation, lean body mass, total body water, cerebral blood flow, creatinine clearance, and liver metabolism (Hamilton and Yonkers, in press). IMI is a tricyclic antidepressant (TCA), and this group of drugs is known to be affected by several sex-related pharmacokinetic factors, including: body composition (females have a greater proportion of body fat compared to males and TCAs are lipophilic); possibly in protein binding (TCAs show a high degree of binding); and effects on hepatic metabolizing enzymes (Yonkers and Hamilton, in press).

Overall, when sex differences are observed, they seem to reveal faster clearance in males, which means slower apparent clearance in females. Similarly, females tend to show greater bioavailability, which means higher fractions of drugs gain systemic circulation. Therefore, optimal dosages in males may be relatively high in females because higher plasma levels tend normally to be found in females (for example, because of greater bioavailability or slower clearance, or both). Unless adequate dosage adjustments are made, females are placed at increased risk for drug toxicity when compared to males (Hamilton et al. 1991; Hamilton and Jensvold, in press; Wilson 1984; Yonkers et al. 1992).

In addition, hormonally related treatments and conditions— including the menstrual cycle and oral contraceptives (OCs)—can affect pharmacokinetics.[1] Here, however, the focus is on evidence of sex-related differences in the outcome of clinical treatment trials for depression. Study outcome studies from 1957–1980 are examined most closely.

Findings from outcome studies available to decision makers in the early 1980s. The first TCA, IMI, received attention in the United States in the late 1950s (Kuhn 1958). The earliest studies included open treatment trials, followed by more rigorously designed (randomized, placebo-controlled, double-blinded) clinical studies in the 1960s. By about the mid 1960s the emphasis in research shifted toward comparing IMI with newer psychotropic drugs. In this way, IMI became the "gold standard" for demonstrating efficacy and safety for treatments of depression (Elkin et al. 1989). The rationale for focusing on antidepressants is that depression occurs most commonly among women compared to men, and women consume more antidepressants than men do.

Identification and selection of studies. A review by Morris and Beck entitled, "The efficacy of antidepressant drugs," appeared in 1974 and became the basis for subsequent reviews.[2] For example, it provides the basis for Baldessarini's discussion of IMI efficacy (1979, 93–94, table 11, 12). Unfortunately, sex differences were not examined in either of these reviews.

The present discussion represents the first comprehensive update of the Morris and Beck review as it relates to IMI.[3] It is also the first systematic review of the literature on outcome studies in humans using IMI (or any other antidepressant) as a treatment for depression to address sex differences.[4]

A computerized search of the Medline database identified articles using IMI in humans for treatment of depression. More recent articles (through 1991) were also searched to obtain citations to papers from 1972 through 1980.[5] Foreign language papers were generally used, especially when numerical data were presented in the form of figures or tables and when they used the Roman alphabet. Using these selection methods, 177 papers on clinical IMI trials from 1957–1980 were further evaluated.

The majority of studies (64 percent) clearly stated that both sexes were included in the research population. In 25 percent of the studies, however, the distribution of subjects by sex was not described, nor were outcome data analyzed by sex. In another 11 percent, single-sex samples were used so that possible sex differences could not be evaluated (generally these consisted of all females, though in one case an all-male sample was used). The characteristics of the studies are summarized in table 12.1.

Few IMI studies are sex-relevant. Even though most studies included women and described the sample by sex, 71 percent failed to focus upon sex either in analyzing or in tabulating the data. Such practices, unfortunately, prevented secondary analyses of these data by sex and prohibited our making definitive conclusions about possible sex differences. Taken together with single-sex studies, this means that sex differences were impossible to assess, even superficially, in at least 82 percent of studies.[6] Of the final sample, only 18 percent ($N = 32$)—or less than a fifth—were "sex-relevant," that is, allowed an examination of possible sex differences in outcome. Characteristics of sex-relevant outcome studies for the treatment of depression with IMI are summarized in table 12.2.[7] In some cases study samples were further assessed by age or diagnostic categories.

The sex difference favors males. Sex differences were first examined by calculating the excess of good-responders in males compared with females (that is, by subtracting the proportion for females from that for males, with a positive percentage representing a male advantage). In some cases sex was discussed, but precise findings by sex and relevant statistics were not reported (Holt, Wright, and Hecker 1960; Abraham 1963; Greenblatt, Grosser, and Wechsler 1964; Klein and Fink 1962; Isaksson et al. 1968; Gerner et al. 1980; Angst et al. 1974). Other studies included pertinent data but did not analyze them by sex (for example, Gram et al. 1976; Reisby et al. 1977; Costa et al. 1980; Perier and Eslami 1971; Kemali et al. 1972; Donnelly et al. 1979; Beckman and Goodwin 1975).

For reasons such as these, data for 64 percent of sex-relevant studies required reanalysis. The methods of analysis were, if anything, conservative (for example, Yates's correction was used for small sample sizes). In one case, the absence of a female advantage was asserted, but the male advantage actually observed received no comment; yet reanalysis of the

TABLE 12.1

A. Characteristics of Imipramine Outcome Studies Having Frequency Data by Sex

Study	Year	Dose (mg/d)		Duration of Trial (weeks)	Diagnosis	Age (years)	
		Average	Usual			Average	Other
Ball	1959	250	•	4	E	•	•
Straker	1959 younger	102	•	•	E	•	•
Straker	1959 older	"	•	•	"	•	•
Delay	1959	•	•	•	M	•	•
Krakowski	1960	150	•	•	M	43	•
Freyhan	1960	•	75–400	4	E	•	74% >50
MacLean	1960	•	125–400	4	M	•	•
Stoller	1960	•	•	•	M	•	•
Angst	1961	•	•	•	E	•	•
Hohm†	1961 older	•	< 200	4	P	•	> = 50
Hohn	1961 younger	•	"	4	"	•	< 50
Rees	1961	150	•	3	M	49	50% > 50
Fleminger*	1962	•	150–225	•	M	•	range 23–72
Medical Research	1965	200	•	4	E	55	•
Perier	1971	•	150	5	M	43	range 18–70
Mindham	1973	•	75–150	24	E	•	range 25–69
Beckman	1975	•	•	3.5	E	47	range 20–67
Gram	1976	225	•	5	E	47	range 19–64
Reisby	1977 endogenous	225	•	4	E	50	range 23–65
Reisby	1977 non-endogenous	"	•	"	E	43	range 19–64
Glassman*	1977	215	•	4	non-E	•	•
Donnelly	1979	•	225	3.4	unipolar non-delus.	45	•
Kemali	1980	•	150	•	E	37	range 17–55
Costa	1980	130	•	3	E	39	range 21–66

Study	Year/Group	N/Dose		n	Type	median	Age
Raskin*	1974 younger	300	•	3	M	median	< 40
Raskin	1974 older	"	•	"	"	44	> = 40
Raskin*	1975 blacks	•	•	3	M	31	•

C. Studies with P-Values Only (Without Statistics or Frequency Data) by Sex

Study	Year	N/Dose		n	Type	median	Age
Wilson**	1966	•	150–225	4	•	37	
Gerner*	1980	305	300	4	E	68	•

D. Narrative Studies Only (Without Data or Statistical Summaries) by Sex

Study	Year	N/Dose		n	Type	median	Age
Kuhn	1957	•	< 300	•	M	•	•
Holt	1960	•	75–200	16	M	•	80% 25–35
Abraham	1963	•	100	8	M	•	•
Klein	1962	•	75–300	3.5	Depr. in Schiz.	•	most < 30
Greenblatt	1964	•	300 max.	8	M	46	•
Isaksson	1968	•	225	8	E	49	•
Angst	1974	•	150	3	E	•	•

E = Endogenous
M = Mixed
P = Psychotic/manic
*p < 0.05
**p < 0.01
t = trend

data demonstrated a significant sex difference favoring males (Fleminger and Groden 1962).

In 55 percent of the sex-relevant studies, males were found to show more benefit from IMI compared with females. In contrast, females were found to benefit more in only 18 percent of studies, with no sex difference observed in about 27 percent. Few sex differences (18 percent) reached statistical significance. This should not be surprising, however, since potentially confounding pharmacological variables (for example, smoking, menstrual cycle phase, menopausal status, and other contextual factors) were not typically assessed. Such variables may create "noise," tending to obscure observation of clear group differences.

Further Evaluation of Studies

In the discussion that follows, I further evaluate these findings by focusing on six main questions: (1) Are findings that suggest sex/gender differences consistent in the direction of effects? (2) Does the number of differences observed exceed that expected by chance? (3) Does the size of the differences between the sexes appear to be clinically meaningful? (4) What is the likelihood that these studies could have detected sex differences that existed? (5) Are sex-relevant studies at least as well designed as non-sex-relevant studies (if not, then the observed sex difference may be an artifact of poor research)? (6) Are studies showing a better response to IMI in males compared to females at least as well designed as other sex-relevant studies (if not, then the observed sex difference favoring males may be an artifact of poor research)?

Whenever appropriate, I cite studies demonstrating effects of interest. In some cases, I include examples that are related, but which are not otherwise included in table 12.1 (or in the narrower summary statistics). Unlike previous commentaries, the examples are not selected to represent a particular point of view, nor are they a scattered sampling of the population of studies (Nuland 1988); instead, data on either side of the issues are included in a representative manner.

1. Are findings that suggest sex/gender differences consistent in the direction of effects? In all six cases where significance was obtained, the effect was in the direction of greater benefit in males (Fleminger and Groden 1962; Wilson et al. 1966; Raskin 1974; Gerner et al. 1980; Glassman et al. 1977; and in a subgroup of Raskin and Crook 1975, Black males responded to IMI better than Black females). Consistency in these data strongly supports the likelihood that a sex/gender differences exists (table 12.2).

2. Does the number of differences observed exceed that expected by chance? Using the conventional level of significance ($p = 0.05$), such re-

TABLE 12.2.

A. Imipramine outcome studies with frequency data by sex[a]

Study	Year	Response Rates		Number of Subjects		Percent Advantage for Males
		Males	Females	Males	Females	
Ball	1959	0.86	0.70	7	20	16
Straker[b]	1959 younger	1.00	0.50	5	6	50
Straker	1959 older	0.75	0.90	4	11	−15
Delay	1959	0.62	0.59	52	85	3
Krakowski	1960	0.78	0.79	18	52	−1
Freyhan	1960	0.64	0.81	22	48	−17
MacLean	1960	0.67	0.75	12	40	−8
Stoller	1960	0.63	0.48	11	26	15
Angst	1961	0.74	0.63	27	78	11
Hohn[c]	1961 older	0.88	0.40	8	10	48[t]
Hohn	1961 younger	0.50	0.40	2	5	10
Rees	1961	0.50	0.36	6	14	14
Fleminger[d]	1962	0.75	0.43	20	35	32*
Medical Research	1965	0.80	0.66	20	38	14
Perier[e]	1971	1.00	0.76	12	25	24
Mindham	1973	0.88	0.73	5	11	15
Beckman	1975	0.80	0.45	5	11	35
Gram	1976	0.63	0.46	8	11	17
Reisby	1977 endogenous	0.33	0.58	12	24	−25
Reisby	1977 nonendogenous	0.71	0.45	7	22	26
Glassman[f]	1977	0.91	0.42	11	19	49*
Donnelly	1979	0.50	0.50	10	18	0
Kemali	1980	0.33	1.00	3	2	−67
Costa	1980	0.50	0.50	12	8	0
Average		0.70	0.59			10.3

(Continued)

TABLE 12.2. (Continued)

B. Studies with other statistics (without frequency data) by sex

Study	Year	Response Rates Males	Response Rates Females	Number of Subjects Males	Number of Subjects Females	Statistic
Raskin[g]	1974 younger	•	•	21	58	$F = 2.35$*
Raskin	1974 older	•	•	21	59	$F = 2.35$
Raskin[h]	1975	•	•	36	10	$F = 3.55$*
				Blacks	Blacks	

C. Studies with p-values only (without statistics or frequency data) by sex

Study	Year	Response Rates Males	Response Rates Females	Number of Subjects Males	Number of Subjects Females	Statistic (estimated)
Wilson[i]	1966	•	•	8	12	$(t = 2.8)$**
Gerner[j]	1980	•	•	3	6	$(r = 0.6)$*

D. Narrative studies only (without data or statistical summaries by sex)

Study	Year	Response rates Males	Response rates Females	Number of Subjects Males	Number of Subjects Females	Stated Findings
Kuhn[k]	1957	•	•	•	•	F>M
Holt[l]	1960	•	•	•	•	F>M
Abraham[m]	1963	•	•	•	•	F=M
Klein	1962	•	•	•	•	M>F
Greenblatt	1964	•	•	•	•	M>F

| Isaksson[n] | 1968 | | • | • | • | F = M |
| Angst | 1974 | | • | • | • | (no difference) |

a. The highly conservative Yates chi-square correction is used for sparse samples. Data shown here are adapted from a table in Hamilton (unpublished manuscript, submitted). $N = 24$.

b. This finding applies to the younger age group (< 50 years); the older age group (≥ 50) is shown on the line below. The combined sample does not yield significant results (chi-square = 0.02, 1 df, $p = 0.903$).

c. This finding is for older (≥ 50 years) manic-depressives; the younger age group (< 50) is shown on the line below. The combined sample does not yield significant results (chi-square = 2.46, 1 df, $p = 0.117$).

d. The author does not report the advantage for males; instead, the discussion is limited to the observation that findings do not support the existence of a female advantage.

e. Power estimated by the t-test.

f. Sex differences could be examined in a subgroup of 30 patients with unipolar nondelusional depression. According to the authors, "both being male and having a high plasma level predicted a positive clinical response" (Glassman et al. 1977, 201). Hence, possible effects of sex were confounded by plasma levels. The authors report a correlation between sex and outcome, where $r = 0.17$ (if df = 59, the criteria for significance at the 0.05 level [one-tailed] = 0.211; i.e., the correlation is not significant).

g. This finding applies to the younger age group (< 40 years), for "appear depressed" at 25 days, or about 3.5 weeks; the older age group (≥ 40) is shown on the line below. The statistic used is $F = 2.32$, with 2 tail $p = 0.05$.

h. For depression rating. Power estimated by F-test.

i. These data may be confounded by age, since the author reports that the males are younger than females. The author provides these statistics for an independent t-test comparing outcome data for males and females: df = 19 and $p = 0.002$.

j. $N = 159$ for Blacks only.

k. The female advantage in Kuhn's 1957 study, published in German, was cited by Angst (1961); however, supporting data were not given.

l. The author reports a female advantage but does not provide size of the advantage, nor statistics; nor are the data available for reanalysis.

m. The author reports no effect of sex, with reference to Kendall's Tau, although statistics, per se, are not provided; nor are the data available for reanalysis.

n. The author reports no effect of sex, although statistics, per se, are not provided, nor are the data available for reanalysis.

*$p < 0.05$
**$p < 0.01$
t = trend

sults might have been observed in 1.6 cases in 32 (that is, 5 percent of 32) by chance. Since 6 is 19 percent of 32, however, the results are clearly in excess of the 5 percent criterion.

An alternative analytical method would be to correct for multiple comparisons using the Bonferroni test (where the usual level of significance is divided by the number of comparisons, to arrive at a more stringent level of significance; in this instance, .05/32 gives a Bonferroni-adjusted probability of $p = 0.0016$, or 0.002). Use of such a stringent criterion is questionable in this instance, however, because the very design of these studies has probably tended to obscure sex differences.

In addition, whereas Greenblatt, Grosser, and Wechsler (1962) did not confirm a sex difference, per se, females (but not males) were found to respond significantly better to ECT than to IMI (80 percent improved versus 39 percent for ECT and IMI, respectively). Re-analysis shows that chi-square $= 9.64$, df $= 2$, $p = 0.008$, which is at least a trend according to Bonferroni criteria (for a new total of 33 studies, including Greenblatt).

Several of the studies, in fact, tend to suggest an age-sex effect, although possible age-sex interactions could be examined infrequently (in less than 10 percent of the entire sample). For example, Straker (1959) reported data that could be analyzed by age and sex; re-analysis revealed an advantage for males under the age of 50 years, although the finding is not significant. Raskin (1974) also found an advantage for younger males under the age of 40. The F-statistic for an age-sex interaction in Raskin's study is significant beyond the $p = 0.0001$ level, meeting the Bonferroni criteria. In addition, Wilson and colleagues (1966) found a male advantage using a sample confounded by age differences, such that males were younger than females. The t-test in Wilson's study was significant at the $p = 0.002$ level, also meeting the Bonferroni criteria.

Although Hohn et al. (1961) found an advantage for males over the age of 50, this study used a patient population that differed from the other studies suggesting an age-sex effect, that is manic-depression (more recently termed bipolar disorder). The possibility of a differential age-sex effect by diagnosis is difficult to assess, since many of the samples were not well described.

3. *Does the size of the differences between the sexes appear to be clinically meaningful?* Even if we assume that there is an effect of sex, it might be so small as to be clinically unimportant or negligible. For the 24 analyses where frequency data are available by sex, males averaged a good response about 11 percent more often than females (table 12.1, .70 vs. .59). In eight instances, the excess benefit in males was 20 percent or greater. For the seven studies with the best design (where the duration was four

weeks or greater, and the dosage was usually 125 mg or greater, the male advantage averaged 17 percent.

A 15 to 20 percent effect is generally considered meaningful in such clinical studies. When using absolute criteria on standardized rating scales as indices of severity, it should be noted, however, that the degree of residual depression that Wilson and colleagues observed in females was not clinically meaningful.[8]

4. *What is the likelihood that these studies could have detected sex differences that existed?* The chi-square is a statistic having little power. When a 25 percent difference in proportions is expected, 120 subjects are needed in order to have the power to detect 80 percent of findings at the 2-tail, .05 level; for a 10 percent difference, 774 subjects are needed (Borenstein and Cohen 1988). Importantly, the average power to detect sex differences in the sex-relevant studies reviewed was only 24 percent (uncorrected). This almost certainly means that we risk incorrectly rejecting hypothesized sex differences in outcome because the sample sizes have been much too small to reasonably detect differences.

5. *Are sex-relevant studies at least as well designed as non-sex-relevant studies?* One concern is the quality of sex-relevant studies compared to that of non-sex-relevant studies. The present argument is strengthened if sex-relevant studies are roughly as well designed as non-sex-relevant studies. The qualitative characteristics assessed are shown in table 12.3

TABLE 12.3. Proportion of the entire sample of IMI studies through 1980 meeting criteria according to sex-relevant subgroups

Criteria	Not Sex-relevant (N = 145)	Sex-relevant (N = 32)
Placebo control	44	33
Randomized[a]	60	45[t]
Blinded[b]	72	42***
Total dose:		
average > 150 mg/d	19	27
usual > 150 mg/d	47	36
Duration > 4 weeks	69	55
Patients:		
mixed diagnoses	31	48
mainly endogenous	35	33
Used rating scale[c]	74	58[t]

a. chi-square = 2.23, df = 1, p = 0.135
b. chi-square = 10.73, df = 1, p = 0.001
c. chi-square = 3.66, df = 1, p = 0.056
*** $p \leq 0.001$
t = trend

and include: (1) whether studies are placebo-controlled, randomized, and blinded; (2) whether the average or usual dose of IMI (>150 mg/d) and duration of treatment (4 weeks) were adequate; (3) the homogeneity of the patient group(s) studied; and (4) whether a rating scale was used.

Overall, it appears that non-sex-relevant studies ($N = 145$) may be of somewhat higher quality overall compared to sex-relevant studies ($N = 32$). However, only the use of blinded controls is significantly higher in non-sex-relevant studies (chi-square = 10.73, df = 1, $p = 0.001$). A trend also exists for higher use of rating scales in non-sex-relevant studies compared to the sex-relevant. Most differences are not significant, however (thereby supporting the present argument).

6. *Are studies showing a better response to IMI in males compared to females at least as well designed as other sex-relevant studies?* Another comparison, not shown here, is the quality of male-advantaged studies ($N = 18$) compared to other sex-relevant studies ($N = 14$). The present argument is strengthened if male-advantaged studies are roughly as well designed as other sex-relevant studies. Overall, male-advantaged studies more frequently meet criteria suggesting better quality. Using frequency analysis, the effect is significant, however, for only one criterion: use of a rating scale (chi-square = 14.41, df = 1, p = 0.001). In addition, a study that used an especially good design (a mg/kg dosage regimen; Glassman et al. 1977) reported effects in the same direction. Thus, we find support for the present argument.

Summary and Discussion

While not definitive, clinical studies through 1980 provided limited, though relatively consistent, support for the hypothesis that there are sex-related differences in outcome for IMI. Overall, it appears that males respond somewhat better to IMI than do females. In particular, there may be age-sex effects for IMI so that younger males are advantaged compared to younger females.

In a few studies, the effect of sex on outcome appears to be small and may not be clinically meaningful; but overall, the better studies suggest a substantial, clinically meaningful effect of sex, with males averaging about a 17 percent advantage when it comes to rates of good responsivity.

These data had not yet been reviewed comprehensively, nor relevant data reanalyzed in the early 1980s. In general, the failure of psychiatric researchers to adequately review the literature is a problem that should be addressed by leaders in the field (Nuland 1988). However, several researchers had commented on the possible male-advantage in responsivity (Raskin 1974), as had the authors of several reviews on predictors of treatment responsivity (Bielski and Friedel 1976; Donlon 1979). Despite suggestive data and opinion such as these, research on sex differences in psychopharmacology was specifically considered to be a low priority in the NIMH Intramural Research Program during 1982 and 1983 (see HHS, ADAMHA 1984).

Profiles of sex-relevant studies over time, however, only weakly support the hypothesis that policy decisions at NIMH impeded research. The sex-relevance of studies in the United States was compared to those in Europe. Although the United States began with higher rates of sex-relevant IMI research in the late 1950s compared with Europe (50 vs. 33 percent), there was a marked decline in the early 1960s and late 1970s (with a low of 14 percent). American researchers failed to rebound in the late 1970s, as was true in other locales. In fact, in the following decade (from 1981 to 1991), the rate of sex-relevant IMI research in the United States fell even further, to only 11 percent. Perhaps the best restatement would be that policy makers at NIMH failed to take the lead on this issue, and so, for upward of a decade, progress was delayed in the United States and perhaps internationally (see note 5).

The fundamental attribution error apparently contributes to a gross oversimplification in the ways we have been trained to do psychopharmacological and psychiatric research. As we shall see in the next section, a great deal of indirect corroboration for effects of sex on outcome also exists. Possible effects of sex/gender clearly deserve further investigation —and have deserved attention since the late 1970s—but definitive results will be achieved only from more rigorously designed future studies that are specifically aimed at assessing sex/gender differences in psychopharmacology.

Extending the Critique

When sex/gender differences are examined, biological causes are typically assumed (Anderson and McNeilly 1991; Strickland et al. 1991). When sex/gender differences are not observed, it is assumed that findings are accurate even when confounding variables were not controlled or sample sizes were inadequate. Both of these assumptions are incorrect, however, and can be traced back to the fundamental attribution error.

In keeping with current research practices, I presented data on sex/gender differences for antidepressants in the preceding section as if they were "pharmacological" in origin. According to the dominant scientific perspective, if sex differences result instead from "confounding" variables, the findings cannot be construed as being "real" but are termed "artifactual."

In contrast, I will argue that so-called "confounding" effects deserve research attention per se. This section is intended to broaden our thinking on these issues (for definitional issues concerning sex, hormonal, gender, and other effects, the reader is referred to the earlier section on theoretical bases for how the field developed).

As will become clear, it is exceedingly difficult to study and understand sex/gender differences. Previously I used the example of a gender difference in response to drug-induced weight gain. Even if there is no sex difference in rates of weight gain (Frank et al. 1992), the gender factor may nonetheless be important. Garland, Remick, and Zis (1988) have emphasized that undesired weight gain may jeopardize patient cooperation with antidepressant therapy, suggesting that females may in some cases discontinue drug treatments that might otherwise have proved beneficial.

Another contextual effect concerns gender-related perceptions of the experimental or clinical treatment setting (Anderson and McNeilly 1991; Rosenthal 1966; Wuebben, Straits, and Schulman 1974). In studies of systolic blood pressure, for example, there are higher rates of blood pressure elevation in females (Pickering et al. 1988) when measures are obtained by a physician (high status, usually male) as opposed to when it is taken by a laboratory technician (low status, usually female). This effect, called "white coat hypertension" (McCubbin et al. 1991; Pickering et al. 1988; but see also Lerman et al. 1989), may embody a special case of experimenter effects (see Hamilton and Parry 1983). It may also help to explain the lack of evidence for antihypertensive effects on mild blood pressure elevation among White females (Anastos et al. 1991).

Elsewhere (Hamilton 1987), I have discussed implications for the use of social psychological methods in pharmacology research (here, for example, experimentally manipulating differences in power or status and directly assessing gender role orientation and attitudes). There is evidence suggesting an effect of the examiner's sex on symptoms reports in depression research (King and Buchwald 1982).

Other confounding effects may include sex/gender-related differences for these patient characteristics at baseline: (1) illness presentation (for example, diagnostic subtype); (2) other illness characteristics (for example, chronicity, initial severity or prognosis of the illness or condition being treated); (3) comorbidity (which may relate to severity of illness or treatment failures); (4) sex differences in pharmacokinetics (see note 1), for example, perhaps women have plasma levels of IMI or its metabolites that are either too low for optimal drug efficacy or too high for minimization of side effects; (5) neglect of menstrual cycle effects may also result in decreased responsivity to antidepressants and increased likelihood that antidepressants that might have proved beneficial for certain women will be prematurely stopped; or (6) patterns of concurrent drug usage that may influence the course of illness or alter pharmacokinetics (for example, smoking and OCs, where the latter may amplify side effects, leading to greater discontinuation of the drug and apparent lessened responsivity).[9]

Pharmacological treatment trials can also be confounded by sex or gender differences, which arise during the course of a study: (1) as suggested earlier, prevalence or salience of and tolerance to side effects, because these could lead to differential dropout rates; (2) speed of response; (3) spontaneous rates of relapse or remission; (4) placebo response rates; (5) quality of the therapeutic alliance, where patient cooperation with the treatment plan may depend, in part, on the success of the therapeutic relationship (these issues are discussed further in Hamilton and Jensvold 1991, in press); or (6) concurrent life stresses, which are known to interfere with antidepressant responsivity (Lloyd et al. 1981). The latter finding is potentially important for women (Cafferata and Meyers 1990) because females experience higher rates of exposure to chronic stressors such as poverty and victimization (such as ongoing sexual harassment) when compared to males. With regard to antidepressant trials, Raskin (1974) cited studies that document sex differences, demonstrating a variety of such confounding variables.

Confounding or Contextual Factors

Now I will examine more specifically some of the confounding or contextual factors for antidepressants, with a special focus on data available for IMI: illness presentation (along with misdiagnosis or improper treatments), other illness characteristics, patterns of comorbidity, differential side effects or drop-out rates, and speed of response. I conclude with recommendations for more contextualized psychopharmacological research. In contrast to the previous discussion, where I most closely examined IMI outcome studies during the restricted time period of 1956–1980, here I refer to IMI findings through 1991 as well. Findings for other antidepressants are also discussed as examples. Findings for IMI provide indirect evidence supporting the existence of a sex/gender difference in outcome for treatment of depression. Moreover, contextual data suggest the need for improved research design, and it appears that at least part of the sex/gender effect is not strictly "pharmacologic."

Varieties of Illness Presentation: Misdiagnosis and Improper Treatments

We know that depressive illness is a heterogeneous disorder. There is a female excess not only for major depressive disorder (MDD, unipolar), but also for dysthymia (a mild, chronic depression); probably for "atypical" (characterized by reverse vegetative symptoms, leaden-weight sensations, and hostility or rejection-sensitive dysphoria); anxiety; rapid-cycling bipolar; seasonal affective disorder; and others (Hamilton, Parry, & Blumenthal 1988; Parry 1989; Hamilton and Jensvold 1991; Hamilton and Halbreich 1993). It remains unclear whether there may be sex differences in depressive symptoms, as opposed to syndromes (Golding 1988).

For non-bipolar depressions, the type most common in men (though still more common in women) is MDD, which is neutrally labeled "depression" (or, typical depression). So-called "atypical" depressions have been so labeled to contrast with MDD, which can thereby be treated as normative. Thus, atypical depressions—predominating even more in females than MDD—are compared to a relative male norm.

In the same vein, anxious depressions, also predominating in women, are not even recognized in the official nomenclature. Recent epidemiological studies have provided support for the existence of a mixed "anxiety/depression" syndrome (Blazer et al. 1988). Links and Akiskal (1987) have observed that a chronic low-grade subtype of depression may be secondary to an underlying anxiety disorder. Zetin, Sklansky, and Cramer (1984) found that depressed women had higher rates of anxious symptoms compared to men.

The preponderance of anxious and atypical (or "hostile") depressions in women may be important as a determinant of antidepressant responsivity. In Raskin's (1974) analysis, the differential effect for women by age may be related to age differences in depressive symptoms, with older women reporting more cognitive impairment and younger women reporting more hostility-related symptoms. According to Raskin, Schulterbrandt, Reatig, and McKeon (1970, 170), Wittenborn reported (at a meeting in 1968) that females under the age of forty-five with paranoid symptoms may respond less well to IMI than those without paranoia. In a review of response predictors, Bielski and Friedel (1976) cited a number of studies suggesting that anxious depressions and gender-related personality traits such as "hysteria" have a poor response to TCAs.

There is, thus, a problem with studying antidepressant responsivity using samples that differ in the presenting characteristics of depression by sex: interpretation of the results is confounded. Yet these studies may inadvertently provide clues to clinically significant sex differences in treatment responsivity *by diagnosis*. More recent studies support the idea that MAOIs are particularly useful in atypical depressions (Quitkin et al. 1988; Stewart et al. 1989) and perhaps in dysthymic disorder (Howland 1991; where the response rate in controlled trials for TCAs averaged 26 percent compared to MAOIs, 56 percent). Raskin (1974) observed a sex difference favoring females in responsivity to the MAOI phenelzine.

We also know that depressive episodes can be precipitated in vulnerable women by reproductive events associated with hormonal changes (Hamilton et al. 1988; Parry 1989): puberty; premenstrual changes, including premenstrual exacerbations of other affective disorders; postpartum disorders; infertility-related depressive symptoms or syndromes (Bell 1981; Paulson et al. 1988); and possibly surgical-menopause-related depression (Avis, Posner, & McKinlay 1989). Women generally appear to have more recurrences of (non-bipolar) depressions compared with men (Van Scheyen 1973).

And finally, Dworkin and Adams (1984) found that women are twice as likely as men to receive antidepressants *even when they are not diagnosed as depressed* (nearly 11 percent versus 5 percent). That is, an antidepressant is prescribed when it may be inappropriate. These data come from a large study in the United States (involving $N = 1,752$ subjects at public sector community mental health clinics in Houston in 1983).

Hohmann (1989) also observed a sex/gender-related bias in the way antidepressants are prescribed to women in the United States, with a rate of 82 percent instead of the expected rate of 67 percent (based on the expected 2:1 female-to-male ratio, this represents an excess of 15 percent). Even when controlling for other significant factors, sex/gender remained an independent predictor for prescribing antidepressants. One implication is that women are more often needlessly exposed to medication side effects. In the medical/scientific community, it is generally understood that the bulk of overprescription of antidepressant medications is the responsibility of physicians other than psychiatrists and psychopharmacologists). Alternatively, physicians might informally be treating anxious depressions with IMI (Zetin, Sklansky, and Cramer 1984).

Occurrence of Other Illness Characteristics

Winokur (1974) was among the first to recognize that the efficacy of antidepressant therapy cannot be easily separated from the course of illness. Certain illness characteristics might be associated with a poor response to treatment independent of purely pharmacological effects. If a sex/gender-related factor (such as chronicity for example) occurred in an antidepressant treatment trial, then observed sex differences in outcome might be the result of that factor alone, or else they might result from a poorer drug response, per se. In a long-term follow-up study, females were three times more likely than males to show a chronic course (25 percent versus 9 percent, respectively). Fry (1960) and Cooper and Fry (1969) also observed greater chronicity, or persistence of depression, in females.

More recent studies have tended to confirm that females show a higher rate of persistence of depression (non-recovery) than do males (Dunn and Skuse 1981), although this may be age-related. For example, Sargeant et al. (1990) found greater persistence of depression only for females over the age of 30 years (29 percent versus 15 percent). However, data are mixed, since Mann, Jenkins, and Belsey (1981) did not find an effect of sex on outcome.

Burke, Burke, Rae, and Regier (1991) found that the peak age of onset of major depression occurs earlier for females (ages from 15 to 19 years) than for males (from 25 to 29 years). There is evidence that an early age of onset may be associated with a more severe, protracted course (Kovacs et al. 1984).

These studies are difficult to interpret, especially when subjects have received treatments for depression. When treated, it is unclear whether females show a more chronic course owing to non-responsivity to medication (which may be related to sex/gender) or whether the natural history of depression in females is different from males regardless of treatment (this is a version of the "chicken-egg" dilemma: we don't know which came first or is causal).

Patterns of Comorbidity

Comorbidity refers to the co-occurrence of two or more disorders. The treatment course of depression can be complicated by the co-occurrence of non-affective conditions, including other psychiatric diagnoses and physical illness. Comorbid conditions that are especially salient to depressions occurring in women include panic disorder (especially with agoraphobia, and possibly without); multiple personality disorder (MPD); post–traumatic stress disorder (PTSD); borderline personality disorder (BPD); and bulimia. These disorders are known to complicate or exacerbate the course of depressive illness and data suggest that each occurs more often in women than in men; comorbidity with panic disorder or a personality disorder is specifically thought to impair treatment responsivity (APA 1987; Helzer, Robins, and McEvoy 1987; Weissman and Merikangas 1986; Dube et al. 1985; Van Valkenburg et al. 1984; Breier, Charney, and Heninger 1984; Grunhaus 1988; Grunhaus, Rabin, and Greden 1986; Docherty, Fiester, and Shea 1986; Pfohl, Stangl, and Zimmerman 1984; Shea et al. 1987; Widiger and Hyler 1987). The major difficulty in interpreting these studies is similar to that involved with chronicity.

Some have observed that several of these salient comorbid disorders (MPD, PTSD, BPD) are associated with a history of victimization. A task force report, *Women and Depression*, issued by the American Psychiatric Association (McGrath, Keita, Strickland, and Russo 1990) emphasized that a context-relevant, gender-sensitive assessment will attend to victimization (Brown 1990). Even though victimization-related disorders such as these may also complicate depressions occurring in men, the preponderance of these comorbid conditions in women adds special relevance for women.

Davidson and Pelton (1986) studied patients with atypical depression and panic attacks using TCAs (including IMI, up to 150/d) and MAOIs (including phenelzine, up to 90 mg/d). Percent change on the Hamilton Depression Rating Scale score was the outcome measure. In these patients, MAOIs were significantly more effective in depressed women (56 percent change as an index of female responsivity versus 31 percent in males); whereas TCAs were superior in men (57 percent responsivity in males versus only 29 percent in females).

In addition, specific data confirm that mania complicated by an antecedent or concomitant non-affective psychiatric illness or by a serious or potentially life-threatening medical illness, predicts a more negative outcome for women when compared to men (Black et al. 1988). The odds of recovery at discharge for patients with co-morbidity were nearly 19 percent for females versus 52 percent for males—that is, a 2.7–fold *lower* rate of recovery for females.

Differential Side Effects and Dropout Rates

With the exception of an early study (Ogilvie and Ruedy 1967), women have been shown to suffer more negative side effects from pharmacotherapy in general than have men (Bottiger, Furhoff, and Holmberg 1979; Domecq et al. 1980; Hurwitz 1969). Given predicted, observed trends for pharmacokinetic effects (lower apparent clearance and a tendency toward higher plasma concentrations, especially in older women) and women's 30 percent lesser average weight, it is apparent that women are sometimes given, not just the "same" absolute daily dosage of drugs (mg) as men, but a higher relative dosage, as expressed in mg/kg. In theory, this relationship predisposes women to higher side-effect and dropout rates than men. In addition, nearly 25 percent of women of reproductive age use OCs (Mishell 1989), which affect the clearance of drugs metabolized by the liver, so that higher side-effect rates are also predicted.

Most antidepressant treatment trials report dropout rates of 15–35 percent (Weissman et al. 1981). Without regard for sex, Porter (1970, 778) found that 74 percent of dropouts were taking IMI rather than placebo, suggesting that IMI side effects are an important reason to terminate treatment (given approximately equal sample sizes for the two groups, rates of about 50 percent would have been predicted). Sex/gender differences in dropout rates in antidepressant trials occasionally have been observed directly. In the following discussion, first I shall describe studies of IMI and then summarize data for other antidepressants.

Mindham et al. (1973) found a significant female excess for dropouts of 15 percent in an IMI study (dropout rates 28 percent in females versus 13 percent in males [chi-square = 5.47, df = 1, $p = 0.019$]; where, in this instance, physicians requested that women discontinue the medication, presumably because of the side effects). Raskin (1968, cited in Schulterbrandt, Raskin, and Reatig 1974) found that females were overrepresented among IMI side-effect-related terminators (the rate among females was 85 percent, whereas a rate of only 65 percent was expected using female base rates in the study population). In Schulterbrandt and colleagues (1974), women on a high dose of IMI (300 mg/d) were overrepresented by 3 percent among IMI side-effect-related terminators, although the effect is not significant (note that the observed dropout rates of only 5 percent versus 2 percent are unusually low [$N = 201$, with 8 dropouts)]; chi-square = 0.414, df = 1, $p = 0.520$). Raskin (1974) also observed a 3 percent higher rate of dropouts among females (again, with unusually low dropout rates of 7 percent versus 4 percent) in another IMI study, but the sex difference also failed to reach significance (chi-square = 0.49, df = 1, $p = 0.503$).

Rickels, Raab, DeSilverio, and Etemad (1967, 677) found a significant sex difference in dropout rates in a study of another TCA, protriptyline, also with a female excess (36 percent versus 12 percent; chi-square = 4.10, df = 1, $p < 0.05$). Suggestive evidence exists that women may experience more side effects in response to other TCAs than do men (Schmidt et al. 1986). In this study, women had more side-effect-related terminations for CMI (where my reanalysis assumes that the sex of subjects reflects the usual rates of depression in males and females, resulting in approximate discontinuation rates of 13 percent for females and 5 percent for males).[10]

Taken together, these data suggest that women typically will have higher dropout rates in antidepressant trials than will males. Data that assess the link between sex and dropout rates are mixed, however. Other investigators commenting on dropouts have not found sex differences in rates of completion (Uhlenhuth and Park 1964; Rickels, Ward, and Schut 1964; Frank, Carpenter, and Kupfer 1988, 43; Kocsis et al. 1989, 257; Sotsky et al. 1991, 1001), although sample sizes were not always adequate to detect effects. Since most studies have not reported rates of completion, it is difficult to weigh the direct and indirect evidence, and the data, therefore, remain inconclusive. In theory, it is important to clarify this issue, since higher rates of dropouts among women would, in effect, widen the gender gap for those benefiting from IMI (from about 20 percent to as much as 35 percent).

Patients with anxious depressions—which appear to predominate in women—are thought to be extremely sensitive to TCA-induced side effects, often misinterpreting them as signs of anxiety or impending physical illness (Fogelson, Bystritsky, and Sussman 1988). Evidence exists that TCAs may, in fact, increase anxiety during the first few weeks of treatment rather than diminish it. This effect may interfere with treatment trials, especially for women. Effects such as these may lead to higher dropout rates for women unless specific measures are taken to counteract the initial increase in anxiety—by concurrent use of anxiolytics.

Rates of discontinuation have been found to be higher for phenelzine than for IMI (Agosti et al. 1988). Since women are thought to be over-represented among those having atypical dysthymic depressions, preferentially responding to MAOIs, the higher dropout rates for phenelzine bear special significance for women.

Speed of Response

Initial trials of medication are recommended for a duration of at least four to six weeks (Quitkin et al. 1984). Frank, Carpenter, and Kupfer (1988) observed a sex difference in the speed of response to an acute treatment regimen (combined pharmacologic and psychotherapeutic) in a sample of patients with recurrent depression. The men were significantly more likely to show a rapid, sustained clinical response than the women; this response was seen in 49 percent of male completers and 32 percent of females (chi-square = 4.80, df = 1, $p = 0.029$). This outcome occurred despite the lack of differences in baseline clinical characteristics and level of severity of depression. If replicated, differences in speed of responsivity may have clinical implications, such as scheduling longer initial trials of medication in women.

Discussion

With these findings, it is important to reexamine table 12.1, further assessing characteristics of the studies that demonstrate a significant male advantage in IMI outcome in terms of diagnoses, duration, and medication dosages. Most of these studies used heterogeneous groups of depressed patients. This means that sex differences may be an artifact of having more females with atypical, dysthymic, or anxious depressions and more males with endogenous depression. However, the male advantage is less likely to be entirely an artifact: Gerner, Estabrook, Steuer, and Jarvik (1980) observed the male advantage even among a more homogeneous group of patients having endogenous depression.

The duration of treatment in these studies is usually four weeks or less. This means that sex/gender differences may be an artifact of a slower speed of response in females. Studies of longer duration may wash out sex differences by allowing females to catch up to males in terms of responsivity. However, the male advantage is less likely to be entirely an artifact: Perier and Eslami (1971) observed a male advantage ($p = 0.17$) in a study of five weeks' duration. And finally, the male advantage holds across a broad range of dosages (150–305 mg/d) and ages (17–90 years).

A new gold standard for sex/gender-sensitive psychopharmacology research emerges from consideration of these issues. Males and females must be equivalent at baseline for a series of issues: diagnostic subtype, chronicity, severity, comorbidity, and patterns of concurrent drug usage affecting pharmacokinetics (smoking, caffeine, alcohol, OCs and so on). Pharmacokinetics must be carefully assessed using sex/gender sensitive methods (this issue is discussed elsewhere, see Hamilton and Jensvold, in press; Hamilton and Yonkers, in press; Yonkers and Hamilton, in press). Gender-role orientation and other social constructs should be measured directly. And data on outcome (using both absolute and proportional indices), pharmacokinetics, side effects, dropouts, speed of response, and placebo responding should be presented by sex and, in some cases, by gender.

In the worst hypothetical case, an excess of females among those suffering side effects may lead females to reject a drug that might otherwise have proved beneficial. Claims that an effective drug has been developed are obviously shallow if there is an unwillingness to take the drug among the population most affected by the condition being treated. In the past, some of women's concerns—such as weight gain—have been poorly understood, leading some physicians to discount the intensity of these women's depressive illnesses. Such attitudes (representing a failure to understand the gender bias in cultural norms) may be painful or damaging to individual women seeking treatment and may have a chilling effect on gender-sensitive psychopharmacological research.

With rare exceptions (Angst et al. 1974; Winokur 1974; Links and Akiskal 1987; Sherwin 1991), sex/gender as a research variable is absent from discussions of antidepressant treatment efficacy, "treatment refractory" depression, and affective comorbidity. This omission is glaring and problematic. Despite the relative neglect of sex/gender as a focus of systematic study, several lines of evidence suggest that women are likely to be overrepresented among those with treatment refractory depression.

Historically, certain types of depression in females may not respond well to those antidepressants selected for development, based on screening procedures in all-male samples. By initially screening for safety and efficacy only in males, drugs that might have been more effective or better tolerated in females than males, or drugs that might have been enhanced by estrogen, may be precluded or excluded from further investigation. The potential bias introduced by single-sex drug screening is like that of a sieve—that is, once one screens something out using a certain criterion (size of a grid for example), whatever is excluded on the first pass will not be further utilized or investigated (Hamilton 1985). While speculative, Raskin's (1974) observation that IMI works better in men than women may be one classic example of this sieve-like effect.

Despite increasing evidence that MAOIs may be of greatest benefit to females, many clinicians are reluctant to use MAOIs. Concerns persist about the need for adherence to dietary restrictions and avoidance of certain medication to minimize risk for hypertensive crises, a side effect that is potentially life-threatening. On the other hand, these concerns may have been inflated relative to the potential benefits. It is unfortunate, for example, that confusion about dietary requirements abounds (a puzzling array of recommended diets exist, ranging in size and detail from brief to voluminous). Since women apparently have the most to gain from use of these drugs, one wonders whether part of the caution in using MAOIs results either from a general reluctance to believe that women are reliable historians or from a more specific reluctance to believe that women (who are so often dieting) can be trusted to adhere to special dietary requirements. In either case, sex/gender-based stereotypes may interfere with appropriate pharmacotherapy for certain depressions in women.

Since 1980, another three IMI sex-relevant outcome studies were identified (pharmacokinetic studies unrelated to clinical outcome were assessed separatedly in Hamilton and Jensvold, in press). Of these, one showed no sex differences (Frank et al. 1990), one showed a non-significant trend favoring females (Kocsis et al. 1986); and one demonstrated a sex difference in which males were advantaged (Liebowitz et al. 1988).

More recently, there have been three reports suggesting that sex, along with other demographic variables, is *not* a predictor of antidepressant responsivity (Croughan et al. 1988; Paykel et al. 1988; Kocsis et al. 1989; Sotsky et al. 1991). Again, however, sample sizes were not always sufficient to detect effects (see note 9). Moreover, the relationship between sex/gender and treatment responsivity may be complex. As noted earlier, sex/gender differences may be masked when we fail to concurrently assess effects of hormonal status and other potentially confounding variables. Even when recent findings are considered, the bulk of the evidence concerning IMI still points to meaningful sex/gender-related differences.

Although other antidepressants have not been reviewed exhaustively, evidence exists that the male advantage is not limited to IMI, or to TCAs (Gerner et al. 1980). On the other hand, the male advantage for IMI and other TCAs may be specific to treatment of depression, since a female advantage has been observed in several outcome studies of pain (Blumer and Heilbronn 1984; Edelbroek et al. 1986).

Despite relatively consistent findings, sex/gender-related considerations are rarely recognized as a priority in psychopharmacological research for depression. They are not integrated into medical school and residency courses in psychopharmacology or psychiatry, nor are they highlighted in continuing medical education programs, nor integrated into treatment guidelines (APA, 1993).

Is It Any Longer Reasonable to Ever Make an Exception for Females in Psychopharmacology Research?

Findings from IMI outcome studies have for many years failed to support the neglect of sex/gender-related differences in psychopharmacological research. An increasingly strong rationale has existed for precise study of sex/gender differences, and one might expect a great deal of interest in and support for this area of inquiry. This has not been the case until, perhaps, quite recently, so we must then explore why the investigational and therapeutic research protocols have developed as they have and why they have resisted modification. Even though policy has recently shifted and women will now be included more often in clinical trials and data will be analyzed by sex more frequently, it remains important to understand why and how the field developed as it did—especially before addressing whether it is ever appropriate to make an "exception" with regard to women in psychopharmacological research.

Implicit biases may help to account for gaps in knowledge about women and drugs. Even the most concerned scientists are not immune to cultural stereotypes about gender roles. The fundamental attribution error, for example, probably operates as an invisible value-laden bias, tending to reinforce and sanction sexism in research (via gender-blind and other acontextual methods). Whereas sex/gender-related biases are not unexpected and could operate unintentionally (a true blind spot), other more neutral explanations must be considered further before accepting sexism as an explanation.

Two major rationales have historically been offered for the exclusion of women from early phases of pharmacological research: (1) menstrual cycle–related effects and (2) extra protection for women and unborn children. Both of these are related to a third reason: (3) the sample size or number and timing of observations are increased. None of these three reasons can explain, however, why data collected from both sexes were not analyzed by sex.

Reevaluation of Reasons for Current Practices

The Menstrual Cycle

In conjunction with other apparently plausible explanations, it has been claimed that women cannot be included in research because their participation might add variance that could obscure finding significant drug effects. Variance caused by the menstrual cycle is assumed thereby to be substantial. It is ironic, therefore, that possible menstrual cycle–related effects have been used as a rationale to exclude women from research. Instead, the suspected presence of such substantial effects should have provided the rationale to include, not exclude, women, precisely because of assumed menstrual effects.

Taken together, explanations related to the menstrual cycle amount to double-talk. That is, proponents of the status quo have tried to have it both ways simultaneously: "There are no important sex differences, so it does not matter if we decide to study males preferentially. And even if it did matter, as with presumed menstrual cycle effects, then it is simply too complicated (or expensive) to include women."

Extra Protection for Women and Unborn Children?

It was also suggested that women were actually being offered an advantage in terms of "extra protection," not a disadvantage. Unfortunately, this position failed to take into account that the "protection" offered to women and to unborn children was, in fact, just a delay in being exposed to drugs (Kinney et al. 1981). Once a drug is released, little if any protection is offered to women and unborn children. Once drugs are marketed, in fact, women may be exposed to overtreatment and undertreatment with certain drugs and to needless side effects because of the research community's failure to have adequately selected and tested drugs in women from the beginning of a research project (Hamilton 1991).

The extra protection rationale is considerably weakened by the fact that certain women in the United States had been given a synthetic hormonal medication, diethylstilbesterol (DES), during pregnancy. First, DES was made available as an anti-miscarriage drug—that is, it was specifically given to pregnant women—even after evidence suggested by the 1950s that it was ineffective and by the early 1970s that it was in fact unsafe. Thereafter, DES was offered in the 1970s as a "morning-after" pill—again to women who believed they were or might be pregnant—even though little evidence of its efficacy existed and DES was considered to have serious side effects. Specifically, use of DES was considered unsafe if a birth occurred (Weiss 1983). The link between maternal use of

DES and cancer in offspring had been observed by 1971 (Weiss 1983; Ruzek 1979, 38–42; Corea 1985, 274–84, 291–93; Gillam and Bernstein 1987). Thus, even if special protection has been given to women, it has been non-uniformly practiced and ambivalently implemented, at best.[11]

Moreover, public policy remains oddly unformulated on a related issue that would, in fact, have offered women reasonable and equivalently good protection when compared with men. There is no federal requirement whatsoever that predictable drug interactions with oral contraceptives be prospectively investigated. The neglect is striking because as many as 25 percent of women of reproductive years use oral contraceptives and there is considerable evidence of multiple and sizable effects on pharmacokinetics and drug interactions (Hamilton and Parry 1983; Teichmann 1990).[12] It is also striking because the omission persists even when women are the high-prevalence users of target drugs and when the predicted side effects are potentially serious (see Gallant 1989, unpublished manuscript, and discussion in Hamilton 1987).

The blanket exclusion of women of reproductive years from the earliest phases of drug testing appears to have been based on the erroneous assumption that all women are equally and always at risk for pregnancy. Yet the possibility of pregnancy could not possibly be the sole reason for the exclusion or "underinclusion" of women, because certain women have always been available for testing without risk of pregnancy. As one example, even drugs that are used and tested at ages when women are postmenopausal (cardiac drugs for example) have not necessarily included women in representative proportions (Gurwitz, Col, and Avorn 1992).

The goal clearly should have been to include women who have the least risk of pregnancy in order to make participation in earlier phases of drug testing reasonably safe—that is, to select women who have had tubal ligations or hysterectomies, those without heterosexual partners, as well as postmenopausal women. Whereas recruiting such women may prove costly in some respects, it certainly need not be prohibitively so.[13]

What is so striking about financial considerations is that the costs are implicitly considered justified for males but not for females. The traditional rationale for drug testing is partly to help guide decision making about use of the drug once it is released. In the later phases of drug testing, and especially once drugs are marketed, women ultimately are exposed to most drugs at least as often as men, and perhaps more often (Kinney et al. 1981; Rossiter 1983; Braude 1986; Baum et al. 1988). Yet women use drugs without the availability of the same quality of data drawn from early studies (such as dose-ranging and side-effect profiles) to guide clinical decision making. Some would observe that if the data were worth getting for anyone, then they would be worth getting for everyone, at least for drugs where the existence of sex or other demographic differences are probable.

A variant of the financial rationalization just described is the assertion that women are more difficult to recruit and retain in clinical trials. This may result partly from the differences inherent in gender roles: women have more child-care and elder-care responsibilities and often have less access to transportation. These are practical issues, however, that could be addressed if we as a society chose to do so.

Sex Biases in Research?

Why then did decision makers at NIMH decide in the early 1980s that the study of sex differences in psychopharmacology was not a priority, despite a strong basic science rationale and supporting clinical evidence? Since the most common rationales—menstrual effects and extra protection (along with financial concerns)—possess limited credibility, the most generous alternative interpretation of psychopharmacology's relative insensitivity to sex/gender is that pharmacological research must be viewed developmentally. According to the developmental perspective, the field has just matured to the point where it is essential to investigate further sex/gender-related effects. That is, the field as a whole is moving toward more individualized, or optimized, dosages. Hence, recognition of sex/gender differences is just one of many issues now being investigated to more finely tune pharmacotherapy projects.

It appears likely, however, that early high interest in IMI sex differences was spurred by concerns that men were disadvantaged—that is, that the female enjoyed an advantage in responsivity. When Fleminger and Groden (1962) found that men were not disadvantaged, they figuratively dropped the ball, failing to note the opposite reality: that males were advantaged and females disadvantaged. Apparently, the latter did not elicit as much concern in the world of pharmacological research.

And, finally, developmental hypotheses are weakened by the length of time that we have, in fact, known that sex/gender differences are possible. Yet the leaders in research failed to systematically follow up on plausible findings and inferences. A paper appearing in 1974 noted the "possible clinical significance" of hormone effects on the brain (Greengrass and Tonge), and one year later "oestrous cycle" variations in rat brain monoamines (MAO enzymes) were recognized explicitly as a possible "basis for interactions between hormones and psychotropic drugs." This applied specifically to MAOIs (Fludder and Tonge 1975), the type of antidepressant often deemed most effective for depressive subtypes predominating in females. Put another way, cyclic variations in sex steroid hormones in rat brains could be expected to modify the brain substrate for behavior and the actions of psychotropic drugs (that is, sex differences in response to these drugs are predicted).

At about the same time, another research group documented effects of sex steroids on rat brains (Wirz-Justice, Hackman, and Lichtsteiner 1974). By 1976, Wirz-Justice and Chappius-Arndt wrote that "the modification of the pharmacological response to a given drug by endocrinological status, whatever the mechanism of action, must also be considered" (p. 425), a statement referring specifically to menstrual cycle effects on an antidepressant, CMI.

By the early to mid 1970s, sex differences in response to antidepressants and other psychotropics had been both predicted and observed clinically. Given the higher rate of depression in females, and Raskin's 1974 report that the first-line antidepressant IMI appeared, ironically, to be more effective in males, these data might have prompted a strong rationale for study of possible sex differences in clinical trials involving antidepressants in the early 1980s. In the absence of sex/gender biases, for example, one would have expected to see policy makers designate sex-differences research a priority and investigators swiftly follow up on preliminary findings. However, the specialty has yet to become a priority for funding and many, if not most, findings of potential importance have not been followed up systematically.

Given the common lag time for technology transfer, a seven-to-ten-year delay in follow-up might have been understandable (Williams 1982). This could have resulted in research initiatives as early as 1981. The actual eighteen-year lag from 1974 to 1992 defies credibility, especially if one assumes a neutral explanation. Given more rapid progress in the study of age and ethnic effects in pharmacology, the time lag for the study of sex differences appears so long as to confirm, prima facie, the existence of bias.[14]

One remaining alternative cause is that women report more symptoms overall as compared with men, and this may be viewed as problematic if a researcher's goal is rapid FDA approval for a new drug. For example, Rickels, Raab, DeSilverio, and Etemad (1965) reported that women show much higher symptom reports even on placebo than do men (32 percent versus 3 percent; chi-square $= 8.54$, df $= 1$, $p = 0.010$). Baseline sex differences in symptoms reporting may be hard to differentiate from drug-induced side effects. Thus, concern about females having higher overall rates of symptoms may have been an underlying unstated reason for women having been largely neglected. Even this reason is untenable as a neutral explanation, however, because methods have long existed for controlling for response biases such as these (use of within-person z-scores, for example).

Women in Science: An Index of Sexism? The main alternative to the hypotheses already presented is that some type of non-rational bias (such as sexism) has been operating silently in clinical pharmacology and psychopharmacology research. It is important to recognize that the participation of women in science at NIMH has been problematic. The policy decision made at NIMH in the early 1980s occurred in a setting that was particularly unreceptive to women in science: for example, no woman had finished the initial two-year fellowship program at the premier intramural campus in Bethesda; no women M.D.s had ever been promoted through the ranks and received tenure; and the NIMH intramural work environment has been and continues to be described as hostile toward women (Wagner 1991; Cotton 1992; Solomon 1993). I can only conclude that sexism is one part of the bias that has impeded research on sex/ gender and psychopharmacology in the United States for as long as eighteen years. More specifically, there was, at best, a lack of leadership on the issue.[15]

A Workable Alternative

A more sex/gender-sensitive psychopharmacology would enhance contextual research and clinical practice in psychiatry. The ultimate goal is to optimize pharmacotherapy for women by maximizing therapeutic benefits and minimizing untoward side effects. The magnitude of certain sex-related effects suggests that this effort will not result merely in fine-tuning but may be much more profound. For example, recognition of sex/gender-related effects might lead to advances so that another 10–20 percent of women would do well on IMI (or vice versa: that response to MAOIs might be enhanced in males).[16]

Although data remain limited, some sex/gender-related effects are increasingly recognized as having clinical significance. Recommendations for incorporating sex into treatment practices have included (1) using a lower dose of another TCA, amitriptyline, for women over age 50 (Preskorn and Mac 1985); (2) using a lower dose of IMI for women chronically taking oral contraceptives (Abernethy, Greenblatt, and Shader 1984; APA 1993); and (3) using a higher dose premenstrually for women with symptomatic breakthroughs and lowered plasma levels during that cycle phase (Conrad and Hamilton 1986; Kimmel et al. 1992; Jensvold et al. 1992).

Some women may benefit from initial co-treatment with axiolytics to decrease early dropouts caused by side effects. Women may respond more slowly to TCAs, necessitating longer treatment trials (Frank, Carpenter, and Kupfer 1988). MAOIs should more often be considered first-line treatments for women with atypical, dysthymic, or anxious depressions (Davidson and Pelton 1986; Quitkin et al. 1988; Stewart et al. 1989; Howland 1991).

Should Women Always Be Included in Research or Should Exceptions Ever Be Made?

Having reconsidered why the field developed as it has, we now return to the ultimate question: Should exceptions ever be made for women in psychopharmacological research? Before recent policy changes, the question would have taken the form of "when to include women." Now, however, we are confronted with a new form of the question: Whether women can ever be excluded? or instead, Must women (almost) always be included? (See note 11.)

Some have concluded that women should always be included in psychopharmacological research. For example, legislation is pending before the U.S. Congress that would require women to be included in clinical trials, with very few exceptions.

Others have suggested that decisions about the inclusion of women or other subgroups should be made "scientifically," on a case-by-case basis. Given the specter of sexism in research, however, the individualized or targeted approach could only be effective in an atmosphere both specifically accepting that women's health needs are deserving of study and explicitly recognizing that sex/gender effects in pharmacology exist.

Hamilton (1991) outlined a method for targeting drugs for intensive sex/gender-related study (e.g., drugs used to treat serious illness, those with a low therapeutic to toxic ratio, those with serious or potentially fatal side effects, those known to show sex difference in animal studies or to be affected by hormones). Using this method, antidepressants clearly would be targeted for scrutiny. It is significant, however, that the method suggests that women need not always be included in clinical trials.

Offering a Contextual Approach to Evaluation, Treatment, and Research

The etiology of sex differences—when they are serendipitously observed—will remain unclear, and data in large part uninterpretable, when effects of context are neglected. A more complex methodology is required to clarify the possible role of sex/gender in psychopharmacology.

An Ideal Methodology

Goals and recommendations for an ideal methodology would urge that researchers:

- more often specifically design studies to assess sex- and gender-related differences;
- report summary data and findings by sex, age, and by an age-sex breakdown;
- more often take into account menstrual and menopausal status and use of hormonal medications, and in some cases indices of gender;
- match groups defined by sex on age, severity and type of depression, chronicity, age of onset;
- match groups defined by sex on other confounding variables affecting pharmacokinetics, such as smoking;
- further assess and report by sex rates of dropouts, spontaneous remission, placebo response, and speed of recovery;
- increase study of types of depression that are normative in females or that demonstrate a reproductive-related patterning of illness episodes;
- study more intensively special patterns of comorbidity that predominate in the high-risk population, women;
- increase screening for drugs with higher efficacy in females as compared with males (as well as the opposite), and preparations for enhancement with sex steroid hormones;
- assess variables that may be related to sex differences in pharmacokinetics; for example, mg/kg dosing, percentage of body fat, premenstrual symptoms, "yo-yo dieting";
- increase attention to and analysis of menstrual cycle–related effects, including timing of initiating trials and baseline reporting of premenstrual symptoms (to separate these from drug-induced side effects, for example);
- study more systematically and prospectively, drug-hormone interactions, especially use of OCs and postmenopausal hormone replacement therapy;
- study true gender-related and other contextual effects, using social psychological methods;
- follow up more quickly and systematically on sex/gender-related findings;
- incorporate more rapidly well-replicated findings into medical (especially psychiatric) education and into quality-assurance and practice guidelines, as has been accomplished for age-related effects.

Implications of an Improved Methodology for the Future of Women's Mental Health

Sex and gender are critical variables in psychotropic drug research. In view of women's ancient role in "pharmacology" or its precursors—

using medicinal plants for healing and control of reproduction (Kolata 1994; Rubel and Hass 1990, but see also M. Green, cited in Kolata, 1994), for example, and their early participation as pharmacists in this country (Higby and Gallagher 1992)—lack of attention to the use of drugs for and by women in the United States is particularly inappropriate and ironic.

As sex-differences research in psychopharmacology receives greater attention, it will be critical to avoid business as usual (albeit with a new focus on sex and gender), as guided by the implicit theory of biological primacy. Instead, more appropriate contextually sensitive and gender-related research theories and methods must be further developed and implemented. A more contextualized approach to research in psycho-pharmacology would ultimately improve the quality of research in psychiatry generally, because it would focus attention on a variety of confounding, though potentially informative, contextual factors.

Improved pharmacotherapy for women holds considerable promise for advancing women's mental health. In addition to optimizing drug treatment for women using psychotropic drugs, advancing methods of sex/gender-sensitive psychopharmacological research will have implications for improving research for other classes of drugs as well. Because pharmacotherapy is such a critical treatment modality in modern medicine, sex/gender-sensitive methods in clinical pharmacology undoubtedly will play an important role in generally improving women's health.

Appendix
Clinical studies of Imipramine, 1957–1980.

Sex-relevant studies

Ball, J. 1959. Brit Med J 2:1052. Freyhan, von F. 1960. *Nervenarzt* 31:112. Krakowski, A. 1960. *Med Times* 88:709. MacLean, R. 1960. *Med J Austral* 1:414. Stoller, A. 1960. *Med J Austral* 1:412. Kuhn, von R. 1957. *Schweiz Med Wschr* 87:1135. Straker, M. 1959. *Canad Med Assn J* 80:546. Delay, J. 1959. *Canad Psychiat Assn J* 4S:100. Holt, J. 1960. *Am J Psychiat* 117:533. Angst, A. 1961. *Psychopharmacologia* 2:27. Abraham, H. 1963. *Brit J Psychiat* 109:286. Hohn, R. 1961. *J Psychiat Res* 1:76. Greenblatt, M. 1964. *Am J Psychiat* 120:935. Medical Research Council (Clin psychiat committee) 1965. *Brit Med J* 1:881. Rees, L. 1961. *J Ment Sci* 107:552. Fleminger, J. 1962. *J Ment Sci* 108:101. Klein, D. 1962. *Am J Psychiat* 119:432. Wilson, I. 1966. *Psychosomat* 7:251. Isaksson, A. 1968. *Acta Psychiat Scand* 44:205. Raskin, A. 1974. *J Nerv Ment Dis* 159:120. Mindham, R. 1973. *Psychol Med* 3:5. Gram, L. 1976. *Clin Pharm Therap* 19:318. Costa, D. 1980. *Psychopharm* 70:291. Glassman, A. 1977. *Arch Gen Psychiat* 34:197. Reisby, N. 1977. *Psychopharm* 54:263. Perier, M. 1971. *Ann Med-Psychol* 1:581. Gerner, R. 1980. *J. Clin Psychiat* 41:216. Kemali, D. 1972. *Arch Neurolog* 27:57. Donnelly, E. F. 1979. *Neuropsychobiol* 5:94. Angst, J. 1974. *Pharmakpsychiat* 7:211. Beckmann, H. 1975. *Arch Gen Psychiat* 32:17. Raskin, A. 1975. *Arch Gen Psychiat* 32:643.

Others Reviewed (non-sex-relevant)

Reznikoff, L. 1960. *Am J Psychiat* 116:1110. Barker, P. 1960. *J Ment Sci* 106:1447. Bruce, E. 1960. *Am J Psychiat* 117:76. Ruskin, D. 1959. *Dis Nerv Sys* 20:391. Mann, A. 1959. *Canad Psychiat*

Assn J 4:38. Klein, D. 1966. *Canad Psychiat Assn J* SS:S146. Hoff, H. 1959. *Canad Psychiat Assn J* 4S:S55. Saucier, J. 1959. *Canad Psychiat Assn J* 4S:S148. Malitz, S. 1959. *Canad Psychiat Assn J* 4S:S152. Doust, J. 1959. *Canad Psychiat Assn J* 4S:S190. Kenning, I. 1960. *Canad Psychiat Assn J* 5:60. Miller, A. 1960. *Canad Psychiat Assn J* 5:150. Blair, D. 1960. *J Ment Sci* 106:891. Holdway, V. 1960. *J Ment Sci* 106:1443. Lehmann, H. 1958. *Canad Psychiat Assn J* 3:155. Azima, H. 1959. *Canad Med Assn J* 80:535. Leyberg, J. 1959. *J Ment Sci* 105:1123. Sloane, R. 1959. *Canad Med Assn J* 80:540. Wittenborn, J. 1962. *J Nerv Dis* 135:131. Uhlenhuth, E. 1964. *J Psychiat Res* 2:101. Rickels, K. 1964. *Am J Med Sci* 247:328. Dally, P. 1961. *Lancet* 1:18. Oltman, J. 1961. *Am J Psychiat* 117:929. English, D. 1961. *Am J. Psychiat* 117:865. Agin, H. 1965. *Psychosom* 6:320. Ainslie, J. 1965. *Arch Gen Psychiat* 12:368. Agnew, P. 1961. *Am J Psychiat* 118:160. Ashby, W. 1961. *J Ment Sci* 107:S47. Bassa, D. 1965. *Am J Psychiat* 121:1116. Daneman, E. 1961. *Dis Nerv Sys* 22:213. Edwards, G. 1965. *Brit J Psychiat* 111:889. Fryer, D. 1963. *J Chron Dis* 16:173. Friedman, C. 1961. *J Ment Sci* 107:948. Haydu, G. 1964. *J Nerv Ment Dis* 139:475. LaFave, H. 1965. *Am J Psychiat* 122:698. Leitch, A. 1963. *Psychopharmacologia* 4:72. Martin, M. 1963. *Brit J Psychiat* 109:279. Overall, J. 1962. *Clin Pharm Therap* 3:16. Richmond, P. 1964. *Brit J Psychiat* 110:846. Robin, A. 1962. *J Ment Sci* 108:217. Rose, J. 1964. *Am J Psychiatr* 121:496. Roulet, N. 1962. *Am J Psychiat* 119:427. Seager, C. 1962. *J Ment Sci* 108:704. Snow, L. 1964. *Psychopharmacologia* 5:409. Spear, F. 1964. *Brit J Psychiat* 110:53. Waldron, J. 1965. *Brit J Psychiat* 111:511. Robin, A. 1964. *Brit J Psychiat* 110:419. Hutchinson, J. 1963. *Brit J Psychiat* 109:536. Kiloh, L. 1961. *Brit Med J* 1:168. Wilson, I. 1964. *Psychosom* 5:88. Friedman, A. 1966. *J Psychiat Res* 4:13. Karkalas, Y. 1970. *Psychosom* 11:107. Porter, A. 1970. *Brit Med J* 1:773. Rose, J. 1969. *Dis Nerv Sys* 30:186. Straker, M. 1966. *Canad Med Assn J* 94:1220. Kessel, A. 1970. *Am J Psychiat* 126:938. Walter, C. 1970. *Proc R Soc Med* 64:282. Wilson, I. 1963. *J Neuropsychiat* 4:331. Hasan, K. 1971. *Curr Ther Res* 13:327. Heller, A. 1971. *Am J Psychiat* 127:1092. Glassman, A. 1975. *Am J Psychiat* 132:716. Beaini, A. 1980. *J Aff Dis* 2:89. Rousaville, B. 1980. *J Aff Dis* 2:73. Quitken, F. 1978. *Am J Psychiat* 135:570. Neki, J. 1971. *E Afr Med J* 48:708. Miller, W. 1973. *Curr Ther Res* 15:700. Rickels, K. 1973. *Brit J Psychiat* 123:329. Sathananthan, G. 1973. *Curr Ther Res* 15:919. Kline, N. 1973. *Curr Ther Res* 15:484. McClure, D. 1973. *Canad Psychiat Assoc* 18:403. Schorer, C. E. 1973. *Psychopharmacolog* 28:115. Rapp, W. 1973. *Acta Psychiat Scand* 49:77. Mendels, J. 1973, *Am J Psychiat* 130:1022. Narayanan, H. 1973. *Ind J Med Sci* 27:1. Rosenblatt, S. 1974. *Arch Gen Psychiat* 30:456. Tsegos, I. 1974. *Curr Med Res Opin* 2:455. Schulterbrandt, J. 1974. *Psychopharmacolog* 38:303. Thorell, L. 1974. *Acta Psychiat Scand* 50:508. Covi, L. 1974. *Am J Psychiat* 131:191. Levinson, B. 1974, *S Afr Med J* 48:873. Stryewski, W. 1975. *Archiv Immunolog Ther Exper* 23:803. Smith, R. 1975. *Curr Ther Res* 18:346. Watanabe, S. 1975. *Arch Gen Psychiat* 32:659. Woggon, B. 1975. *Arch Psychiat Nervenkr* 221:157. Kessell, A. 1975. *Med J Austral* 1:773. Koluch, J. 1975. *Activ Nerv Sup* 17:231. Woodward, A. 1975. *Dis Nerv Sys* Mar:125. Perel, J. 1976. *Neuropsychobiol* 2:193. Davidson J. 1976. *Am J Psychiat* 133:952. Sathananthan G., 1973. *Arch Gen Psychiat* 33:1109. Simpson, G. 1976. *Arch Gen Psychiat* 33:1093. Lehman, H. 1976. *Curr Ther Res* 19:463. Nandi, D. 1976. *Brit J Psychiat* 128:523. Singh, A. 1976. *Curr Ther Res* 19:451. Pecknold, J. 1976. *Psychopharm Bull* 12:26. Zung, W. 1976. *Psychopharm Bull* 12:50. Murphy, J. 1976. *The Practitioner* 217:135. Woggon, B. 1977. *Int. Pharmacopsychiat* 12:38. Angst, J. 1977. *Arch Psychiat Nervenkr* 224:175. Nies, A. 1977. *Am J Psychiat* 134:790. Goldberg, H. 1977. *Dis Nerv Sys* Oct:785. dElia, G. 1977. *Acta Scand* 55:10. Davies, B. 1977. *Med J Austral* 1:521. Bhanji, A. 1977. *Europ J Clin Pharmacol* 12, 349. Forrest, A. 1977. *Brit J Pharmac* 4:215 S. Pichot, P. 1978. *Brit J Clin Pharac* 5:87 S. Perry, G. 1978. *Brit J Pharmac* 5:35 S. Van Kammen, D. 1978. *Am J Psychiat* 135:1179. Amin, L. 1978. *Psychopharm Bull* 14:39. Muscettola, G. 1978. *Arch Gen Psychiat* 35:621. Holden, J. 1979. *Curr Med Res Opin* 6:338. Kellams, J. 1979. *J Clin Psychiat* 40:390. Logue, J. 1979. *J. Clin Pharmac* (Jan.): 64. Beckmann, H. 1979. *Arch Psychiat Nervenkr* 227:49. Avery, D. 1979. *Am J Psychiat* 136:559. McCawley, A. 1979. *Am J Psychiat* 136:841. Chouinard, G. 1979. *Acta Psychiat Scand* 59:395. Santonastaso, P. 1979. *Acta Psychiat Scand* 60:137. Linberg, D. 1979. *Acta Psychiat Scand* 60:287. Escobar, J. 1980. *J. Clin Pharmacol* (Feb./Mar.): 124. Eilenberg, D. 1980. *New Zealand Med J* (Feb.): 92. Feighner, J. 1980. *J Clin Psychiat* 41:250. Fifkin, A. 1980. *J Clin Psychiat* 41:124. Gershon, S. 1980. *J Clin Psychiat* 41:100. Elwan, O. 1980. *J Int Med Res* 8:7. Al-Yassiri, M. 1980. *Psychopharmacol* 19:1191.

Foreign Language Journals
Svestka, J. 1979. *Ceskoslovenska Psychiatrie* 75:316. Floru, L. 1979. *Pharmakopsychiat* 12:313. Kuhne, G. 1978. *Psychiat Neurol Med Psychol* 30:104. Faltus, F. 1978. *Ceskoslovenska Psychiatrie* 74:61. Kuhne, G. *Zeitschrift für arztliche fortbildung-Jena* 70:835. Benkert, V. O. 1976. *Drug Res* 26:1162. Angst, J. 1975. *Int Pharmacopsychiat* 10:65. Carolei, A. 1975. *Clinica Terapeutica* 75:469. Beckman, V. H. 1974. *Drug Res* 24:1010. Angst, J. 1974. *Arch Psychiat Nervenkr* 219:265. Rizzitelli, F. 1973. *Arch Neurologia* 28:580. Anonymous 1971. *Activitas Nervosa Superior* 13:166. Peter, L. 1972. *J Med Lyon* 53:549. Ose, E. 1971. *Tidsskrift for den Norske Laegeforening* 91:2388. Smidt, E. 1972. *Nordisk Psykiatrisk Tidsskrift* 26:414. Vinarova, E. 1971. *Activitas Nervosa Superior* 13:162. Dencker, S. 1971. *Nordisk Psykiatrisk Tidsskrift* 25:463 (see also above, under sex-relevant studies, Kuhn 1957).

Examples of Articles Excluded
Articles concerning all schizophrenic patients. Leuthold, C. 1961. *Am J Psychiat* 118:354. Overall, J. 1964. *J Am Med Assn* 189:605.
Non-Patients. Dimascio, A. 1968. *Am J Psychiat* 124S:55.
Data Redundant. Freyhan, F. 1959. *Canad Psychiat Assn J* 4S:S86. Greenblatt, M. 1964. *Curr Psychiat Ther* 4:134. Greenblatt, M. 1962. *Am J Psychiat* 119:144. Raskin, A. 1970. *Arch Gen Psychiat* 23:164. Wilson, I. 1967. *Psychosom* 8:203. Levine, J. 1974. *Pharmacopsychiat* 7:217. Woggon, B. 1977. *Psychopharmacol Bull* 15:29. Floru, L. 1979. *Drug Res* 26:1170. Kuhne, G. 1979. *Psychiat Neurol Med Psychol* 31:203. Pull, C. 1978. *Acat Psychiat Belg* 78:827. Mantero, M. 1975. *Minerva Medica* 66:4098. Irwin, P. 1978. *Brit J Pharmac* 5:43S.
Articles that are not depression-outcome studies. Caron, L. B. 1973. *Int J Clin Pharm Th Tox* 7:37. Geissman, M. 1972. *Bordeaux Med* (Jan.): 115.

NOTES

1. Some of the synthetic steroid hormones in oral contraceptives (OCs) such as ethinyl estradiol—but not conjugated, natural estrogens, which are commonly used post-menopausally—can further reduce clearance of drugs metabolized primarily by oxidative pathways, including the TCA imipramine (IMI). Abernethy, Greenblatt, and Shader (1984) found that when IMI was used in combination with OCs, absolute bioavailability increased by 63 percent. For chronic long-term OC users, these authors recommend that IMI dosages be decreased to about two-thirds of that given to OC-free women to decrease risk for toxicity.

In contrast to the general tendency of females to show greater bioavailability and slower clearance (higher plasma levels), at least some women show an opposing effect premenstrually—that is, lower plasma levels of antidepressants such as lithium (Conrad and Hamilton 1986), desipramine and trazodone (Kimmel et al. 1992), and nortriptyline and fluoxetine (Jensvold et al. 1992). The steady-state plasma concentrations of these drugs have dropped by as much as 53 percent premenstrually, when a constant dose was used (Kimmel et al. 1992). The direction of change for lithium is unclear, since a premenstrual increase (Kukopulos, Minnai, and Muller-Oerlinghausen 1985) and a decrease (Conrad and Hamilton 1986) have been observed. In some cases, dosages have been pragmatically increased premenstrually to maintain adequate blood levels and treatment response. When unrecognized, such menstrual effects will contribute to decreased efficacy of treatments for a small but significant group of women.

The magnitude of sex-related effects for psychotropics can be as great as those observed for age (Ochs et al. 1981; Divoll et al. 1981), where the age effects are recognized as clinically relevant. Pharmacodynamic studies in animals provide additional strong theoretical support for hypothesized sex-related effects.

2. This review, covering the period from 1958 to 1972, cited fifty studies on IMI versus a placebo, and another eleven on IMI versus another TCA (excluding those on desipramine, a metabolite of IMI). Studies were said to be summarized only if they were randomized, controlled, and blinded trials.

3. Because the Morris and Beck (1974) paper remained so influential through the late 1970s and into the early 1980s, I have used it as the starting point for the present review. My method included obtaining papers cited therein and also tracking other references to the original papers cited. Of the fifty papers on IMI and placebo cited by Morris and Beck (1974), eight were ultimately found to be not relevant to the treatment of depression, per se (some were studies of alcoholic depression, neurological illness, or were limited to schizophrenics, or involved non-patient volunteers). Another six were inaccessible because of publication in obscure journals. Unlike Morris and Beck (1974), twenty-eight "open" trials from the early study period they reviewed were included in the final subsample, which totals sixty-four.

4. Another review (Yonkers et al. 1992) claims to be a review of "all English-language articles" on gender differences in psychopharmacology, but it is not. Although the focus is said to be on pharmacokinetics and pharmacodynamics, outcome studies are somewhat haphazardly included (perhaps because these are thought to indicate dynamic effects). Only one of the sex-relevant studies of IMI identified in the present paper was included. On the basis of this incomplete "review," clear findings concerning antidepressants were not found. Oddly, it was also observed in the abstract that women may respond better to some of the newer non-cyclic antidepressants, although no such findings were cited in the text. As a review article, the essay is also curious, in that it fails to cite any previous reviews—a marked departure from the standards of scholarship in most social sciences, and according to Nuland (1988), medicine.

Although earlier reviews had not been comprehensive, they did not claim to be. In addition, the purpose of authors of earlier reviews had been to highlight these issues, using selected examples to stimulate the interest of researchers and policy makers.

5. Did the field develop differently over time in the United States compared to Europe, as assessed by the proportion of sex-relevant studies during successive five-year periods (if not, then the argument that policy decisions in the United States impeded research is somewhat weakened)?

The proportion of sex-relevant studies in the entire sample was examined for successive five-year intervals. Because of the focus on policy decisions in the United States, sex relevance was examined separately for the United States and Europe. For the entire sample, about 39 percent of studies were conducted in the United States and 43 percent in Europe, with 18 percent done elsewhere. Overall, the proportion of sex-relevant studies was somewhat lower in the United States than in Europe (39 percent versus 49 percent, respectively), although the effect of region was not significant (chi-square = 1.54, df = 1, $p = 0.215$).

An L-shaped graph forms when the proportion of sex-relevant studies in the United States is plotted for successive five-year time periods, with the highest point occurring between 1956 and 1960 (with a rate of 50 percent) and the lowest points occurring between 1961 and 1965 and again between 1976 and 1980 (with rates of 16 percent and 14 percent, respectively). The plot for Europe is similar, except that the high point, also occurring in 1956–1960, was lower (33 percent) compared to that in the United States. Profiles for sex-relevant studies in the United States and Europe are thus similar over time, although the deterioration in research practices in the United States is greater relative to initial practices.

If rates of sex-relevance for psychotropics differed from non-psychotropics, policy decisions at the NIMH might, nonetheless, be implicated. However, rates of sex-relevance in the United States for the psychotropic IMI during the latter period are roughly similar to those reported more generally in clinical pharmacology, as sampled by the January issues of *Clinical Pharmacology and Therapeutics* from 1976 to 1980 (based on the method of Levey 1991, the rates are 14 percent versus 6 percent for IMI versus more general pharmacological reports).

And finally, if the rates of sex-relevance for IMI differ from those for psychological research, that is, non-pharmacological, then drug policy decisions at NIMH might also be implicated. The period between 1971 and 1991 was examined for IMI because a comparable analysis exists for selected psychological research during that period (Woolsey 1993, 38). Rates for IMI were only 13 percent, contrasting markedly with the rates of sex-relevant research in developmental psychology of 79 percent and social psychology of 48 percent during the same period. As hypothesized, the lower rates for IMI compared to psychological research that is non-pharmacological may reflect differing attitudes toward women by those in psychiatry (the medical specialty most concerned with clinical trials of psychotropics in humans) and those in psychology, or differences in rates of participation of women among researchers in these two fields, or both. (These proportions were originally calculated including Akiskal et al. 1980, which included study of secondary amines. The findings are similar even when this case is excluded.)

6. That is, $.71 \times .64 = .45$, so that about 45 percent of the total describe both sexes in the sample but allow no analysis or conclusions by sex; and another 11 percent are single-sex; 25 percent do not describe the sample by sex. The total is rounded to 82 percent.

7. Data were described by race in only five of the 177 IMI outcome studies (3 percent); of these, three were single-race studies. In only two studies (1 percent) were studies race-relevant. In one study, Whites responded more positively than Blacks, and in another, race had no effect on outcome.

8. Another quantitative analytical method option would be to assess statistical "effect sizes" in these studies. I have not used this method here because such analyses were infrequent in the early 1980s and would not be likely to have been available to decision makers during the time period of interest. Such an analysis is in progress—albeit covering the broader time period from 1957 through 1991—and will appear elsewhere (Hamilton and Jensvold, submitted).

9. There has been a great deal of concern about under-treatment of depressive disorders. It has been emphasized that the dose of IMI recommended in textbooks is either too low or too high. I suggest that it is more often too low (in the case of women with premenstrual exacerbations of illness) or too high (as in the case of older women or women on OCs) because of sex-related factors for females than for males.

Sex-related differences in plasma concentrations are most likely to be clinically meaningful for antidepressants with a low therapeutic index such as nortriptyline. Low plasma concentrations can be related to lack of efficacy, and high concentrations to increased side-effects or toxicity, potentially leading in either case to dropouts and to lack of benefit from treatment (although the latter would only easily become apparent in *effectiveness* studies, and not in pure, controlled trials, which rarely report dropout rates by sex).

10. Harding (1986) studied psychotropic dosages in Saskatchewan, Canada. The aver-

age total dose (calculated by multiplying strength by number of units) of AMI was nearly 5 grams for women over 70 years of age compared to 4.3 for males of similar age. This may have resulted from longer periods of treatment for women. Alternatively, perhaps dosages were pushed higher in some women due to their relative non-responsivity (to IMI, for example) compared to men; if so, this practice may be associated with greater toxicity and side effects, along with higher dropout rates among women.

11. As this chapter goes to press, new developments were summarized in Hamilton 1994.

12. Legislation requiring inclusion of women in clinical trials was passed by the U.S. Congress in June 1993.

13. At least two versions of the developmental perspective are plausible: the simpler "no bias" and the more complex "benign neglect" explanations. Proponents of benign neglect hypotheses make this type of argument: "We didn't have any definitive reason to study effects of sex in clinical trials because sex differences had not been conclusively proved to exist. And besides, women have always been adequately represented in clinical antidepressant trials, even if we didn't look for sex differences."

Although the developmental view has some merit, it presents several problems. There is the circular nature of the argument. That is, the status quo (relative inattention to research on sex differences) is used to justify its very existence: "Absent conclusive studies, you can't prove sex differences exist; therefore, we can justify continuing to neglect sex as a research variable in future studies, since it is inappropriate to gather extraneous data." Moreover, this view sets up a straw-man argument, perhaps to deflect attention from the real dispute. It is not enough simply to include women in clinical trials: at issue is whether we are analyzing and reporting the data by age and sex, and when appropriate, designing studies in such a way as to elicit possible sex/gender differences. Group differences are likely to be masked if we compare males and females of different ages, especially when we combine data from women before and after menopause, on and off OCs, and with and without premenstrual complaints.

If sex really did not matter, then why not have selected all males in one study and non-pregnant (for example, hysterectomized) females in the next? That is, we simply could have alternated. The fact that we did not alternate selection procedures by sex, historically, weakens seriously the contention that women have been systematically excluded from research projects for gender-neutral reasons.

14. In law, a hypothetical procedure exists for evaluating the credibility of an argument that one might consider making. Credible arguments are called "blushable," meaning that an attorney could go before a judge in good faith and present a proposed argument credibly, without blushing. A blushability test assumes concern about the appearance of credibility. The developmental, menstrual, and extra protection hypotheses clearly do not meet the blushability test.

15. Regarding this hypothesis, I examined women's participation as authors of research reports. My analysis suggests a limited relationship between who participates in science (having female co-authors) and characteristics of the work that is done, such as sex relevance. Authors were identified as female or male by inspection of first names, with rates of female co-authorship calculated in two ways: relative to the number of papers where first names are available (which is probably an overestimate) and relative to the total number of papers (which is probably an underestimate).

Overall, women were included as co-authors (rarely, if ever, as first authors) in 31 percent of papers providing first names, but in only 15 percent of the total. I plotted the proportion of female co-authors against time in five-year intervals. I found that the proportional representation of women as identifiable co-authors of IMI papers follows a similar time course to rates for sex-relevant IMI studies, at least in the 1950s and 1960s. But the representation of women as co-authors demonstrates a more U-shaped curve, ultimately, with the lowest point occurring in 1966–1970 (none) both in the United States and in Europe.

Hence, the proportion of sex-relevant IMI studies does not appear to be strictly related to the proportion of studies having female co-authors; instead, there is a more complicated relationship, so that the decline in rates of sex-relevant IMI studies is partially correlated with the decline in female co-authors, but only from 1961 through 1970. We have yet to see a rise in rates of sex-relevant IMI studies that might correspond to the rise in female co-authors that occurred from 1971 to 1980.

The initial drop in the proportion of sex-relevant studies immediately precedes or coincides with the rise of the feminist movement in the United States in the 1960s. That the decline in the early 1960s may represent a general trend is suggested by other data. For example, a similar decline is observed by examining the number of articles on women and health appearing over time in selected history journals (Leavitt 1984, p. 5). In Leavitt, the nadir occurs between 1959 and 1962, but there is a U-shaped curve, signifying rising numbers of articles on women and health in the 1970s. In marked contrast, a rise in sex-relevance in the 1970s does not occur in IMI studies, although it remains possible that a rise may yet occur after a considerable lag time (studies in Europe, for complex reasons, have followed a pattern similar to that in the United States).

As this chapter goes to press, M. Jensvold (1994, pers. comm.) has begun to explore the connections between sexism at NIH and women's health research.

16. It is unclear whether the female advantage of MAOIs balances the male advantage for IMI. It is possible that females will benefit as much or more than males from some of the newer antidepressants. However, a sex difference favoring males has been reported for trazodone (Gerner et al. 1980).

REFERENCES

Abernethy, D. R., Greenblatt, D. J., and Shader, R. I. 1984. Imipramine disposition in users of oral contraceptive steroids. *Clin Pharmacol Ther* 35:792–97.

Abraham, H. C., Kanter, V. B., Rosen, I., and Standen, J. L. 1963. A controlled clinical trial of Imipramine (Tofranil) with outpatients. *Brit J Psychiat* 109:286–93.

Agosti, V., Stewart, J. W., Quitken, F. M., et al. 1988. Factors associated with premature medication discontinuation among responders to an MAOI or a tricyclic antidepressant. *J Clin Psychiat* 49:196–98.

Akiskal, H. S., Rosenthal, T. L., Haykal, R. F., Lemmi, H., Rosenthal, R. H., and Scott-Strauss, A. 1980. Characterological depression. *Arch Gen Psychiat* 37:777–83.

American Psychiatric Association (APA).

1987. *Committee on Nomenclature and Statistics: diagnostic and statistical manual of mental disorders.* 3d ed. Revised (DSM-III-R). Washington, D.C.: APA.

1993. Practice guideline for major depressive disorder in adults. *Am J Psychiat* 150:1–26. Supplement.

Anastos, K., Charney, P., Charon, R. A., Cohen, E., Jones, C. Y., Marte, C., Swiderski, D. M., Wheat, M. E., and Williams, S. 1991. Hypertension in women: what is really known? *Annals of Internal Medicine* 115:287–93.

Anderson, N. B., and McNeilly, M. 1991. Age, gender, and ethnicity as variables in psychophysiological assessment: sociodemographics in context. *Psychological Assessment: A Journal of Consulting and Clinical Psychology* 3(3):376–84.

Angst, J. 1961. A clinical analysis of the effects of Tofranil in depression. *Psychopharmacologia* 2:381–407.

Angst, J., Baumann, U., Hippius, H., and Rothweiler, W. 1974. Clinical aspects of resistance to imipramine therapy. *Pharmakpsychiat* 7:211–16.

Avis, N. E., and Posner, J. G., and McKinlay, J. B. 1989. Menopause and depression. Paper presented at the annual meeting, American Psychological Association, New Orleans, Louisiana. August.

Baldessarini, R. J. 1979. *Chemotherapy in psychiatry*. Cambridge, Mass.: Harvard University Press.

Baum, C., Kennedy, D. L., Knapp, D. E., Juergens, J. P., and Faich, G. A. 1988. Prescription drug use in 1984 and changes over time. *Medical Care* 26:105–14.

Beckmann, H., and Goodwin, F. K. 1975. Antidepressant response to tricyclics and urinary MHPG in unipolar patients. *Arch Gen Psychiat* 32:17–21.

Bell, J. S. 1981. Psychological problems among patients attending an infertility clinic. *J Psychosom Res* 25:1–3.

Belmont Report. 1979. *Ethical principles and guidelines for the protection of human subjects of research*. Washington, D.C.: U.S. Department of Health, Education and Welfare. April 18.

Bennett, J. C. 1993. Inclusion of women in clinical trials—policies for population subgroups. *New Engl J Med* 329:288–92.

Bielski, R. J., and Friedel, R. O. 1976. Prediction of tricyclic antidepressant response. *Arch Gen Psychiat* 33:1479–89.

Black, D. W., Winokur, G., Bell, S., Nasrallah, A., and Hulbert, J. 1988. Complicated mania: comorbidity and immediate outcome in the treatment of mania. *Arch Gen Psychiat* 45:232–36.

Blazer, D., Swartz, M., Woodbury, M., Manton, K. G., Hughes, D., and George, L. K. 1988. Depressive symptoms and depressive diagnosis in a community population. *Arch Gen Psychiat* 45:1078–84.

Blumer, D., and Heilbronn, M. 1984. Antidepressant treatment for chronic pain: treatment outcome of 1,000 patients with the pain-prone disorder. *Psychiatric Annals* 14:796–800.

Borenstein, M., and Cohen, C. 1988. *Statistical power analysis: a computer program*. Hillsdale, N.H.: Lawrence Erlbaum.

Bottiger, L. E., Furhoff, A. K., and Holmberg, L. 1979. Fatal reactions to drugs. *Acta Med Scand* 205:451–56.

Braude, M. C. 1986. Drugs and drug interactions in the elderly woman. In *Women and drugs: a new era for research*, ed. B. A. Ray and M. C. Braude, pp. 58–64. NIDA Research Monograph 65.

Breier, A., Charney, D. S., and Heninger, G. R. 1984. Major depression in patients with agoraphobia and panic disorder. *Arch Gen Psychiat* 41:1129–35.

Brett, A. S. 1989. Treating hypercholesterolemia: how should practicing physicians interpret the published data for patients? *N Engl J Med* 321:676–80.

Brown, L. S. 1990. Taking account of gender in the clinical assessment interview. *Professional Psychology Research and Practice* 21:12–17.

Burke, K. C., Burke, J. D., Rae, D. S., and Regier, D. A. 1991. Comparing age at onset of major depression and other psychiatric disorders by birth cohorts in five U.S. community populations. *Arch Gen Psychiat* 48:78–95.

Cafferata, G. L., and Meyers, S. M. 1990. Pathways to psychotropic drugs: understanding gender differences. *Medical Care* 28:285–300.

Conrad, C. D., and Hamilton, J. A. 1986. Recurrent premenstrual decline in serum lithium concentration: clinical correlates and treatment implications. *J Am Acad Child Psychiat* 26:852–53.

Cooper, B., and Fry, J. 1969. A longitudinal study of psychiatric morbidity in a general practice population. *Brit J Prev Soc Med* 23:210–17.

Corea, G. 1985. *The hidden malpractice.* Updated edition. New York: Harper and Row.

Costa, D., Predescu, V., Visan-Ionescu, I., and Ciurezu, T. 1980. Endogenous depression and imipramine levels in the blood. *Psychopharmacology* 70:291–94.

Cotton, P.
1990. Is there still too much extrapolation from data on middle-aged White men? *J Am Med Assn* 263:1049–50.

1992. Harassment hinders women's care and careers. *J Am Med Assn* 267(6):778–83.

Croughan, J. L., Secunda, S. K., Katz, M. M., Robins, E., Mendels, J., Swann, A., and Harris-Larkin, B. 1988. Sociodemographic and prior clinical course characteristics associated with treatment response in depressed patients. *J Psychiat Res* 22(3):227–37.

Davidson, J., and Pelton S. 1986. Forms of atypical depression and their response to antidepressant drugs. *Psychiatry Research* 17:87–95.

Deaux, K. 1993. Commentary. Special section: Sex or Gender? *Psychological Science* 4:125–26.

Divoll, M., Greenblatt, D. J., Harmatz, J. S., and Shader, R. I. 1981. Effect of age and gender on disposition of temazepam. *J Pharmaceut Sci* 70:1104–7.

Docherty, J., Fiester, S., and Shea, T. 1986. Syndrome diagnosis and personality disorder. In *Psychiatry Update,* ed. R. Hales and A. Frances, pp. 315–55. *American Psychiatric Association's Annual Review.* Washington, D.C.: American Psychiatric Press.

Domecq, C., Naranjo, C. A., Ruiz, I., and Busto, U. 1980. Sex-related variations in the frequency and characteristics of adverse drug reactions. *Int J Clin Pharmacol Ther Toxicol* 18(8):362–66.

Donnelly, E. F., and Murphy, D. L., Waldman, I. N., and Goodwin, F. K. 1979. Prediction of antidepressant responses to imipramine. *Neuropsychobiology* 5:94–101.

Donlon, P. T. 1979. Factors influencing clinical response to psychotropic drugs. *International Pharmacopsychiat* 14:135–48.

Dube, S., Kumar, N., Ettedgui, E., et al. 1985. Cholinergic REM induction response: separation of anxiety and depression. *Biol Psychiat* 20:408–18.

Dunn, G., and Skuse, D. 1981. The natural history of depression in general practice: Stochastic models. *Psych Med* 11:755–64.

Dworkin, R. J., and Adams, G. L. 1984. Pharmacotherapy of the chronic patient: gender and diagnostic factors. *Community Mental Health Journal* 20(4):253–61.

Edelbroek, P. M., Linnsen, C. G., Zitman, F. G., Rooymans, H. C. G., and de Wolf, F. A. 1986. Analgesic and antidepressive effects of low-dose amitriptyline in relation to its metabolism in patients with chronic pain. *Clin Pharmacol Ther* 39:156–62.

Elkin, I., Shea, T., Watkins, J. T., Imber, S. D., Sotsky, S. M., Collins, J. F., Glass, D. R., Pilkonis, P. A., Leber, W. R., Docherty, J.P., Fiester, S. J., and Parloff, M. B. 1989. National Institute of Mental Health treatment of depression collaborative research program. *Arch Gen Psychiat* 46:971–82.

Fausto-Sterling, A. 1992. *Myths of gender: biological theories about women and men.* 2d ed. New York: Basic Books.

Feighner, J. P. 1980. Trazodone, a triazolopyridine derivative, in primary depressive disorder. *J Clin Psychiat* 41:280–55.

Fingl, E., and Woodbury, D. M. 1975. General principles. In *The pharmacological basis of therapeutics,* ed. L. S. Goodman and A. Gilman, pp. 1–46. 5th ed. New York: Macmillan.

Fleminger, J. J., and Groden, B. M. 1962. Clinical features of depression and the response to imipramine ("Tofranil"). *J Ment Sci* 108:101–4.

Fludder, M. J., and Tonge, S. R. 1975. Variations in concentration of monoamines in eight regions of rat brain during the oestrous cycle: a basis for interactions between hormones and psychotropic drugs. *J Pharmacol Pharmacother* 27(suppl) 2:39p.

Fogelson, D. L., Bystritsky, A., and Sussman, N. 1988. Interrelationship between major depression and anxiety disorders. *Psychiat Ann* 18:158–67.

Food and Drug Administration (FDA). 1977. General considerations for the clinical evaluation of drugs. HEW (FDA) 77-3040. Washington, D.C.: U.S. Government Printing Office.

Frank, E., Carpenter, L. L., and Kupfer, D. J. 1988. Sex differences in recurrent depression: are there any that are significant? *Am J Psychiat* 145:41–45.

Frank, E., Kupfer, D. J., Buhari, A., McEachran, A. B., and Grochocinski, V. J. 1992. Imipramine and weight gain during long-term treatment of recurrent depression. *J Aff Dis* 26:65–72.

Frank, E., Kupfer, D. J., Perel, J., Cornes, C., Jarrett, D B., Mallinger, A. G., Thase, M. E., McEachran, A. B., and Grochocinski, V. J. 1990. Three-year outcomes for maintenance therapies in recurrent depression. *Arch Gen Psychiat* 47:1093–99.

Fry, J. 1960. What happens to our neurotic patients? *The Practitioner* 185:85–89.

General Accounting Office (GAO). 1992. Report to congressional requesters. *Women's health.* FDA needs to ensure more study of gender differences in prescription drug testing, 1992. U.S. Superintendent of Documents, GAO/HRD-93-17, Washington, D.C.

Gallant, S. 1989. Sex, stress, and responses to phenylpropanolamine and caffeine. (Unpublished manuscript, Medical Psychology, Uniformed Services University of the Health Sciences, Bethesda, MD 20814.)

Garland, E. J., Remick, R. A., and Zis, A. P. 1988. Weight gain with antidepressants and lithium. *J Clin Psychopharmacol* 8:323–30.

Gerner, R., Estabrook, W., Steuer, J., and Jarvik, L. 1980. Treatment of geriatric depression with trazodone, imipramine, and placebo: a double-blind study. *J Clin Psychiat* 41:216–20.

Gillam, R., and Bernstein, B. J. 1987. Doing harm: the DES tragedy and modern medicine. *The Public Historian* 9(1):57–82.

Glassman, A. H., Kantor, S., and Shostak, M. 1975. Depression, delusions, and drug response. *Am J Psychiat* 132:716–19.

Glassman, A. H., Perel, J. M., Shostak, M., Kantor, S. J., and Fleiss, J. L. 1977. Clinical implications of imipramine plasma levels for depressive illness. *Arch Gen Psychiat* 34:197–204.

Golding, J. M. 1988. Gender differences in depressive symptoms: statistical considerations. *Psychology of Women Quarterly* 12:61–74.

Gram, L. F., Reisby, N., Ibsen, I., et al. 1976. Plasma levels and antidepressive effect of Imipramine. *Clin Pharmacol Ther* 19:318–24.

Greenblatt, M., Grosser, G. H., and Wechsler, H.
    1962. A comparative study of selected antidepressant medications and EST. *Am J Psychiat* 119:144–53.
    1964. Differential response of hospitalized depressed patients to somatic therapy. *Am J Psychiat* 120:935–43.

Greengrass, P. M., and Tonge, S. R.
    1974. Suggestions on the pharmacological actions of ethinyloestridial and progesterone on the control of monoamine metabolism in three areas from the brains of gonadectomized male and female mice and the possible clinical significance. *Archives of International Pharmacodynamics* 211:291–303.

Grunhaus, L. 1988. Clinical and psychobiological characteristics of simultaneous panic disorder major depression. *Am J Psychiat* 145:1214–21.

Grunhaus, L., Rabin, D., and Greden, J. F. 1986. Simultaneous panic and depressive disorder: response to antidepressant treatments. *J Clin Psychiat* 47:4–7.

Gurwitz, J. H., Col, N. F., and Avorn, J. 1992. The exclusion of the elderly and women from clinical trials in acute myocardial infarction. *J Am Med Assn* 268:1417–22.

Hamilton, J. A.
1985. Avoiding methodological and policy-making biases in gender-related research. In *Report of the Public Health Service Task Force on women's health issues.* Vol. 2, pp. IV 54–64. Superintendent of Documents. Washington, D.C.: U.S. Government Printing Office.
1986. An overview of the clinical rationale for advancing gender-related psychopharmacology and drug abuse research. In *Women and drugs: a new era for research,* ed. B. A. Ray and M. C. Braude, pp. 14–20. National Institute on Drug Abuse, Monograph 65. Superintendent of Documents. Washington, D.C.: U.S. Government Printing Office.
1987. Cognitive-mediated and socio-environmental effects in pharmacology: beyond placebo controls. *Social Pharmacology* 1(4):305–22.
1989. Reproductive pharmacology: perspectives on gender as a complex variable in clinical research. *Social Pharmacology* 3:181–200.
1992a. Biases in women's health research. *Women and Therapy* 12:91–101.
1992b. Special report. Medical research: the forgotten 51 percent. *Medical and Health Annual,* pp. 317–22. Encyclopaedia Britannica. Chicago.
1993. Feminist theory and health psychology: tools for an egalitarian, woman-centered approach to women's health. *J Wom Health* 2:49–54.
1994. Going to extremes. *Women's Review of Books* 11:15–16.
Hamilton, J. A., ed. 1991. Clinical pharmacology panel report. In *Forging a women's health research agenda,* ed. S. J. Blumenthal, P. Barry, J. Hamilton, and B. Sherwin. Conference proceedings, pp. 1–27. Washington, D.C.: National Women's Health Resource Center.
Hamilton, J. A., and Alagna, S. W. 1988. Toward a clinical research perspective. In *The premenstrual syndrome,* ed. L. H. Gise, N. G. Kase, and R. I. Berkowitz, pp. 35–46. New York: Churchill-Livingstone.
Hamilton, J. A., and Conrad, C. D., 1987. Toward a developmental psychopharmacology: the physiological basis of age, gender, and hormonal effects on drug responsivity. In *Basic handbook of child psychiatry,* ed. J. D. Noshpitz, vol. 5, pp. 66–81. New York: Basic Books.
Hamilton, J. A., Grant, M., and Jensvold, M. J. In press. Sex and treatment of depressions: when does it matter? In *Psychopharmacology of women,* ed. M. J. Jensvold, V. Halbreich, and J. Hamilton. Washington, D.C.: American Psychiatric Press.
Hamilton, J. A., and Halbreich, U. 1993. Special aspects of neuropsychiatric illness in women: with a focus on depression. *Ann Rev Med* 44:355–64.
Hamilton, J. A., and Hirschfeld, R. M. A. 1984. An additional recommendation on reporting depression. *Am J Psychiat* 141(9):1134–35.
Hamilton, J. A., and Jensvold, M. J.
1991. Pharmacotherapy for complicated depressions in women. *Psychiatric Times* 8(5):1, 47–49, 51–54.
In press. Feminist psychopharmacology. In *Psychopharmacology from a feminist perspective,* ed. J. A. Hamilton, M. J. Jensvold, E. Rothblum, and E. Cole. *Women and therapy.*
Hamilton, J. A., and Parry, B. 1983. Sex-related differences in clinical drug response: implications for women's health. *J Am Med Wom Assn* 38:126–32.
Hamilton, J. A., Lloyd, C., Alagna, S. W., Phillips, K., and Pinkel, S. 1984. Gender, depressive subtypes, and gender-age effects on antidepressant response: hormonal hypotheses. *Psychopharmacology Bulletin* 20(3):475–80.
Hamilton, J. A., Parry, B. L., and Blumenthal, S. J. 1988. The menstrual cycle in context. I: Affective syndromes associated with reproductive hormonal changes. *J Clin Psychiat* 49:474–80.
Hamilton, J. A., and Yonkers, K. A. In press. Sex differences in pharmacokinetics. Part 1:

Physiological basis for effects. In *Psychopharmacology of women: sex, gender, and hormonal considerations*, ed. M. J. Jensvold, U. Halbreich, and J. Hamilton. Washington, D.C.: American Psychiatric Press.

Harding, J. 1986. Mood-modifiers and elderly women in Canada: the medicalization of poverty. In *Adverse effects: women and the pharmaceutical industry*, ed. K. McDonnell, pp. 51–86. Toronto: Women's Educational Press.

Helzer, J. H., Robins, L. N., and McEvoy, L. 1987. Post-traumatic stress disorder in the general population. *N Engl J Med* 317:1630–34.

HHS, ADAMHA, no. A1-83, p. 4. April 2, 1984. Rockville, Md.

Higby, G. J., and Gallagher, T. C. 1992. Pharmacists. In *Women, health, and medicine in America: a historical handbook*, ed. R. D. Apple, pp. 489–508. New Brunswick, N.J.: Rutgers University Press.

Hilts, P. J. 1993. FDA ends ban on women in drug testing. *New York Times*, March 24.

Hohmann, A. A. 1989. Gender bias in drug prescribing in primary care. *Medical Care* 27:478–90.

Hohn, R., Gross, G. M., Gross, M., and Lasagna, L. 1961. A double-blind comparison of placebo and imipramine in the treatment of depressed patients in a state hospital. *J Psychiat Res* 163:76–91.

Holt, J. P., Wright, E. R., and Hecker, A. O. 1960. Comparative clinical experience with five antidepressants. *Am J Psychiat* 117:533–38.

Howland, R. H. 1991. Pharmacotherapy of dysthymia: a review *J Clin Psychopharmacol* 11:83–92.

Hurwitz, N. 1969. Predisposing factors in adverse reactions to drugs. *Brit Med J* 1:536–39.

Institute of Medicine. 1994. Report of the committee on ethical and legal issues relating to the inclusion of women in clinical studies: changes needed to encourage researcher to enroll more women in clinical studies. Press release. Washington, D.C.: National Academy of Sciences. February 24.

Isaksson, A., Larkander, O., Morsing, C., Ottosson, J. O., and Rapp, O. 1968. A comparison between imipramine and protriptyline in the treatment of depressed out-patients. *Acta Psychiat Scand* 44:205–23.

Jensvold, M. J., Reed, K., Jarrett, D. B., and Hamilton, J. A. 1992. Menstrual cycle-related depressive symptoms treated with variable antidepressant dosage. *J Wom Health* 1(2):109–15.

Jones, E. E., and Harris, V. A. 1967. The attribution of attitudes. *Journal of Experimental Social Psychology* 3:1–24.

Jones, J. H. 1981/82. *Bad blood: the Tuskegee syphilis experiment—a tragedy of race and medicine*. New York: The Free Press.

Julius, S., Mejia, A., Jones, K., Krause, L., Schork, N., van de Ven, C., Johnson, E., Petrin, J., Abed-Sekkarie, M., Erik-Kjeldsen, S., Schmouder, R., Gupta, R., Ferraro, J., Nazzaro, P., and Weissfeld, J. 1990. "White coat" versus "sustained" borderline hypertension in Tecumseh, Michigan. *Hypertension* 16:617–23.

Karasu, T., and Workgroup. 1992. Practice guidelines for the treatment of major depression. Draft. Personal communication.

Kemali, D., Pacini, A., Vacca, L., and Rinaldi, L. 1972. Thymoleptic activity of a new antidepressant. *Acta Neurologica* 27:57–67.

Kimmel, S., Gonsalves, L., Youngs, D., and Gidwani, G. 1992. Fluctuating levels of antidepressants premenstrually. *J Psychosom Ob and Gyn* 13:277–80.

King, D. A., and Buchwald, A. M. 1982. Sex differences in subclinical depression: administration of the Beck Depression Inventory in public and private disclosure situations. *Journal of Personality and Social Psychology* 42:963–69.

Kinney, E. L., Trautman, J., Gold, J. A., Vesell, E. S., and Zelis, R. 1981. Underrepresentation of women in new drug trials. *Annals of Internal Medicine* 95:495–99.

Klein, D. F., and Fink, M. 1962. Psychiatric reaction patterns to imipramine. *Am J Psychiat* 119:432–38.

Kocsis, J. M., Hanin, I., Bowden, C., and Brunswick, D. 1986. Imipramine and amitriptyline plasma concentrations and clinical response in major depression. *Brit J Psychiat* 148:52–57.

Kocsis, J. H., Mason, B. J., Frances, A. J., Sweeney, J., Mann, J. J., and Marin, D. 1989. Prediction of response of chronic depression to imipramine. *J Aff Dis* 17:255–60.

Kolata, G. 1994. In ancient times flowers and fennel for family planning. *New York Times (Science Times)*, March 8.

Kovacs, M., Feinberg, T. L., Crouse-Novak, M. A., Paulauskas, S. L., and Finkelstein, R. 1984. Depressive disorders in childhood: I, II. *Arch Gen Psychiat* 41:229–37, 643–49.

Krakowski, A. J. 1960. Depression therapy with imipramine hydrochloride. *Medical Times* (London) 88:709–17.

Kuhn, von R.
  1957. Uber die Behandlung depressiver Zustande mit einem Iminodibenzylderivat (G 22355). *Schweiz MedWschr* 87:1135–40.
  1958. The treatment of depressive states with G22355 (Imipramine hydrochloride). *Am J Psychiat* 115:459–64.

Kukopulos, A., Minnai, G., and Muller-Oerlinghausen, B. 1985. The influence of mania and depression on the pharmacokinetics of lithium. *J Aff Dis* 8:159–66.

Leaf, A. 1989. Management of hypercholesterolemia: are preventive interventions advisable? *N Engl J Med* 21:680–84.

Leavitt, J. W., ed. 1984. *Women and health in America*. Madison: University of Wisconsin Press.

Lerman, C. E., Brody, D. S., Hui, T., Lazaro, C., Smith, D. G., and Blum, M. J. 1989. The white-coat hypertension response: prevalence and predictors. *Journal of Internal Medicine* 4:226–31.

Levey, B. A. 1991. Bridging the gender gap in research. (Commentaries). *Clin Pharmacol Ther* 50:641–46.

Liebowitz, M. R., Quitken, F. M., Stewart, J. W., McGrath, P. J., Harrison, W. M., Markowitz, J. S., Rabkin, J. G., Tricamo, E., Goetz, D. M., and Klein, D. F. 1988. Antidepressant specificity in atypical depression. *Arch Gen Psychiat* 45:129–37.

Links, P. S., and Akiskal, H. S. 1987. Chronic and intractable depressions: terminology, classification, and description of subtypes. In *Treating resistant depression*, ed. J. Zohar and R. H. Belmaker, pp. 1–21. New York: PMA Publishing.

Lloyd, C., Zisook, S., Click, M., and Jaffe, K. E. 1981. Life events and response to antidepressants. *J Human Stress* 7:2–15.

McCubbin, J. A., Wilson, J. F., Bruehl, S., Brady, M., Clarke, K., and Kort, E., 1991. Gender effects on blood pressures obtained during an on-campus screening. *Psychosomatic Medicine* 53:90–100.

McGrath, E., Keita, G. P., Strickland, B. R., and Russo, N. F., eds. 1990. *Women and depression: risk factors and treatment issues*. Washington, D.C.: APA. Mann, A. H., Jenkins, R., and Belsey, E. 1981. The twelve-month outcome of patients with neurotic illness in general practice. *Psychol Med* 11:535–50.

Marinier, R. L., Pihl, R. O., Wilford, C., and Lapp, J. E. 1985. Psychotropic drug use by women: demographic, lifestyle, and personality correlates. *Drug Intelligence and Clinical Pharmacology* 19:40–45.

Marshall, E. 1994. New law brings affirmative action to clinical research. *Science* 263:602.

Merkatz, R. 1993. Ethical issues and women as subjects in pharmacological protocols. Paper presented at "Toward a new psychobiology of depression in women: treatment and gender." National Institutes of Mental Health, Bethesda, Md., November 4.

Merkatz, R. B., Temple, R., Sobel, S., Feiden, K., and Kessler, D. A. 1993. Women in clinical trials of new drugs: a change in Food and Drug Administration policy. *New Engl J Med* 329:292–96.

Mindham, R. H. S., Howland, C., and Sheperd, M. 1973. An evaluation of continuation therapy with antidepressants in depressive illness. *Psychol Med* 3:5–17.

Mishell, D. R. 1989. Contraception. *N Engl J Med* 320:777–87.

Moeller, J. F., and Mathiowetz, N. A. 1989. Prescribed medicines: a summary of use and expenditures by Medicare Beneficiaries (National Medical Expenditure Survey Research Findings 3, DHHS Publication Number [PHS] 89-3448), National Center for Health Services Research and Health Care Technology Assessment.

Morris, J. B., and Beck, A. T. 1974. The efficacy of antidepressant drugs. *Arch Gen Psychiat* 30:667–74.

Nuland, S. B. 1994. The pill of pills: listening to Prozac. *New York Review of Books* 41:4–8.

Ochs, H. R., Greenblatt, D. J., Divoll, M., Abernethy, D. R., Freyerabend, H., and Dengler, H. J. 1981. Diazepam kinetics in relation to age and sex. *Pharmacology* 23:24–30.

Ogilvie, R. I., and Ruedy, J. 1967. Adverse drug reactions during hospitalization. *Canad Med Assn J* 97:1450–57.

Parry, B. L. 1989. Reproductive factors affecting the course of affective illness in women. *Psychiatric Clinics N Am* 12:207–20.

Paulson, J. D., Haarman, B. S., Salerno, R. L., and Asman, P. 1988. An investigation of the relationship between emotional maladjustment and infertility. *Fertility and Sterility* 49(2):258–62.

Paykel, E. S., Hollyman, J. A., Freeling, P., and Sedgwick, P. 1988. Predictors of therapeutic benefit from amitriptyline in major depression. *J Aff Dis* 14:83–95.

Perier, M., and Eslami, H. 1971. Clinical evaluation of antidepressant effects of doxepin. *Annales Medico-Psychologies* 1:581–87.

Pfohl, B., Stangl, D., and Zimmerman, M. 1984. The implications of DSM-III personality disorders for patients with major depression. *J Aff Dis* 7:309–18.

Pickering, T. G., James, G. D., Boddie, C., Harshfield, G. A., Blank, S., and Laragh, J. H. 1988. How common is white coat hypertension? *J Am Med Assn* 259:225–28.

Porter, A. M. W. 1970. Depressive illness in general practice. *Brit Med J* 1:773–78.

Preskorn, S. H., and Mac, D. S. 1985. Plasma levels of amitriptyline: effects of age and sex. *J Clin Psychopharm* 46:276–77.

Quitkin, F. M., Rabkin, J. G., Ross, D., and McGrath, P. J. 1984. Duration of antidepressant drug treatment. *Arch Gen Psychiat* 41:238–45.

Quitkin, F. M., Stewart, J. W., McGrath, P. J., Liebowitz, M. R., Harrison, W. M., Tricamo, E., Klein, D. F., Rabkin, J. G., Markowitz, J. S., and Wager, S. G. 1988. Phenelzine versus imipramine in the treatment of probable atypical depression. *Am J Psychiat* 145:306–11.

Raskin, A. 1974. Age-sex differences in response to antidepressant drugs. *Journal of Nervous and Mental Diseases* 159:120–30.

Raskin, A., and Crook, T. H. 1975. Antidepressants in Black and White inpatients. *Arch Gen Psychiat* 32:643–49.

Raskin, A., Schulterbrandt, J. G., Reatig, N., and McKeon, J. J. 1970. Differential response to chlopromazine, imipramine, and placebo. *Arch Gen Psychiat* 23:164–73.

Reisby, N., Gram, L. F., Bech, P., Nagy, A., Petersen, G. O., Ortmann, J., Isben, I., Dencker, S. J., Jacobsen, O., Krautwald, O., Sondergaard, I., and Christiansen, J. 1977. Imipramine: clinical effects and pharmacokinetic variability. *Psychopharmacology* 54:263–72.

Reitman, D. (cited by C. Hooper). 1990. Some drug trials show gender bias. *J NIH Research* 2:47–48.

Rickels, K., Raab, E., DeSilverio, R., and Etemad, B. 1967. Drug treatment in depression: antidepressant or tranquilizer? *J Am Med Assn* 201(9):675–81.

Rickels, K., Ward, C. H., and Schut, L. 1964. Different population, different drug responses. *Am J Med Sci* 247:328–35.

Rosenthal, R. 1966. *Experimenter effects in behavioral research.* New York: Appleton-Century-Crofts.

Ross, L. 1977. The intuitive psychologist and his shortcomings: distortions in the attribution process. In *Advances in experimental social psychology,* ed. L. Berkowitz. Vol. 10. New York: Academic Press.

Rossiter, L. F. 1983. Prescribed medicines: findings from the National Medical Care Expenditure survey. *Am J Public Health* 73(11):1312–15.

Rubel, A. J., and Hass, M. R. 1990. Ethnomedicine. In *Medical anthropology: contemporary theory and method,* ed. C. F. Sargent and T. M. Johnson, pp. 115–31. New York: Praeger.

Ruzek, S. B. 1979. *The women's health movement: feminist alternatives to medical control.* New York: Praeger.

Sargeant, J. K., Bruce, M. L., Florio, L. P., and Weissman, M. M. 1990. Factors associated with one-year outcome of major depression in the community. *Arch Gen Psychiat* 47:519–26.

Schmidt, L. G., Grohmann, R., Muller-Oberlinghausen, B., Ochsenfahrt, H., and Schonhofer, P. S. 1986. Adverse drug reactions to first- and second-generation antidepressants: a critical evaluation of drug surveillance data. *Brit J Psychiat* 48:38–43.

Schulterbrandt, J. G., Raskin, A., and Reatig, N. 1974. True and apparent side effects in a controlled trial of chlorpromazine and imipramine in depression. *Psychopharmacologia* 38:303–17.

Shea, T., Glass, D., Pilkonis, P., Watkins, J., Docherty, J., et al. 1987. Frequency and implications of personality disorders in a sample of depressed outpatients. *J Personality Disorders* 1:27–42.

Sherwin, B. B. 1991. Estrogen and refractory depression. In *Advances in neuropsychiatry and psychopharmacology,* ed. J. D. Vander, pp. 209–18. New York: Raven Press.

Solomon, A. 1993. Snake pit. *Mirabella* (April): 140–44.

Sotsky, S. M., Glass, D. R., Shea, T., Pilkonis, P. A., Collins, J. F., Elkin, I., Watkins, J. T., Imber, S. D., Leber, W. R., Moyer, J., and Oliveri, M. E. 1991. Patient predictors of response to psychotherapy and pharmacotherapy. *Am J Psychiat* 148:997–1008.

Stewart, J. W., McGrath, P. J., Quitkin, F. M., Harrison, W., Markowitz, J., Wager, S., and Liebowitz, M. R. 1989. Relevance of DSM-III depressive subtype and chronicity of antidepressant efficacy in atypical depression. *Arch Gen Psychiat* 46:1080–87.

Straker, M. 1959. Imipramine (Tofranil): a safe, effective antidepressant drug in private practice. *Canad Med Assn J* 80:546–49.

Strickland, T. L., Raganath, V., Lin, K-H., Poland, R. E., Mendoza, R., and Smith, M. W. 1991. Psychopharmacologic considerations in the treatment of Black American populations. *Psychopharmacology Bulletin* 27(4):441–48.

Teichman, A. T. 1990. Influence of oral contraceptives on drug therapy. *Am J Ob and Gyn* 136:2208–13.

Travis, C. B., and Moore, P. L. 1988. Psychotropic drugs: treatment issues. In *Women and health psychology: mental health issues,* ed. C. B. Travis. Hillsdale, N.J.: Lawrence Erlbaum.

Tuana, N., ed. 1989. *Feminism and science.* Bloomington: Indiana University Press.

Uhlenhuth, E. H., and Park, L. C. 1964. The influence of medication (imipramine) and doctor in relieving depressed psychoneurotic outpatients. *J Psychiat Res* 2:101–22.

U.S. Public Health Service. 1985. Report of the Task Force on Women's Health Issues. Vol. II, pp. IV, 54–64. Superintendent of Documents. Washington, D.C.: U.S. Government Printing Office.

Van Scheyen, J. D. 1973. Recurrent vital depressions. *Psychiatrica, Neurolgia, Neurochirurgia* 76:93–112.

Van Valkenburg, C., Akiskal, H. S., Puzantian, V., et al. 1984. Anxious depressions: clinical, family history, and naturalistic outcome, comparisons with panic and major depressive disorders. *J Aff Dis* 6:67.

Wagner, R. 1991. Sexual discrimination, harassment found in research and academia. *Psychiatric Times* 8(11):65–66, 68–70.

Weiss, K. 1983. Vaginal cancer: an iatrogenic disease. In *Women and health: the politics of sex in medicine,* ed. E. Fee, pp. 59–75. Farmingdale, N.Y.: Baywood.

Weissman, M. M., and Merikangas, K. R. 1986. The epidemiology of anxiety and panic disorders: an update. *J Clin Psychiat* 47:11–17. (Supp. 6)

Weissman, M. M., Klerman, G. L., Prusoff, B. A., Sholomskas, D., and Padkan, N. 1981. Depressed outpatients: results one year after treatment with drugs and/or interpersonal psychotherapy. *Arch Gen Psychiat* 36:51–55.

Widiger, T., and Hyler, S. 1987. Axis I/Axis II interactions. In *Psychiatry,* ed. R. Michels and J. Cavena. Philadelphia: J. B. Lippincott.

Williams, T. I. 1982. *A short history of twentieth-century technology.* Oxford: Clarendon Press.

Wilson, I. C., Rabon, A. M., Merrick, H. A., Knox, A. E., Taylor, J. P., and Buffaloe, W. J. 1966. Imipramine pamoate in the treatment of depression. *Psychosomatics* 7:251–53.

Wilson, K. 1984. Sex-related differences in drug disposition in man. *Clinical Pharmacokinetics* 9:189–202.

Winokur, G. 1974. Genetic and clinical factors associated with course in depression. *Pharmakopsychiat* 7:122–26.

Wirz-Justice, A., and Chappius-Arndt, E. 1976. Sex specific differences in chlorimipramine inhibition of serotonin uptake in human platelets. *Eur J Pharmacol* 40:21–25.

Wirz-Justice, A., Hackman, E., and Lichtsteiner, M. 1974. The effect of pestradiol dipropionate and progesterone on monoamine uptake in rat brain. *J Neurochemistry* 22:187–89.

Wittes, B., and Wittes, J. 1993. Research by quota: group therapy. *The New Republic,* April 5, pp. 15–16.

Woolsey, M. L. 1993. Social responsibility as a topic for psychological research, 1971–1991. Dissertation, Department of Psychology, Social and Health Sciences, Duke University, Durham, N. C.

Wuebben, P. L., Straits, B. C., and Schulman, G. I. 1974. *The experiment as a social occasion.* Berkeley, Calif.: The Glendessary Press.

Yonkers, K. A., and Hamilton, J. A. In press. Sex differences in pharmacokinetics. Part 2: Effects on selected psychotropics. In *Psychopharmacology of women: sex, gender, and hormonal considerations,* ed. M. J. Jensvold, U. Halbreich, and J. Hamilton. Washington, D.C.: American Psychiatric Press.

Yonkers, K. A., Kando, J. C., Cole, J. O., and Blumenthal, S. 1992. Gender differences in pharmacokinetics and pharmacodynamics in psychotropic medication. *Am J Psychiat* 149:587–95.

Zetin, M., Sklansky, G. J., and Cramer, M. 1984. Sex differences in inpatients with major depression. *J Clin Psychiat* 45:257–59.

Zimmerman, M. K. 1987. The women's health movement: a critique of medical enterprise and the position of women. In *Analyzing gender: a handbook of social science research,* ed. B. B. Hess and M. M. Ferree, pp. 442–71. Beverly Hills, Calif.: Sage Publications.

Training for Culturally Appropriate Mental Health Services

C LINICAL education in the core mental health professions is based on various theoretical models and associated diagnostic and treatment methods that generally are assumed to apply to all human beings. But as professionals are well aware by now, many of the accepted truisms of clinical training and practice are based on unsupported theory or on studies conducted on highly restricted populations, and much research has been limited to White, middle-class males. Deficits in test standardization have raised questions regarding the accuracy of diagnoses across cultures.

In recent years instructors have learned that it is appropriate to mention that gender, social class, race, ethnicity, or cultural background should be taken into account. New waves of immigrants and refugees have generated discussion of the mental health implications of translocation and acculturation, as well as relations of new groups with both mainstream and minority groups of the host culture. However, curriculum materials are lacking and guidelines are vague about how this knowledge should be applied. A few research and training programs are oriented toward the needs of specific ethnic groups, as well as to special initiatives from the National Institute of Mental Health (NIMH) for training minority students in the core professions. In the main, however, preparation for work with culturally diverse populations is very loosely embedded, and often nonexistent, in the curricula of most professional training programs (Lefley 1985b).

There are many reasons for this generalized avoidance. Even among those clinicians who are sensitive to cultural pluralism, there is a problem in disentangling socioeconomic and minority status from ethnocultural

351

heritage, and in assessing exactly how these elements may impinge on a particular case. Moreover, there is increasing and compelling research evidence that major mental disorders (such as schizophrenia, endogenous depression, or bipolar disorder) are biologically based, and this is reflected in most state-of-the-art textbooks used in clinical training (Talbott, Hales, and Yudofsky 1988). Thus, in treating serious mental illnesses some clinicians have viewed psychosocial variables as incidental to primary somatic therapies and have paid little attention to rehabilitation. Many practitioners ignore or minimize critical variables affecting the intensity and course of illness. These include (1) the symbolic meaning of mental disorder to the patient and its impact on self-image and functioning (Estroff 1989); (2) social-environmental stresses that may trigger decompensation; and (3) the importance of cultural worldview, kinship structure, and support systems in averting chronic disability (Lefley 1990).

Among the unfortunate consequences of institutional racism have been failures of professional training programs to recognize the type and degree of mental health and mental illness problems in ethnic minority populations, and to equip their trainees with effective tools to assess and to help alleviate them. This chapter begins with data that suggest the scope and variability of these problems including the potential impact of clinical misinterpretation or bias. We then go on to describe a community mental health program that developed an innovative culturally sensitive model of mental health delivery to ethnic minority populations, recognizing and tapping community resources for strengths and supports. We indicate how the program then generated training for mental health professionals and other human service providers in culturally appropriate service delivery, and produced research data demonstrating the efficacy of the service model and the cost-benefit of cross-cultural training. Finally, we propose some generalized guidelines for academic training programs and for mental health service providers that may facilitate the delivery of culturally sensitive and effective care for racial or ethnic minority populations.

The Scope of the Problem

The following information is derived from epidemiological surveys and national statistics of the federal government. The picture begins with epidemiological data that show few differences among populations in the distribution of major mental disorders. Minor ethnic variations in lesser diagnostic conditions seem tied to social rather than endogenous factors. These racial or ethnic uniformities in the major disorders—those for which people are typically hospitalized—are then viewed against statistics that show great disparities in racial or ethnic distributions of admissions to mental hospitals and strangely inverse relationships between admissions and lengths of stay. We then present research findings that indicate a possible connection between these profiles and problems in evaluation, diagnosis, and treatment of clients from different cultural and socioeconomic backgrounds.

The Epidemiological Picture

The most logical and parsimonious premise is that mental disorders, particularly those presumed to be biogenic, are evenly distributed across populations. There is evidence in the literature, however, that such disorders may be triggered or exacerbated by environmental stress (Talbott, Hales, & Yudofsky 1988), and that cultural stressors, both internal and external, may affect their intensity and duration (Lefley 1990). It may be expected, then, that populations suffering economic and social pressures might have an even distribution of disorders in terms of lifetime prevalence, but that they manifest possible differences in both acute psychotic episodes and in chronicity of disorders.

In past years our global picture of the distributions of mental disorders in the United States—and in the world as well—were gleaned from an assortment of studies that were disparate in sampling, instrumentation, diagnostic standardization, and methodological rigor. Most were based on treated cases or hospital statistics, although these figures are obviously subject to admissions policies and service utilization patterns. But today's data are derived from the Epidemiologic Catchment Area Survey (ECA), the largest and most scientific study of psychiatric disorders ever undertaken. Tapping thirty of the major psychiatric disorders listed in the Diagnostic and Statistical Manual (3rd edition) of the American Psychiatric Association (1980; DSM-III) the ECA administered standardized interviews in five sites to systematic samples of almost twenty thousand Americans (Robins and Regier 1991). Although Williams (1986) has cited some sampling flaws with respect to African Americans, noting in particular the artifact of differential rate of imprisonment of poor African American males and the omission of this population from the catchment area samples, this is nevertheless the best database we have at this point in time.

The results indicated that one or more of these thirty psychiatric disorders had been experienced at some time in their lives by 32 percent of American adults, and 20 percent had an active disorder. They also showed that African Americans had a significantly higher rate of both lifetime (38 percent) and active (26 percent) disorder than did Whites or Hispanics. The lifetime and active prevalence rates were, respectively, 32 percent and 19 percent for Whites, 33 percent and 20 percent for Hispanics.

A closer look, however, indicated that many of these differences washed out when the data were controlled for socioeconomic status. For example, in schizophrenia, the lifetime rate for Blacks (2.1 percent) was significantly higher than the rate for non-Hispanic Whites (1.4 percent) and for Hispanics (0.8 percent). However, when the data were controlled for age, gender, marital status, and (most important) socioeconomic status, the significant difference between Black and White prevalence rates disappeared. The researchers note: "Hence, the higher rates which appear for the black population may well be explained by the confounding variables of lower socioeconomic status and higher rates of marital separation or divorce, which are independently associated with higher rates of schizophrenia" (Keith, Regier, & Rae 1991, 41).

The researchers found little ethnic variation in bipolar disorder, but a significantly higher prevalence of major depression among Whites than among Blacks and Hispanics. Hispanics were highest in dysthymia, with Blacks lower than either group in both major depression and dysthymia. The authors note, "this lower rate of depressive disorders in blacks is especially interesting since a number of studies have reported that blacks have more depressive symptoms (not syndromes as defined by DSM-III) than whites. . . . Perhaps black suffer more from mild forms of distress, but less from clinical depression" (Weissman et al. 1991). This finding is particularly significant since for many years the older research literature suggested that African Americans did not have diagnosable depressive symptoms, ignoring generalized distress in the search for major psychiatric disorder (Jones and Gray 1986).

The ECA also dispelled some myths. The data indicated that "the disorders associated with criminality, drug and alcohol abuse and antisocial personality, were not higher in blacks than whites, despite the overrepresentation of blacks in prisons and jails" (Robins, Locke, and Regier 1991, 352). In fact, only two disorders, both fairly uncommon in clinical practice, appeared to show significant differences for race or ethnicity. One was somatization disorder, the presentation of multiple physical complaints without known organic causes. Here the lifetime prevalence was significantly higher for Blacks than for all other groups (2.29 versus 1.99), "but the effect of sex is more dramatic, with women reporting an average of 2.76 symptoms versus 1.21 symptoms for men" (Swartz et al. 1991, 230).

The other disorder was severe cognitive impairment in older persons.

Older Blacks had significantly more cognitive impairment than older Whites. This may have been partially due to health-related organic factors. However, the researchers point out that the instrument used, the Mini-Mental State Examination, has been shown to be strongly correlated with education and social status. They suggested that the finding may have been due in large part to a history of unskilled employment and poor education in the world in which older African Americans were reared (Robins, Locke, & Regier 1991).

The Treatment Picture

The ECA results suggest that there would be little difference among groups with respect to their needs for treatment and hospitalization. Here the picture changes dramatically, however. For many years now government statistics have shown that admission rates to inpatient psychiatric services were significantly higher for non-Whites (Blacks and other races) than for Whites, for both women and men. This pattern has never deviated and continues in the most recent data (NIMH 1990). The currently reported admissions for all inpatient facilities show a rate of 1,074 for non-Whites versus 594 for Whites, per 100,000 population, with males continuing to have higher admission rates than females in most facilities that serve the most seriously disabled patients. In contrast, there is almost no racial difference in admissions for outpatient care (889 White versus 886 non-White, per 100,000 population).

A distinction exists between admissions, which may be brief encounters involving speedy discharge, and patients who are in beds receiving care. Here the differences are even more dramatic. The total for all inpatients under care shows a rate of non-Whites (126.8) more than double that for Whites (56.5). Non-Whites were higher than Whites in both admissions and maintenance for partial hospitalization. But again, no racial differences were evident for outpatients under care (576 White versus 588 other races).

With respect to patients served in state mental hospitals, a longitudinal study showed that for both discharged and resident patients, the cohorts were largely adult (92 percent over age 18), predominantly male (61 percent) and disproportionately Black. Black patients accounted for 22–32 percent, far above their expected frequencies based on general population distributions.

The most recent report of national mental health statistics (NIMH 1990) repeated the earlier practice of using racial differentiation only (White and all other races). However, the earlier 1987 report (NIMH 1987), gave data for other racial and ethnic groups. This report showed that, relative to population distributions, African Americans and American Indians had significantly higher admission rates than other racial and ethnic groups to all inpatient facilities, including state and county mental hospitals, private psychiatric hospitals, general hospitals, and Veterans Administration medical centers. Rates per 100,000 population were as follows: 931.8 for Blacks; 818.7 for American Indians or Alaska Natives; 550.0 for non-Hispanic Whites; 451.4 for Hispanics (who could be of any race); and 268.1 for Asians. The rates for African Americans were thus two-thirds higher than for Whites, more than double the rates of Hispanics, and two and one-half times greater than those for Asians (NIMH 1987, table 3, p. 76).

These distributions, however, showed inverse patterns with levels of disability. Among inpatients, including those diagnosed with schizophrenia (the most frequent diagnosis), groups with the lowest admission rates (Asians, Hispanics, and Whites) have had considerably higher median inpatient stays than African American or American Indian patients (ibid., table 3.5, p. 80). The rates of admissions, in fact, are almost directly inverse to the patients' apparent needs for hospital care.

Numerous issues arise in observing these relationships. Do these patterns reflect cultural differences in service utilization patterns? For persons diagnosed with schizophrenia (the primary diagnosis requiring hospitalization), Hispanics and Asians had median stays of 54 and 52 days respectively, considerably less than the respective 32 days and 20 days for African Americans and American Indians (ibid.). It has been suggested that the former groups are more likely to keep the patients at home and to present them for hospitalization only at an advanced stage of illness. Snowden and Cheung (1990) note that data are lacking on differential access and on ethnic differences in help-seeking patterns or the use of alternatives to inpatient services. They also suggest that two other areas require far more attention from researchers: proceedings leading to involuntary commitment, and bias in diagnosis. Bias in admitting practices, they point out, may include not only "overeagerness for confinement of Blacks and Native Americans," but may also be reflected in "minimizing bias" in judging the behavior of Asian Americans and Whites (354).

To what extent are these patterns artifacts of interviewing, assessment, and admitting practices that may reflect cultural bias or misunderstanding? There is a large literature on various aspects of diagnosis, such as the use of assessment instruments and interviewing techniques, language, psycholinguistics, and clinician-patient relationships that may be problematic in cross-cultural diagnosis (Adebimpe 1984; Jones and Gray 1986; Lefley 1986b; Kinzie and Manson 1987; Pavkov, Lewis, and Lyons 1989; Westermeyer 1987; William 1987). It has been demonstrated that race and sex of patient and psychiatrist can influence diagnosis even when clear-cut DSM-III criteria are used (Loring and Powell 1988). Diagnostic clarity is often confounded by cultural differences in the behavioral manifestations of psychosis (Chu et al. 1985; Fabrega, Mezzich, and Ulrich 1988; Mukherjee et al. 1983). There is also an emerging literature on racial or ethnic differences in response to medications, with difficulties in assessing the relative contributions of biological and cultural factors (Lin, Poland, and Lesser 1986).

Treatment has also been a long-standing issue. There is now a substantial literature on the cross-cultural applicability of therapeutic models developed largely in nontraditional industrialized nations with middle-class patients, and focusing on individuals and individual growth. Alternative models—building on family strengths and involving kinship networks and other support systems—are deemed more culturally appropriate for traditional, family-oriented cultures (Lefley 1986b, 1990). In the African American community (as noted by Griffith, Young, and Smith 1984), religion has been a core social and spiritual resources. The church provides collective support, opportunities for self-expression and for helping others, and a reference point for meaningfulness in life. Religious belief systems have rarely been considered part of the treatment armamentarium, and yet they may offer the most therapeutic medium of all. By and large, the treatments offered by the mental health service delivery system rest on chemotherapy and psychotherapy and only recently have begun to focus on rehabilitation skills for deinstitutionalized patients. Modes of addressing the needs of persons from ethnic minority groups with a multiplicity of environmental problems, or linking with existing culturally acceptable modes of treatment, have been largely unaddressed.

Roles of Mental Health Professionals

Many of these problems are a function of a ubiquitous racism that has permeated all dimensions of society, from extraordinary social stressors impinging on vulnerable individuals to the failure of the system to provide adequate remedies. In fact, the mental health system itself has demonstrated numerous barriers, failing to provide accessible and appropriate service (Bestman 1981). Societal discrimination and its sequelae of poverty, unemployment, interrupted education, and social disintegration lead not only to poor mental health and demoralization. They are also known correlates of biologically based mental illnesses (Robins, Locke, and Regier 1991). Whereas diathesis for schizophrenia and other major disorders may be evenly distributed across racial or ethnic groups, these conditions may be triggered or exacerbated by environmental stress.

Institutional racism has also affected the professional community and reduced the pool of potential helpers. Despite affirmative action policies aimed toward encouraging professional training for students from ethnic minority groups, the inheritance of years of discriminatory policies persists. It will be many years before there are enough practitioners from these groups to serve the number of clients who need services. Mental health professionals continue to be predominantly of non-Hispanic, White, middle-class background.

Although there is continuing discussion in the literature on whether it is preferable for clients to be served (typically in psychotherapy) by clinicians of matching ethnicity, numerous studies provide empirical evidence that a social and cultural gap between service providers and clients may affect each level of the preventive, diagnostic, and therapeutic process. A sample of many problems from the research literature includes basic communication difficulties and bias in interviewing; linguistic and psycholinguistic barriers in evaluation; serious diagnostic errors in assessing psychopathology; failure to understand differential response patterns on screening instruments; underrecording or misinterpretation of symptoms; misunderstanding of culturally normative behaviors; misinterpretation of psychodynamics; failure to differentiate between adaptive and maladaptive behavior; advice that runs counter to cultural mores; and treatment goals that may alienate clients from a needed support system (for overviews, see Lefley 1986b; Lefley and Bestman 1984).

In recent years a number of books relating to service delivery to specific ethnic populations have been published. Most focus or have chapters on major minority groups such as African Americans, American Indians and Alaska Natives, Asians and Hispanics, but also deal with generalized cross-cultural practice and training (see Comas-Diaz and Griffith 1987; Lefley and Pedersen 1986; Pedersen et al. 1989; Sue and Sue 1990; Wilkinson 1986).

The modes of applying this knowledge, however, are subject to debate. The mental health field is filled with a variety of therapeutic theories and approaches, but practitioners generally fall into two camps. One group, from psychoanalytic to family systems theorists, subscribes to universalistic paradigms of human behavior and family transactions. A number of theoreticians and practitioners, from minority as well as mainstream cultures, consider the psychoanalytic or psychodynamic paradigm the most elegant explanatory model, applicable across cultures and responsive to the needs of individual clients regardless of their particular life situations. For these clinicians, cultural information is used to understand linguistic references, behaviors, or diagnostic profiles, which they realize they may misinterpret, but the basic therapeutic model remains the same.

At the other extreme are eclectic practitioners who view insight therapies as too time-consuming and often alien to the lives and needs of many of their clients. They prefer brief, here-and-now counseling and may use comprehensive environmental interventions to deal with reality problems or to ease social pressures. They tend to work with families and social networks as much as possible, realizing that clients from ethnic minority groups are likely to come from more traditional, sociocentric cultures. They may focus on family strengths and use psychoeducational and social network designs rather than deficit-model therapies in working with families. For clients with and without families, there is an aim of individual skill-building and strengthening interpersonal support systems rather than focusing on psychodynamic insights. In some cases, this may involve interventions at the community level (Bestman 1981, 1986b).

Mindful of the scope of the problems of service delivery to racial or ethnic minorities, a pioneering program based on the eclectic model was developed by a multidisciplinary group of social scientists and clinicians (including the authors) at the University of Miami School of Medicine. In the following section, we describe our reconceptualization and expansion of therapeutic modalities, focusing on the development of culturally appropriate mental health services for ethnically diverse communities experiencing poverty, minority group status, and/or translocation as refugees or entrants. Examples are given of intervention techniques at individual and community levels, together with evaluation data on acceptance and effectiveness of the program.

A Culturally Sensitive Community Mental Health Model

In March 1974, the University of Miami–Jackson Memorial Community Mental Health Center (CMHC) was funded by the NIMH to serve a catchment area rich in ethnic diversity in inner-city Miami. Almost 85 percent of the population was of African American, Caribbean, and Central or South American origin. This was also a federally designated poverty area with a multiplicity of social problems and needs. The program developed to meet these needs began as a branch of the Department of Psychiatry of the University of Miami and after seven years became freestanding as New Horizons CMHC, the name it is known by today.

The model for the CMHC derived from a comprehensive three-year research effort, the Health Ecology Project (Weidman 1978), which had studied health systems, beliefs, and behaviors of five major ethnic groups in the catchment area: African Americans, Bahamians, Cubans, Haitians, and Puerto Ricans. Interviews and daily health calendars maintained by over five hundred families indicated many stressors and a high degree of emotional distress. Although there was occasional use of indigenous healers, clinical mental health treatment was almost never solicited. Field data from the Health Ecology Project together with emergent diagnostic and therapeutic problems among ethnic patients in the hospital system strongly suggested that a CMHC established along traditional lines would be neither maximally effective nor optimally utilized. Further, while all groups suffered from multiple socioeconomic and environmental stressors, the indications were that in many cases culturally specific therapeutic interventions might be required to deal with different ethnic groups living within the same poverty area (see Bestman 1986a; Lefley and Bestman 1984).

The CMHC that was developed reflected the prevailing community mental health ideology of the day: the vistas of service were broad. To a greater extent than many other centers, the program served and continues to serve seriously and persistently mentally ill people, particularly the deinstitutionalized population whose needs were highly visible in a poor inner-city area. The mission, however, was to provide fully accessible, culturally appropriate services to all community residents, and to alleviate environmental stressors by helping residents receive their fair share of adaptive resources.

With this in mind, the CMHC developed five teams of indigenous mental health workers to serve African American, Bahamian, Cuban, Haitian, & Puerto Rican populations. Corresponding with the demographics of the catchment area, we subsequently added two teams to serve primarily Anglo and African American elderly. In each ethnic community, the team had an advisory board that helped with needs assessment, staffing, and developing services. Combining applied research, community development, and clinical functions, each team was led by a social scientist, typically at the Ph.D. level, and each had a clinical social worker and a part-time psychiatrist and psychologist, together with four or five trained paraprofessionals. Almost all staff, of all levels and disciplines, were of matching ethnicity to the populations served.

Team functions included needs assessment, action-oriented research to bring needed resources into communities, such as day care or hot meals programs, social services, and consultation and education responsive to communities' definition of their needs. After the teams came to be viewed as a viable helping resource, nine neighborhood "mini-clinics" were established in each of the ethnic communities. These provided aftercare, outpatient and day treatment; they dispensed consultation and education, and functioned as neighborhood centers for the local population. Crisis intervention and inpatient services were provided at Jackson Memorial Hospital, our affiliated teaching hospital that served the entire county.

Levels of Intervention

The program model dealt with mental health problems at both the microcosmic and macrocosmic levels, with at least four levels of intervention. The teams might work with a client within a concentric matrix of first the individual, then the family, neighborhood support systems, and community resource networks. Long before the term *case managers* entered our lexicon, paraprofessional team members, called neighborhood workers, fulfilled a case management role in linking clients with needed financial, medical, vocational, and social resources. In addition to clinic-based services, teams were involved in home visits and in establishing a network of information, referral, and social service coordination for clients. They tapped family networks, churches, and ethnic organizations; they found jobs, medical aid, child care; and they met a range of basic survival needs for their clients. A study analyzing the model of intervention found that successful environmental interventions significantly predicted favorable therapeutic outcome (Lefley 1979).

The teams were also involved in collective actions at neighborhood and community levels. Led by social scientists, the teams acted as initiators and coordinators of projects to bring new resources into their communities or to strengthen existing ones; they conducted surveys to provide supportive data for community-requested programs, linked consumer groups with appropriate service agencies, and helped residents learn how to utilize agencies to ameliorate specific neighborhood problems. Examples included organizing elderly residents to develop and administer a multiservice center, and to eliminate stressors such as drug-dealing through community action. The Puerto Rican team organized an initiative to bring a community school for adult education into its area. The Bahamian team developed a summer employment team for low-income Black teenagers. The Black American team helped organize a tenants council to improve service in a housing project. The Cuban team attracted $450,000 in community development funds into a low-income area, developed crime prevention programs, and became active in multi-ethnic coalition building. And the Haitian team became involved in massive advocacy efforts for the Haitian community. A special project evolved when it was found that numerous Haitian children were not attending school because their parents were illegal aliens and could not enroll their children since the schools demanded student documentation. In the first year following negotiations with the school system, the Haitian team was able to enroll 750 Haitian children in school with no required documentation.

Program evaluation subsequently demonstrated the efficacy of these combined approaches. Empirical data demonstrated that when compared with normative statistics then available from other centers, this CMHC had a high minority utilization rate (80 percent) and significantly lower no-show and dropout rates then other CMHCs. For example, cultural inaccessibility often results in minority members failing to keep appointments, with reported no-show rates ranging from 40 percent to 56 percent for African American and Hispanic patients (Hertz and Stamps 1977). Our mean no-show rate was 9.7 percent. Dropout rates of ethnic minority clients ranging from 42 to 50 percent were reported for over 14,000 CMHC clients (Sue 1977). For the same time period, this CHMC's highest annual dropout rate was 12 percent. Other data on client satisfaction, and outcome measures based on goal-attainment scaling and recidivism rates, similarly demonstrated the effectiveness of the program model (see Lefley and Bestman 1984).

Developing Cross-Cultural Training

Social scientists and clinicians on the ethnic teams were called "culture brokers"—a professional role in the health care delivery system described by Weidman (1983) as involving a bridging, interpretive, collaborative, and teaching function at the interface of the hospital and community and within the two systems. As faculty members in the Department of Psychiatry, culture brokers had combined academic, applied social scientist, and service provider roles. Hospital linkages facilitated an exchange of transcultural clinical information with medical as well as mental health staff. Culture brokers educated both mental health professionals about cultural beliefs and practices and community members about what to expect and how they might benefit from professional clinical interventions.

In the course of treating our multiethnic clientele in the hospital and mini-clinics; in ongoing supportive contacts and home visits with families; and in consultation and intervention in the schools, criminal justice system, and other community agencies, a body of information emerged that was relevant to the application of culturally appropriate care. Two training projects were subsequently funded by the NIMH to transmit this information to other practitioners. The first focused on enhancing the cultural sensitivity of mental health professionals working with clients from minority groups. The second addressed the needs of a range of human service workers in providing culturally appropriate care to clients from refugee and entrant groups. Both training projects were funded by the NIMH and conducted through the joint efforts of the University of Miami School of Medicine Department of Psychiatry in conjunction with faculty and staff of the New Horizons CMHC.

The Cross-Cultural Training Institute for Mental Health Professionals (CCTI)

Following a national needs assessment, the CCTI was developed to provide intensive eight-day continuing education workshops to mental health practitioners currently working in agencies serving low-income, culturally diverse populations. The curriculum began with the exploration of one's own cultural value orientations and assumptions in multicultural groups. A focus on cultural self-awareness was based on the premise that the trainee's self-understanding will lead to a greater ability to understand and adjust to another culture.

Training staff were primarily African American and Hispanic faculty members from the CMHC and Department of Psychiatry but included other academicians, practitioners, folk healers, community aides, and various consultants. The curriculum involved a synthesis of didactic, transactional, experiential, and cultural immersion techniques, as well as operationalized action plans for transfer of training. Lecture materials focused on contemporary culture in historical perspective, such as Afrocentric cognitive systems, religion, worldview and value systems, family structure and interactions, child rearing, age and sex roles, supernatural beliefs and alternative healing, and interracial, intercultural communication. Normative behavior, lifestyles, support systems, cultural stressors and coping mechanisms, adaptive strategies for survival, and the interrelationships of ethnic minority status and mental health were explored. Particularly important were cultural immersion, which was used throughout the eight days and involved systematic participant observation in ethnic neighborhoods; visits to restaurants, bars, and botanicas; street encounters; church participation; visits to ethnic community clinics; and even visits to clients' homes, with group processing of reactions.

Practicum experiences included videotaped role-playing and simulation of therapeutic encounters with clients and families of other cultures. Each trainee was videotaped interacting with a role-playing minority "client" before and after training. This yielded one of the behavioral measures used in evaluating the project.

The CCTI ultimately trained 174 mental health professionals representing 97 agencies and institutions throughout the United States. Trainees were selected to insure an ethnic mix for mutual sharing of cultural expertise and representation of administrators as well as clinicians to provide support for knowledge sharing, inservice cultural training, and structural changes in the home agencies.

The CCTI had an extremely comprehensive evaluation component. Short-term evaluation applied participant feedback in rating the workshops but also used objective measures of changes in knowledge and skill levels; reductions in cognitive, social, and attitudinal distance; understanding of values; and behaviorally demonstrated therapeutic effectiveness with a person of another culture.

Long-term evaluation looked at effects on clinical and administrative practice, agency changes and spin-off effects, and impact on cultural accessibility in terms of minority utilization and dropout rates. A cost-benefit analysis determined the savings obtained by reducing clients' failure to keep scheduled appointments. And a twelve-to-eighteen-month follow-up was obtained of the long-range impact of the training on participants' own work, self-concept, perceptions of deficits in their own professional education, and views of the parameters of good mental health care. (More detailed curriculum and evaluation materials may be found in Lefley and Pedersen 1986.)

Significant increases in learning occurred on all cognitive measures, as well as significant changes in social distance, which varied as a function of the ethnicity of the trainee (Lefley 1985a). With training, participants' perceptions of the values and worldview of a contrast culture moved closer to those of persons representing that culture. Videotaped vignettes of interviewing skills with a client from a different cultural background—rated blind by over one thousand community viewers stratified for African American, Hispanic, and Anglo backgrounds--indicated a significant increase in therapists' skills and sensitivity after training, with controls for practice effects.

Reports of the long-range subjective impact months after CCTI training indicated changes in participants' work, self-concept as professionals, cultural self-awareness, assessment of cultural deficits with suggestions for improving standard clinical training, and more community-oriented views of good mental health care. The following are just a few examples of their comments.

On self-concept as a person and as a professional:

"Surprisingly to myself, I became more aware of my own motivations and drives." "I take more pride in my own culture and background. I feel less alienated from my past." "My self-concept as a person has changed since I realized my liberal 'color blindness' reflected good will but a lot of fear and ignorance too. In the year since CCTI I have come to know some friends and colleagues in a much fuller, honest way." "My sense of professional competency has increased as a result of having obtained a wider scope and appreciation of cultural diversity."

Effects of the training on clinical performance:

"I have become more comfortable working with minority clients . . . more open to using alternative forms of treatment." "My therapeutic stance now allows for cultural differences to emerge without being defined as 'pathologically' different." "More aware of my own 'differentness' to the client . . . more willing to work within someone else's framework, less demanding that they work within mine." "It has taught me to be more aware of all subgroups—people in wheelchairs as well as those of other races."

"My work as a clinician has changed as a result of the CCTI training experience of myself and our administrative staff, in that we all provide more linkage/brokerage services to our clients so that exacerbating stresses are reduced, thereby resulting in our clients being more in control of vital resources and rising in their functional level. I also provide more services in the field, including support, brokerage with landlords, transportation to hospitals, and promoting peer support networks in apartment complexes."

Long-range evaluation of action plans indicated that many agencies had implemented goals involving ethnic needs assessments, community liaison and outreach, affirmative action plans, ethnic representation on boards, continuing education, special services, and quality assurance. There were multiple spin-off effects, ranging from total restructuring and decentralization of an urban CMHC to improve its services to ethnic minorities, to replication of cross-cultural training at the home site.

Perhaps the most significant findings, however, were those that suggested an impact on clients. Comparison of agency utilization rates, using a prior six-month period for baseline percentages and controlling for projected increase, indicated the following: (1) an increase in minority utilization, both in clinician and agency caseloads; (2) a significant reduction in agency dropout rates, overall (p = .001) and for specific ethnic groups. This could not be attributed to the passage of time alone, since normative data from the NIMH Annual Biometry Inventory on all federally funded CMHCs indicated remarkable stability in dropout rates, with less than .02 percent deviation over a two-year period. Finally, (3) a cost-benefit analysis suggested a projected mean annual savings of $152,930 based on only one output unit—the last scheduled appointment. (A more detailed analysis may be found in Lefley 1986a.)

The Mental Health Human Services Training Center (MHHSTC)

In many areas of the country, massive immigration has been accompanied by mental health problems in both the entrant and resident populations. During the early 1980s Dade County, Florida, had seen a number of massive upheavals in its social structure. These included (1) the steady immigration of people from Latin America and the Caribbean who gradually changed the social, economic, cultural, and linguistic patterns of the areas; (2) upheavals on the part of the native African American population, manifested in rioting related to perceived police brutality and other discrimination; (3) a massive strain on the infrastructure created by the entry, in one year of approximately 125,000 Cuban and 60,000 Haitian newcomers; (4) escalating drug traffic; and (5) a variable but apparently escalating crime rate.

Any community faced with such massive social changes will drain the resources of its caretakers—principally the police, schools, and other human service providers. Immigrants are by definition at risk for emotional problems, since they face uprooting, loss, separation from loved ones, an unfamiliar culture, and unpredictable futures, as well as antagonism from economically threatened native-born residents and sometimes from prior immigrants as well.

At this time the NIMH awarded approximately $5 million in refugee funding to the mental health centers in South Florida communities that were most affected by the influx of newcomers. This led to a significant increase in the number of new mental health care workers addressing the needs of refugees. There was thus a need for training to (a) provide intensive skill-building in transculturally oriented mental health interventions, and (b) provide training in Cuban and/or Haitian culture to all human service, health, mental health, and public agency service personnel. MH-HSTC was funded to serve these purposes.

As in the CCTI, project staff were representative of the multicultural populations of South Florida. Human service providers were requested to complete a learning needs assessment survey, which was used to develop the curriculum. Training methods included a demographic overview of Cuban and Haitian refugees in the United States; a brief immersion experience to promote transcultural understanding and sensitivity of mental health workers; alternative healing systems; review of values, attitudes, and lifestyles of refugees, of stresses affecting refugees, and similar issues. The training consisted of three programs. Program I—Employee Orientation—offered one week (40 hours) pre-service training to personnel recently hired or assigned to Cuban or Haitian refugee services. The trainees would ideally enter Program I within their first two months of employment. This program attracted both professional and paraprofessional staff including agency administrators, psychologists, social workers, nurses, policemen, vocational rehabilitation counselors, and others from a variety of agencies. Didactics, field observations in New Horizons clinics, audiovisual presentations, role-playing, small group discussion and sharing, and cultural immersion were offered to a total of 630 participants, who also received continuing education credits.

Program II was delivered in two cycles of sixteen weeks each. This program addressed skill-building through participation in role-playing sessions that were videotaped for productive feedback. Cultural immersion experiences in Cuban and Haitian communities were provided, as well as guest lectures by Cuban and Haitian community leaders and mental health professionals. This program was completed by fifty trainees who received continuing education credits.

Program III consisted of fifteen transcultural workshops conducted throughout Southeast Florida with the participation of community leaders, mental health and other human service workers, public services policy makers, and administrative personnel. This program reached 948 trainees. All programs were rated above 4.13 on a scale of 1 to 5.

A number of policy implications emerged from the training experiences. First was the importance of integrating and dovetailing the disbursement of funds to agencies providing human services and the appropriate transcultural understanding of those persons charged with delivering services. The need for providing timely training in cultural sensitivity to service providers was highlighted. Second was the importance of ensuring that this integrative function be placed simultaneously in the mental health and human service sectors and also in sectors providing other types of governmental intervention with entrants. We found, for example, that police officers as well as health care personnel (nurses, physicians, orderlies, housekeepers) were sorely in need of this information and the attitude-adjustment training that the Center provided. A third finding was the importance of having senior- and managerial-level personnel undergo this type of training. We found that although lower-level staff might become sensitized as to how they could provide more culturally appropriate services to entrants, they often felt hampered by insensitive supervisors and policy makers. Another policy imperative related to the importance of inter-institutional cooperation among senior universities, community junior colleges, community mental health centers, and other agencies to provide academic and financial leverage, training personnel, a praxis element, and academic credit useful for those workers who were below the baccalaureate level.

This project also highlighted the importance of active participation of credential-awarding bodies in curriculum development, training delivery, and quality control. Another element often neglected in development of policies and guidelines pertaining to training is the actual trainee. Recommendations were that during policy formulation at the national and regional levels, the input of former trainees, as well as those awaiting training, should be solicited on experiences, needs, expectations, and ideas of what would be most beneficial. Regarding the specific mandate of the MHHSTC to train human service providers to work with entrants, we suggest that policy makers and training providers should actively seek the meaningful participation of those persons about whom the training and development are given—the entrants themselves—as educators. In fact, there is currently a movement in all areas of mental health training to involve consumers as educators, so that they may share their experiences and needs with those who serve them.

Conclusion

We have described a community mental health center that developed a model program to deliver culturally appropriate and sensitive services, and the training efforts that derived from the experiences, knowledge, and techniques acquired in this program. The program led to two training institutes and some comprehensive research findings that seem to indicate that even short-term, intensive cross-cultural training can transfer to practice. Our findings, however, highlight the deficits in standard professional education in preparing clinicians to work effectively with clients from diverse cultural and socioeconomic backgrounds.

Although it is evident that cultural training may lead to greater sensitivity and effectiveness, there are also dangers of misapplication of irrelevant data, of stereotypes, and overgeneralizations. Therefore, many questions remain about how best to train clinicians to deliver culturally appropriate mental health services to members of ethnic minority groups. We have still not resolved many questions—such as models for disentangling minority, socioeconomic, or migrant status from ethnocultural issues; the significance of ethnic matching of therapists and clients; and the relative importance of cultural information as compared with the therapist's overall attitude toward other human beings. We might indeed ask: Is cultural knowledge essential for the provider to be perceived as a viable helping resource? Do respect and empathy provide what is needed, or must they be combined with (and be reflected in) cultural expertise? Or is credibility the main issue—that is, the client's belief that he or she will be helped by the therapeutic intervention?

These are critical issues, because it is obvious that therapists cannot become total experts in all the cultures likely to be reflected by their clientele. An analysis of the literature by Sue and Zane (1987) suggests that clients' perception of two interrelated processes, credibility and giving, are essential for therapeutic efficacy in cross-cultural counseling and psychotherapy. This was supported empirically in the CCTI research findings. In evaluating the videotapes of trainees' interactions with a client from another cultural or socioeconomic group before and after training, over a thousand raters used a twenty-item rating scale that had been developed by a multicultural group of clinical staff. A principal components factor analysis with varimax rotation found that a single factor accounted for 85 percent of the variance; credibility as helper, that is, perception of the therapist as someone with problem-solving abilities (Lefley 1989). Sue and Zane (1987) point out that small pieces of cultural knowledge, which make the client comfortable, can convey to the client a problem-solving capability and an ability to give something viewed as directly beneficial.

Our trainees for the most part were concerned and empathic mental health practitioners and human service providers, eager to obtain knowledge and to become culturally competent. In the CCTI findings, we know that our training in cultural sensitivity must have generalized to more sensitive practice overall because dropout rates were reduced for all ethnic groups, including Anglo clients. The implication is clear that the clinicians and administrators became more attentive to the needs of their clients; this was manifested in the fact that more clients viewed the agency as a viable helping resource and came back for services.

The agencies, however, expanded their view of service delivery. They included ethnic groups on their governance boards, took affirmative action policies, and decentralized some of their services to benefit their ethnic constituencies. They implemented the notion of community intervention (Bestman 1986b) to improve the lives of their constituents.

It was evident also that clinicians expanded their view of the parameters of mental health services for individual patients. Emulating the experiences of the training staff, they began to see therapeutic interventions as far more than simply psychotherapy, pharmacotherapy, or work with the immediate family. They began to view the clients and their families as part of a much larger system, one that might impose stressors but that could also, alternatively, offer adaptive resources and cultural strengths. They began to see the role of mental health professionals as one of tapping a multiplicity of resources to alleviate problems and foster rehabilitation of their clients.

In training for culturally sensitive care, we believe that a variety of approaches can be used, ranging from the use of cultural data in insight-oriented therapies to developing appropriate acculturation classes for refugees. For the majority of clients affected by the stressors of racism, however, we suggest that the treatment of choice is a multifaceted approach that offers case management for basic survival needs and recognizes the extent to which psychological problems may be reactive to external stressors of economics and racism. Treatment plans may thus aim toward the enhancement of coping capabilities through the development and utilization of adaptive community resources. In this context, culturally sensitive treatment deals with reality problems, builds on cultural strengths, enhances cultural pride, and aims at developing adaptive behavior in the client's environment of choice.

Ideally, training in cultural sensitivity should begin in one's earliest years and continue throughout the entire lifetime. This would make better persons and better clinicians of us all. For specific application in clinical interventions, however, culturally sensitive professional training should begin at the pre-service level and become a continuing and integrated component of all inservice training and continuing education. In the context of training for work with specific populations, it is important to ensure that representatives of the target groups—whether they be members of ethnic minority groups, refugees, migrants, or long-term mental health consumers—are always involved in curriculum development and as participant trainers. Whenever possible, supervisors, administrators, and policy makers should be included in cultural sensitivity training for their staff. It is also extremely important to effect an attitude change on the part of persons who credential training programs and who evaluate the performance of human service workers, including professionals. We suggest that credentialing bodies and mental health administrations begin to review clinical training curricula in the colleges and universities in terms of their relevance to the needs of the populations they serve.

REFERENCES

Adebimpe, V. R. 1984. American Blacks and psychiatry. *Transcultural Psychiatric Research Review* 21:81–111.
American Psychiatric Association (APA).
    1980. *Diagnostic and statistical manual of mental disorders.* 3d. ed. (DSM-III). Washington, D.C.: APA.
    1987. *Diagnostic and statistical manual of mental disorders.* 3d. ed. revised (DSM-III-R). Washington, D.C.: APA.
Bestman, E. W.
    1981. Blacks and mental health services. In *Community mental health: a sourcebook,* ed. W. H. Silverman. New York: Praeger.
    1986a. Cross-cultural approaches to service delivery to ethnic minorities: the Miami model. In *Mental health research and practice in minority communities: development of,* ed. M. Miranda and H. Kitano. Culturally Sensitive Training Programs (pp. 199–224) DHHS ADM (86–1466). Washington, D.C.: Government Printing Office.
    1986b. Intervention techniques in the Black community. In *Cross-cultural training for mental health professionals,* ed. H. P. Lefley and P. B. Pedersen, pp. 213–24. Springfield, Ill.: Charles C. Thomas.
Chu, C., Sallach, H. S., Zakeria, S. A., et al. 1985. Differences in psychopathology between Black and White schizophrenics. *International Journal of Social Psychiatry* 31:252–57.
Comas-Diaz, L., and Griffith, E. E. H. 1987. *Clinical guidelines in cross-cultural mental health.* New York: Wiley.
Estroff, S. E. 1989. Self, identity, and subjective experiences of schizophrenia: in search of the subject. *Schizophrenia Bulletin* 15:189–96.
Fabrega, H., Mezzich, J., and Ulrich, R. F. 1988. Black-white differences in psychopathology in an urban psychiatric population. *Comprehensive Psychiatry* 29:285–97.

Griffith, E. E. H., Young, J. L., and Smith, D. L. 1984. An analysis of the therapeutic elements in a Black church service. *Hospital and Community Psychiatry* 35:464–69.

Hertz, P., and Stamps, P. L. 1977. Appointment-keeping behavior re-evaluated. *Am J Public Health* 67:1033–36.

Jones, B. E., and Gray, B. A. 1986. Problems in diagnosing schizophrenia and affective disorders among Blacks. *Hospital and Community Psychiatry* 37:61–65.

Keith, S. J., Regier, D. A., and Rae, D. S. 1991. Schizophrenic disorders. In *Psychiatric disorders in America: the epidemiologic catchment area study*, ed. L. N. Robins and D. A. Regier, pp. 33–52. New York: Free Press.

Kinzie, J. D., and Manson, S. M. 1987. The use of self-rating scales in cross-cultural psychiatry. *Hospital and Community Psychiatry* 38:190–96.

Lefley, H. P.
1979. Environmental interventions and therapeutic outcome. *Hospital and Community Psychiatry* 30:341–44.

1985a. Impact of cross-cultural training on Black and White mental health professionals. *International Journal of Intercultural Relations* 9:305–18.

1985b. Mental health training across cultures. In *Handbook of cross-cultural counseling and therapy*, ed. P. B. Pedersen, pp. 259–66. Westport, Conn.: Greenwood Press.

1986a. Evaluating the effects of cross-cultural training: some research results. In *Cross-cultural training for mental health professionals*, ed. H. P. Lefley and P. B. Pedersen, pp. 265–347. Springfield, Ill.: Charles C. Thomas.

1986b. Why cross-cultural training? applied issues in culture and mental health service delivery. In *Cross-cultural training for mental health professionals*, ed. H. P. Lefley and P. B. Pedersen, pp. 11–44. Springfield, Ill.: Charles C. Thomas.

1989. Empirical support for credibility and giving in cross-cultural psychotherapy. *American Psychologists* 44:1163.

1990. Culture and chronic mental illness. *Hospital and Community Psychiatry* 41:277–86.

Lefley, H. P., and Bestman, E. Q. 1984. Community mental health and minorities: a multiethnic approach. In *The pluralistic society: a community mental health perspective*, ed. S. Sue and T. Moore, pp. 116–48. New York: Human Sciences Press.

Lefley, H. P., and Pedersen, P. B., eds. 1986. *Cross-cultural training for mental health professionals*. Springfield, Ill.: Charles C. Thomas.

Lin, K.-M., Poland, R. E., and Lesser, I. M. 1986. Ethnicity and psychopharmacology. *Culture, Medicine, and Psychiatry* 10:151–65.

Loring, M., and Powell, B. 1988. Gender, race, and DSM-III: a study of the objectivity of psychiatric diagnostic behavior. *Journal of Health and Social Behavior* 29:1–22.

Mukherjee, S., Shukla, S., Woodle, J., et al. 1983. Misdiagnosis of schizophrenia in bipolar patients: a multiethnic comparison. *Am J Psychiat* 140:1571–74.

National Institute of Mental Health (NIMH).
1987. *Mental health, United States, 1987*, ed. R. W. Manderscheid and S. A. Barrett. DHHS Pub. No. (ADM)87-1518. Supt. of Docs. Washington, D.C.: U.S. Government Printing Office.

1990. *Mental health, United States, 1990*, ed. R. W. Manderscheid and M. A. Sonnenschein. DHHS Pub. No. (ADM)90-1708. Supt. of Docs. Washington, D.C.: U.S. Government Printing Office.

Pavkov, T. W., Lewis, D. A., and Lyons, J. S. 1989. Psychiatric diagnoses and racial bias: an empirical investigation. *Professional Psychology: Research and Practice* 20:364–68.

Pedersen, P. B., Draguns, J. G., Lonner, W., and Trimble, J., eds. 1989. *Counseling across cultures*. 3d ed. Honolulu: University Press of Hawaii.

Robins, L. N., and Regier, D. A., eds. 1991. *Psychiatric disorders in America: the epidemiologic catchment area study*. New York: Free Press.

Robins, L. N., Locke, B. Z., and Regier, D. A. 1991. An overview of psychiatric disorders in America. In *Psychiatric disorders in America: the epidemiologic catchment area study*, ed. L. N. Robins and D. A. Regier, pp. 328–66. New York: Free Press.

Snowden, L. R., and Cheung, F. K. 1990. Use of inpatient mental health services by members of ethnic minority groups. *American Psychologist* 45:347–55.

Sue, D. W., and Sue, D. 1990. *Counseling the culturally different: theory and practice*. 2d ed. New York: Wiley.

Sue, S. 1977. Community mental health services to minority groups. *American Psychologist* 32:616–24.

Sue, S., and Zane, N. 1987. The role of culture and cultural techniques in psychotherapy: a critique and reformulation. *American Psychologist* 42:37–45.

Swartz, M., Landerman, R., George, L. K., Blazer, D. G., and Escobar, J. 1991. Somatization disorder. In *Psychiatric disorders in America: the epidemiologic catchment area study*, ed. L. N. Robins and D. A. Regier, pp. 220–55. New York: Free Press.

Talbott, J. A., Hales, R. E., and Yudofsky, S. C. 1988. *The American Psychiatric Press Textbook of Psychiatry*. Washington, D.C.: American Psychiatric Press.

Weidman. H. H.

1978. *Miami health ecology project report: a statement on ethnicity and health*. Vol. 1. Miami: University of Miami School of Medicine.

1983. Research, science, and training aspects of clinical anthropology: an institutional overview. In *Clinical anthropology: a new approach to American health problems?* ed. D. B. Shimkin and P. Golde, pp. 119–53. Lanham, Md.: University Press of America.

Weissman, M. M., Bruce, M. L., Leaf, P. J., Florio, L. P., and Holzer, C. 1991. Affective disorders. In *Psychiatric disorders in America: the epidemiologic catchment area study*, ed. L. N. Robins and D. A. Regier, pp. 53–80. New York: Free Press.

Westermeyer, J. 1987. Clinical considerations in cross-cultural diagnosis. *Hospital and Community Psychiatry* 38:160–65.

Wilkinson, C. B., ed. 1986. *Ethnic psychiatry*. New York: Plenum.

Williams, C. L. 1987. Issues surrounding psychological testing of minority patients. *Hospital and Community Psychiatry* 38:184–89.

Williams, D. H. 1986. the epidemiology of mental illness in Afro-Americans. *Hospital and Community Psychiatry* 37:42–49.

Women's Mental Health: Research Agenda for the Twenty-first Century

EVELOPING a U.S. women's mental health research agenda for the twenty-first century is a formidable task, requiring research approaches that consider the interacting effects of gender and ethnicity in their sociocultural context over the life cycle. Recognition of the need for a national women's mental health research agenda emerged in the 1970s as the women's movement forced widespread examination of the prejudice, stereotyping, discrimination, and devaluation experienced by women. In 1978, the President's Commission on Mental Health (PCMH) officially noted inadequacies in mental health services for women, expressing concern about "the failure of mental health practitioners to recognize, understand, and empathize with the feelings of powerlessness, alienation, and frustration expressed by many women" (PCMH 1978, 7). The report of the PCMH Subpanel on the Mental Health of Women documented the social, economic, and psychological effects of inequality involved in those feelings, stating "the mental health implications of the pervasive sexism that impacts ... women of all ages, socioeconomic and racial/ethnic groups in our society must receive priority attention in policy formation and program implementation" (1025).

The subpanel made numerous recommendations for mental health research, service delivery, and strategies for prevention. Although the specifics of these recommendations have evolved in numerous policy reports over the subsequent decade (Eichler and Parron 1987; Public Health Service Task Force on Women's Health Issues 1985; Russo 1985, 1990), a common theme has persisted: Existing scientific knowledge is inadequate for understanding gender differences in the etiology, diagnosis, treatment, and prevention of mental disorder. Feminist researchers have begun to construct the new knowledge base needed for that understanding.

Feminism involves diverse frameworks, goals, and strategies. Broadly defined, however, feminist researchers seek knowledge to empower women to achieve their self-defined goals and to improve women's status in society. In building the needed knowledge base, feminists have recognized the importance of dealing with the interaction of gender, ethnicity, social class, and other social categories that affect women's lives and create multiple realities for women (for reviews, see Carmen, Russo, and Miller 1981; Green and Russo 1993; O'Connell and Russo 1991; Rieker and Carmen 1984; Russo 1985, 1990; Russo and Green 1992). This chapter builds on feminist efforts, offering ways to construct a women's mental health research agenda designed to serve the needs of women into the twenty-first century.

Gender Differences in Mental Disorder: An Unfinished Portrait

The agenda for the 1990s must address the issues posed by the large, complex gender differences found in mental disorder, gender differences that vary with the sociocultural context in ways traditional biomedical models or intrapsychic perspectives cannot explain. Whether one examines lifetime prevalence rates or six-month prevalence rates, community surveys conducted by the influential NIMH Epidemiological Catchment Area (ECA) Program have found women to have higher rates of depressive disorders (major depressive disorder, dysthymia), anxiety disorders (simple phobia, agoraphobia, panic disorder, obsessive-compulsive disorder), schizophrenia, and somatization disorder. In contrast, men have higher rates of alcohol abuse or dependence, antisocial personality, and drug abuse or dependence (Myers et al. 1984; Robins et al. 1984). Unfortunately, these important studies did not report their findings separately by gender and ethnic minority group.

The need to examine the link between social roles and mental health is found in variation in rates of mental disorder with marital status. Particularly large gender differences by marital status are found in patient populations, with married women having higher admission rates to mental health facilities than married men, and never-married and separated or divorced men having higher admission rates than comparable women (Russo and Sobel 1981; Russo, Amaro, and Winter 1987).

This gender difference holds for both Blacks and Whites (Russo and Sobel 1981; Russo and Olmedo 1983). How it would vary with diagnosis is unknown, however. Given that depressive disorders are the leading diagnosis for women regardless of race, it is likely that the overall gender difference reflects the gender difference for those diagnoses. Other research suggests that such gender differences indeed vary with ethnicity and psychological disorder (Russo, Amaro, and Winter 1987).

Whether such gender differences in service utilization reflect differences in etiology, help-seeking, diagnosis, or treatment decision has yet to be ascertained: the picture is complex. Nonetheless, for affective disorders—disorders that are high prevalence for women—women's higher rates among married and never-married categories appear to be similar whether one is White or Black, Hispanic or non-Hispanic (Russo, Amaro, and Winter 1987; Russo and Sobel 1981).

The difference in rates of affective disorder between married and unmarried women depends on marital quality (Aneshensel 1986). Using ECA data, Weissman (1987) reported that women in unhappy marriages were three times more likely than men to be depressed. The depression rates for both sexes were lower in happy marriages, but the gap was larger: women in happy marriages were nearly five times more likely to experience depression than men in such marriages.

Some authors have suggested that women's higher rates of affective disorder, particularly for unhappily married women, reflect the burdens of childbearing rather than the demands of the marital role (Gater, Dean, and Morris 1989). Number of children has been found to be negatively related to women's self-esteem, even when marital status, education, income, and employment are controlled (Russo and Zierk 1992). Unfortunately, a portrait of the interactive relationships among gender, ethnicity, and marital and parental roles for high prevalence mental disorders in women has yet to be constructed. Although recent government reports are now reporting some data by gender and ethnic minority group, findings are not separated by marital status, parental status, and type of disorder. Thus, the epidemiological information needed to develop a portrait of the relationship of women's gender roles of wife and mother to mental disorder is lacking.

Moreover, all ages are lumped together (Manderscheid and Sonnenschein 1990). The failure to report findings separately for adults and children yields a particularly distorted portrait of male/female differences in community surveys as well as in service utilization. The female excess in mental disorder does not appear until adolescence (Horwitz and White 1987; Kandel and Davies 1982; Nolen-Hoeksema 1990). The gender difference in appearance of mental disorder is likely to vary with ethnicity. In 1975, more than one half of Black males admitted to outpatient facilities were under 18 years of age, compared to 33 percent of White males, 21 percent of Black females, and 16 percent of White females (Russo and Olmedo 1983).

In conclusion, such findings clearly demonstrate that global summaries of epidemiological data are inadequate and misleading. They underscore the importance of building an epidemiological portrait of mental disorder that will clearly identify the interactive relationships among gender, ethnic group, and marital and parental roles, particularly for high prevalence disorders in women such as depressive and anxiety disorders.

Diagnosis and Treatment

The epidemiological findings suggest a paradoxical relationship between gender stereotyping and mental health diagnosis and treatment: women are both overrepresented and underserved in treatment populations (Russo 1984). Thus, women have higher rates of disorders that are congruent with society's view of "femininity" (such as depression and anxiety). For disorders that are incongruent with society's idealized view of "femininity" (such as abuse of illegal drugs or alcoholism), women have traditionally been invisible and neglected. How the lack of congruence between gender-related expectations and definitions of mental disorder affects clinical judgments must be ascertained. Processes that affect such judgments include overpathologizing, or inappropriately perceiving patients whose behavior violates norms as more disturbed; overdiagnosis, or inappropriately applying a diagnosis as a function of group membership; and underdiagnosis, or inappropriately avoiding application of a diagnosis as a function of group membership (Lopez 1989).

Evidence for overpathologizing is found in a classic study by Rosenfield (1982), who reported a greater probability of hospitalization for men and women when their diagnoses were inconsistent with gender role stereotypes. A more recent study found that men diagnosed with major depression and women diagnosed with antisocial personality or alcohol abuse disorders were rated as more severely disturbed and more likely to be recommended for drug treatment than individuals of the opposite sex receiving similar diagnoses (Waisberg and Page 1988).

Overdiagnosis of depression for both Black and White women was found in clinical judgments by male psychiatrists of a case description constructed to reflect undifferentiated schizophrenia with a dependent personality disorder. Female psychiatrists did not exhibit a bias toward overdiagnosing depression in women of either ethnic group—although they did have a tendency to diagnose White female patients as having a brief reactive psychosis (Loring and Powell 1988). In contrast, underdiagnosis is a concern for women who abuse alcohol and drugs, disorders incongruent with society's feminine ideal (Russo 1985).

The overlapping of gender stereotypes and symptoms of psychopathology in depressive and anxiety disorders makes misdiagnosis in women a particular concern (Russo 1984, 1985; McGrath et al. 1990). Depressive and anxiety disorders are heterogeneous diagnostic categories that involve overlapping symptoms, including crying, feelings of sadness and unhappiness, and eating and sleeping disorders (American Psychiatric Association [APA] 1994). High levels of these symptoms have been found in 20–25 percent of community samples (Kaplan et al. 1987).

Misdiagnosis can lead to inappropriate treatment. In particular, inappropriate drug treatment continues to be a major issue, particularly for older women (Russo 1985). Women receive prescriptions for psychotropic drugs at a higher rate than men for a variety of reasons, including gender differences in stressful life events, age, physical illnesses, psychiatric disorders, and help-seeking that leads to exposure to the medical system, which results in more prescriptions (for a more complete discussion, see Hamilton et al., in press; Travis 1988). However, a misdiagnosis of other disorders as depression may also lead to inappropriate drug treatment; drugs developed to treat major depression are not necessarily effective in treating other disorders.

The interacting effects of gender and ethnicity on treatment decisions bear close examination. In a study of 1975 admissions rates to outpatient facilities, Russo and Olmedo (1983) found that treatment for depressive disorders differed markedly by gender and ethnic minority status. For example, Black males were much less likely to receive individual therapy than other patients (26.6 percent of Black males diagnosed with depression received individual therapy, compared to 71.3, 84.1, and 84.4 percent, for similarly diagnosed White females, Black females, and White males, respectively). The processes that result in such differences in treatment must be identified and understood. Unfortunately, these findings do not control for age.

Diagnostic definitions reflect the vision, values, goals, and limited wisdom of the individuals who are given the power to create them. They have changed with time and, like most human concepts, are imperfect reflections of reality. The DSM-IV (APA 1994) is a basic reference for diagnosing mental disorder, and a substantial amount of research rests on DSM diagnostic definitions. Whether the thoughts and behaviors that make up a particular diagnosis are equally indicative of psychopathology across gender, let alone diverse ethnic minority groups, needs to be systematically studied (Comas-Díaz 1987). Basic research is needed on the consistency of patterns of symptoms in these disorders across diverse subpopulations of women and men.

In particular, symptoms of post–traumatic stress syndrome overlap with anxiety and depression, including depressed mood, sleep and appetite disturbance, social withdrawal, lowered self-esteem, and psychomotor retardation or agitation (APA 1994). Given the high prevalence of violence against women (Koss 1990), research that clarifies the relationships among symptoms of depression, anxiety, and other related disorders in subpopulations of women is clearly needed.

Both anxiety and depressive diagnoses are correlated with personality disorders (for a more complete discussion of the implications of this overlap, see McGrath et al. 1990). Misdiagnosis may account for some of that overlap, and the possible misdiagnosis of women who have experienced physical and sexual abuse is a particular concern. Bryer et al. (1987) found that childhood physical and sexual abuse and suicidal symptoms were associated with a high proportion of borderline personality diagnoses. Thus, a number of authors have argued for using post–traumatic stress syndrome rather than personality disorder as the initial diagnosis for abused patients (Gelinas 1983; van der Kolk 1988).

Risk factors may differ for subtypes of anxiety disorders. Weissman, Leaf, and Bruce (1987) found that panic disorders were higher among single mothers than married mothers, for both Black and White women. Those researchers also reported that married mothers had higher risk for obsessive-compulsive disorder than single mothers. This was particularly true for Black married mothers, whose rates were nearly seven times those of Black single mothers. The comparable figure for White mothers was nearly 3 to 1.

These findings, combined with the epidemiological portrait provided above, provide compelling evidence for the need to develop alternatives for understanding the development, diagnosis, and treatment of mental disorder, alternatives that take into account women's diverse social roles and life circumstances. A stress and coping framework provides such an alternative.

Stress and Coping Perspective on Women's Mental Health

Stress plays a pivotal role in the precipitation of psychological distress, particularly for anxiety and depressive disorders (see also Thoits 1984; Brown and Harris 1978). A stress and coping framework considers events in their social and economic contexts, thereby providing a useful model for conceptualizing the conditions that contribute to increased risk for psychological distress and mental disorder among women in diverse circumstances, across ethnic minority group and economic status. This type of perspective reflects the influence of mental health research that has examined the mental health impact of chronic stress and daily hassles in addition to that of major negative life events. Such a framework examines the interaction of sources of stress, coping resources, coping strategies, and social support, all of which may involve biological, psychological, social, cultural, or environmental factors (Hobfoll 1986a; 1986b; Hobfall and Leiberman 1987; Hobfall and London 1986; Hobfall and Walfisch 1984; Kessler, Price, and Wortman 1985; Lazarus and Folkman 1984; Thoits 1987a, 1987b).

A stress and coping model includes recognition of women's strengths as well as problems. This is particularly important when examining mental health issues for ethnic minority women. All too often the study of ethnic minorities has been approached from a perspective that emphasizes pathological and negative aspects of being an ethnic minority, applies White middle-class norms, and reinforces stereotypes (Fine 1985). Such models also avoid stereotyping women as passive victims of their environments. Women can be viewed as active agents who vest meaning and seek control and mastery of their environments by marshaling available resources and choosing among options. Although women may experience hardships, discrimination, violence, and degradation, they can and do survive their experiences and go on to be productive, functioning human beings. Thus, a systematic application of a stress and coping model that incorporates a combination of gender-related physical, psychological, social, and economic factors in examining the mental health implications of negative life events offers promise of creating a women's mental health research agenda to meet the needs of women from diverse ethnic groups.

Stressful Life Events

A stress and coping model envisions stress as a response to negative life events or conditions. Negative life events and life crises clearly contribute to women's higher rates for affective disorders. There is evidence that women experience stressful life events more often than men (Aneshensel, Frerichs, and Clark 1981; Belle 1990; Cleary and Mechanic 1983; Newmann 1984, 1986). Women's experiences of reproductive life events such as menstruation, pregnancy, birth, and menopause entail substantial stress and demonstrate the need for biopsychosocial models of stress and coping. They are also often used to justify women's disadvantaged social, economic, and political status, so that such events affect the lives of all women, even those not directly experiencing a particular event. This literature is extensively reviewed elsewhere, however, so it will not be considered in detail here (McGrath et al. 1990; Russo and Green 1992a).

The rising prevalence of AIDS among women and their families is a new source of stress, particularly for ethnic minority women (Fullilove 1988). Intravenous drug abuse during pregnancy, which can lead to pediatric AIDS, has provided a new and insidious source of chronic stress that disproportionately affects ethnic minority women (Selik, Castro, and Pappaioanou 1988).

Violence, poverty, and multiple roles all contribute to elevated levels of mental disorder in women. In 1987, NIMH developed a women's mental health research agenda that emphasized the mental health effects of stress related to these conditions (Belle 1990; Eichler and Parron 1987; Koss 1990; McBride 1990; Russo 1990). Unfortunately, studies that have used event checklists commonly used to ascertain gender differences in stressful life events have typically failed to include many events associated with common life experiences for women, particularly those linked to violence and poverty (Newmann 1986).

For example, in the sixty-item Life Experiences Survey (Sarason, Johnson, and Siegel 1978; Turner and Avison 1989) there are no questions that ask if a person has experienced forced intercourse, physical or verbal violence, sexual or racial harassment or discrimination, tokenism, occupational exposure to toxic substances, or loss of property due to criminal activity. Thus, although a stress and coping perspective has a great advantage over traditional intrapsychic approaches for developing a body of knowledge that will have relevance for all women, its potential will not be fulfilled until the multiple realities of women's lives are fully investigated and reflected in research protocols and instruments. In particular, the impact of the pervasive physical and sexual abuse of women, effects of poverty, and problems associated with multiple roles must be more fully taken into account in research on the etiology, diagnosis, and treatment of mental disorder (Russo 1990). In conceptualizing life stress associated with such conditions, the differential effects of acute and chronic stress must be examined and the process of their influence understood (Hobfall 1986a; Newmann 1986).

Physical and Sexual Abuse

Physical and sexual abuse of women by intimates is widespread, is found among all segments of society, and often has deadly consequences, particularly for minority women. Over one half of U.S. women who are murdered are killed by a current or former male partner (Browne and Williams 1989), and Black women are more likely than White women to be killed by their spouse (Plass and Strauss 1987). Risk factors include chronic alcohol and drug abuse in the partner, violence in the family of origin, living in central cities, poverty, and unemployment, among others (Harlow 1991; Tolman and Bennett 1990).

Violence and abuse take many forms, including stranger, acquaintance, date, and marital rape; wife battering; sexual harassment; sexual abuse of children; and elder abuse. Types of violence reported by women include being slapped, kicked, thrown bodily, scalded, choked, smothered, bitten, stabbed, and shot (Browne 1987). Needless to say, this violence against women has severe physical and mental health consequences (for a review of this literature see Goodman, Koss, and Russo 1993a, 1993b; Koss et al. 1994). Battered women are also affected by their partner's violence toward their children. One hospital-based study of child abuse victims found that records of 59 percent of the mothers of such victims had evidence of victimization histories. Further, the rate of violence against single mothers was four times the rate against married mothers (McKibben et al. 1989).

Although the issue of violence in pregnancy has been recognized for more than a decade (Gelles 1975), the contribution of such violence to psychopathology has yet to be adequately investigated. Stacey and Shupe (1983) reported that 42 percent of their sample of women entering shelters for battered women said they had been battered during pregnancy, experiencing slaps, kicks, and punches to abdomen and genitals. Stark, Flitcraft, and Frazier (1981) reported that one out of four pregnant battered women reported an escalation of violence during pregnancy. These researchers also suggest that battering during pregnancy entails higher risk for spontaneous abortion, another source of acute stress for women. In this context, a life events scale that asks women and men if they or their partner is pregnant and counts the experience as equal in stress if both respond affirmatively has definite shortcomings.

Abuse itself must be studied in context. It is correlated with different high-risk behaviors in different subpopulations of women. For example, Amaro and her colleagues (1989) found that adolescent mothers who used illicit drugs during pregnancy were more than twice as likely to be exposed to physical abuse than were pregnant adolescents who did not use such drugs (24 percent compared with 9 percent). This difference persisted regardless of maternal race and age. Pregnant adolescent drug users were also more likely to be North American Black (as opposed to foreign born), to have a history of venereal disease and of elective abortion, and to report more negative life events, violent and nonviolent (Amaro, Zuckerman, and Cabral 1989).

Child sexual abuse is a fact of life for both Black and White women (Wyatt 1985). Research has documented a relationship between sexual assault experiences (including childhood sexual abuse) and higher risk for major depressive episodes, substance use disorders, and anxiety disorders (including phobia, panic, and obsessive-compulsive disorder). Gender, Hispanic background, and education did not appear to affect overall probability of developing a disorder after abuse experiences (Burnam et al. 1988). Assault in childhood has been found to result in higher risk for subsequent disorder than assault later in life. Thus, sexual assault contributes to women's higher rates of mental disorder because women are more likely to have assault experiences rather than because they are more "vulnerable" to mental disorder than men.

Carmen and Rieker (1989) provide an insightful model of the victim-to-patient process in which the damage to the self caused by sexual abuse begins a variety of psychological and social processes that can result in numerous forms of mental disorder. They ingeniously link the damaged self of sexual abuse victims to AIDS risk in adolescent runaway, homeless, and mentally ill populations, thereby illustrating the complex web of stressors experienced by these victims. Their model is applicable across ethnicity and class, for it relates the mental health outcomes of the abuse experience to elements of the social context, including ongoing family relationships, that disconfirm and transform the abuse in destructive ways.

Poverty

Low income and low socioeconomic status are consistently found to be related to mental health problems (Belle 1990). One review that examined numerous studies found that the rate of psychopathology in the lowest social class averaged two-and-one-half times that of the highest social class (Neugebauer, Dohrenwend, and Dohrenwend 1980).

There are high levels of poverty among women and children, particularly among ethnic minority communities. In 1987, 30 percent of Black, 25 percent of Hispanic, and 10 percent of White families had incomes below the poverty level (U.S. Bureau of the Census 1989). Although poverty is not necessarily a chronic condition, Blacks and female single heads of households, in particular, are at higher risk for poverty that persists over many years. As Deborah Belle (1990) has described, poverty is associated with uncontrollable and threatening life events and involves higher risk from stressors from financial problems, inadequate housing and homelessness, crime and violence, imprisonment of husbands, dangerous neighborhoods, and illness and death of children. Poor women are also more likely to experience unwanted pregnancy (Russo and Zierk 1992). For ethnic minority women, who are more likely to experience poverty than majority women, these deleterious effects are compounded by exposure to discrimination and discrimination-related harassment and violence.

Although poor women have developed survival strategies that include mutual aid and extended kin networks (Stack 1974), poverty undermines the effectiveness of such strategies (Wolf 1987). The members of poor women's social networks are themselves likely to be poor and stressed, so that belonging to such a network may exact higher social and emotional costs than are repaid (Riley and Eckenrode 1986). Poverty is also associated with marital unhappiness (Zill 1978) and with having husbands who are less likely to serve as confidants (Brown et al. 1975). Poor women must depend on unresponsive, overburdened bureaucratic systems for assistance with basic needs, and their resulting frustration may contribute to feelings of powerlessness that undermine mental health (Belle 1990).

Multiple Roles
     Discrimination, lack of education, urban life, and poverty all create different opportunity structures for women of color and have shaped their family organization in multiple ways (Staples 1987; Zinn 1990). How the roles of worker, wife, and mother are combined varies across ethnic groups, so that the combinations of stressors and coping resources differ for ethnic minority women. All women, however, face issues of pay inequity, sexual harassment, and occupational segregation and discrimination. Sex and race discrimination interact, producing White-female-dominated jobs and minority-female-dominated jobs (Green and Russo 1992). One study found that Mexican Americans and Mexican immigrant women in minority-female-dominated jobs experienced more physical distress and danger at work and were more at risk for economic fluctuations than those working in jobs that were dominated by White women (Segura 1989). Because of a combination of salary discrimination and pay inequity, women earn less than men, and ethnic minority women earn less than majority women.
     Family income and education is correlated with marriage formation and stability (Staples 1987; Zinn 1989). Ethnic minority women are thus more likely to experience the stress of divorce and to be found in female-headed households (Saluter 1989). The powerful effects of poverty on family form are reflected in the large proportion of Black women who never marry, which largely reflects the economic status of Black men (Zinn 1989). Inequality in marital relationships is a source of psychological distress for women and is an issue for both majority and minority families (Golding 1990). How the issue is manifested and dealt with among diverse ethnic groups has not yet been systematically investigated, however.
     Motherhood embodies a social role and status in addition to a biological event. Pregnancy and delivery are stressful life events for both women and men. They can aggravate problems for women with histories of mental disorders (Hamilton, Parry, and Blumenthal 1988) and have been

linked to increased bipolar and psychotic illness in women's partners (Hamilton 1984; Freeman 1951; Towne and Afterman 1955). A woman's psychological response to motherhood reflects her satisfaction with her marital role. As mentioned above, marital role dissatisfaction is an important predictor of postpartum depression (Cox, Connor, and Kendell 1982; Weissman 1987; Whiffen 1988). Mood and behavior changes correlated with pregnancy and delivery can occur for both women and men. These changes can be informed by a stress and coping model that recognizes that neuroendocrine response is associated with social roles, status, and other sociocultural variables (Hamilton 1984).

Motherhood is associated with increased risk of depression for all women, but particularly for poor women (Belle 1990). Family size is associated with lower self-esteem and higher psychological distress, particularly among poor women. Ethnic minority women are more likely to be poor, become mothers during adolescence, and have larger families than other women (Russo and Zierk 1992). The burdens of childbearing for ethnic minority women are compounded by the more complex socialization needs of ethnic children who must be taught how to deal with harassment and other forms of racism (McAdoo and McAdoo 1985).

In summary, women's mental health is a complex topic, impossible to cover completely in any single chapter. Selected types of stressful life events and circumstances are only highlighted here to demonstrate the importance of examining the interrelationships among biological, psychological, and social variables over the life cycle in understanding the multiple realities of women's lives.

Women's Responses to Stressful Life Events

A stress and coping perspective recognizes that exposure to negative life events does not necessarily result in mental disorder. Several studies described below, after controlling for exposure to stressors, have suggested that women are more likely than men to report distress or seek help. Such studies have been used to suggest that women are more emotionally responsive to negative life events than men, because of differences in capacity to deal with stressful circumstances. Both gender-related personal attributes and women's roles and status have been offered as explanations for such gender differences.

Personal Attributes

Some researchers suggest that female sex role socialization can result in maladaptive coping styles and other personal attributes that contribute to risk for mental disorder in response to stress (Abramson and Andrews

1982; Kessler and McLeod 1984; Kessler, McLeod, and Wethington 1985; Nolen-Hoeksema 1987).

When depressed, both men and women are likely to use emotion-focused responses and less likely to use problem-solving coping responses in response to stressful life events (Billings, Cronkite, and Moos 1983). Nolen-Hoeksema (1987) argued that gender differences in depression may be due to women's emotion-focused, ruminative response styles, which may amplify and prolong depressive episodes. In contrast, men's more active response styles may dampen the effects of depressive episodes. A ruminative response set may interfere with instrumental behavior, increasing failure, feelings of helplessness, and the likelihood that an individual will develop a pessimistic, depressive explanatory style.

It has been suggested that the personal attributes of nurturance and caring on the part of women contribute to higher risks for psychopathology. However, several reviews of research have found little relationship between women's mental health and the gender-related personality trait of expressiveness, that is, orientation toward and concern for others (Spence, Helmreich, and Stapp 1974). In the majority of research studies it is instrumentality—that is, a sense of agency or mastery—rather than expressiveness that is associated with better mental health.

The personal attribute of instrumentality, along with perceived control of life events—the obverse of powerlessness—are negatively associated with psychopathology (for reviews, see Bassoff and Glass 1982; Whitely 1985). Wortman and Brehm (1975) suggest that whether or not a person responds to a negative life event with helplessness or a desire to regain control depends on control expectations. Women who are lower in instrumentality, mastery, and/or perceived control may be more likely to have both helplessness expectancies (that is, the expectation that outcomes are not controllable) and negative outcome expectancies (that is, not being able to attain highly valued outcomes or to avoid aversive outcomes). These are postulated to combine to create hopelessness, which leads to depression in response to negative life events (Abramson, Metalsky, and Alloy 1989). The interrelationships among gender and sex roles, ethnic minority status, and expectancies of helplessness and hopelessness have yet to be systematically investigated.

Unfortunately, most studies of the mental health implications of instrumentality and expressiveness have been conducted on predominantly White college student populations. It may be that the trait of expressiveness will not correlate with mental disorder in the absence of a provoking agent, such as relationship loss. In addition, the measures of mental health used have largely emphasized symptoms associated with anxiety, affective, and somatoform disorders, which by definition reflect feelings of helplessness and the lack of feelings of mastery, autonomy, and efficacy.

In conceptualizing causal dynamics between gender-related traits and psychopathology, it should be remembered that personal attributes such as instrumentality and perceived control may be both cause and consequence of stressful life events (Hamilton and Abramson 1983). Ultimately, transactional models will be needed to sort out the interactions among characteristics of the situation and characteristics of the person in creating risk for mental disorder.

Before the excess in women's mental health problems becomes attributed to gender-related psychological characteristics, methods used to identify occurrence of stressful life events must include negative experiences associated with violence, poverty, tokenism, discrimination, and stereotyping. It must be remembered that "responsivity" or "vulnerability" are labels for leftover variance in differences in symptom levels between women and men after accounting for effects of stressful life events (Thoits 1987c). Such labels are not explanations for that variance.

Although women do not appear to be more responsive than men to negative life events in general, they do appear to be differentially responsive to events involving "network crises that have the capacity to provoke distress through the creation of empathic concern" (Kessler, Price, and Wortman 1985, 538). It has yet to be ascertained whether women are more responsive to such events because of gender-related psychological traits, such as expressiveness and nurturance, or because they are fulfilling role expectations held by themselves and others. Caring and nurturing are central aspects of women's gender, gender role, and the sex roles of wife and mother.

Whether intrinsically or extrinsically motivated, the stress of caring for others may indeed be the major contributor to the gender gap in rates of psychopathology that is found for married people regardless of ethnic group (Kessler and McLeod 1984; Russo and Green 1992a, 1992b; Thoits 1986, 1987b). Marriage and family relationships offer opportunities for the mental health benefits of social support as well as for psychological burdens and stressors. Given the emphasis on mutual support and caring in ethnic minority communities (Collins 1989; Lewis 1977/89), ethnic minority women are more likely to experience both the benefits and costs of extended family and kin networks (Greene 1990; Lewis 1977/89).

Women's Roles and Status

In studying gender-related differences in social support, it will be important to separate the contribution of gender-related attributes (such as expressiveness, nurturance) and those of the women's feminine gender, wife, and mother roles. Researchers must keep in mind that women's roles in general, and ethnic minority women's roles in particular, are characterized by lack of access to instrumental resources. Lack of instrumental resources remains a powerful contributor to depression and anxiety.

Women's differential response to crises in interpersonal networks may thus reflect a "cost of subordination" that reflects the normative expectation that women should respond to the needs of others combined with lack of power and resources associated with women's roles and status. Snodgrass (1985) did an experimental study in which she manipulated the status of individuals interacting in small groups. She found that interpersonal sensitivity was an interactive process that was more closely related to the status of the individuals than to their gender, per se.

In discriminatory contexts, the female gender can signify a devalued master status that cuts across other social categories such as ethnic group and age and is found across a variety of situations. Thus, in analyzing women's responsiveness and caring for others, behaviors such as deference, helpfulness, sensitivity, and other behaviors associated with lower status should not automatically be attributed to gender-related psychological traits. As Reid and Comas-Díaz (1990) have eloquently observed, "among the various characteristics which have been identified as contributors to status, gender and ethnicity are undoubtedly the most permanent, most noticeable, and have the most established attributional systems to accompany them" (397).

Similarly, invoking cultural values to explain differences across ethnic groups before considering more proximal factors associated with economics, social context, and the life cycle can result in misleading conclusions and stereotyping. Comparisons among women of diverse ethnic groups are particularly complicated by racial segregation in women's occupations. Just as it is not appropriate to compare the mental health of "working men" to "working women" without controlling for occupational variables related to sex segregation in the workforce, comparing "working women" of diverse ethnic groups is not appropriate without controlling for occupational variables related to segregation of ethnic minority women in the workforce.

Feminist research and theory have provided new conceptual tools for conceptualizing gender and sex roles and thinking about difference among individuals that can inform research on the relationship between women's social roles and mental health. Although sex is a personal characteristic, gender is a dynamic social construct. Gender is a social category tied to the position of women in society, a position that differs by ethnic group (Amaro and Russo 1987). Gender issues are inextricably bound to those of class and ethnic minority group membership, and the experience of gender is heterogeneous (Reid and Comas-Díaz 1990).

In addition to being a salient personal attribute, one's sex is the basis for social cues that engage a host of gender role norms and expectations on the part of others whose actions toward an individual are based on that individual's sex. The defining characteristics of gender, like race, are in the eyes of the beholder, and effects of gender and racial stereotypes and expectations should not be confused with effects of personal attributes. When the personal attributes of women and men are compared, there are many more similarities than differences. It is when perceptions and responses to women and men are compared that large and persistent differences are found (Deaux 1985). Similarly, differences and similarities among individuals across ethnic groups would be expected to differ depending upon whether personal attributes or perceptions of and behaviors toward those individuals are under scrutiny. Thus, women of different ethnic groups may vary in ethnic-related values and motivations. Nonetheless, they must all deal with societal expectations that they fulfill the female sex roles of wife and mother. Women of all ethnic groups must deal with the risk of rape and the potential consequences of unprotected sexual intercourse.

The content, meaning, and interlocking relationships of sex roles differ by ethnic group in unknown ways. Masculine and feminine gender roles are but one kind of social role assigned by sex. Others include marital roles (wife/husband), parental roles (mother/father), offspring roles (daughter/son), and kin roles (aunt/uncle, niece/nephew). Research has yet to fully examine the quality of these roles for women in general, let alone how the privileges, obligations, and mental health implications of such roles vary across ethnic groups (Russo and Green 1992a). Yet conflicts, inconsistencies, stressors, and coping resources associated with women's roles have powerful implications for their mental health. Difficulties for ethnic minority women are compounded by conflicts between role expectations for members of their ethnic group and role expectations for women as defined by the larger society.

Because the meaning of gender and gender roles differs for women in diverse social groups, conceptions of gender and gender roles cannot be limited to those endorsed by the dominant group in society. In particular, feminist women of color in psychology have articulated the inadequacies of White middle-class conceptions of gender and sex roles. In a discussion of some of these contributions to the evolution of feminist psychology, Lillian Comas-Díaz (1991) identified several feminist principles of particular relevance to women of diverse ethnicity—affirming the feminist emphasis on the importance of the sociocultural context to women's mental health and the need to understand women's multiple realities. The priority for the next decade is to translate that recognition into research paradigms that fully explore those multiple realities.

Future Prospects

Building a women's research agenda that will advance understanding of gender differences in psychological distress and mental disorder thus requires refinement of our concepts of gender and sex roles and a more sophisticated examination of women's development, roles, and life circumstances in all of their diversity. This examination must include the multiple intersections of gender, ethnicity, race, class, age, sexual orientation, able-bodiedness, and other social categories that define identity, and that reflect lines of power, status, and resources in U.S. society.

Transforming research on women's mental health so that a body of knowledge develops with relevance to all women requires addressing profound theoretical, methodological, and epistemological issues. The women's mental health research agenda for the twenty-first century must entail a multitude of topics and issues that cannot be touched upon adequately here. Four fundamental points emerge from this discussion, however.

First is the need for a fundamental restructuring of the premises of the dominant conceptualizations of mental health as biologically and intrapsychically based. We must develop paradigms that articulate the mental health consequences of the complex web of negative life events associated with violence, poverty, and social inequality that characterize women's lives, especially those of ethnic minority women. Although narrow intrapsychic and biological approaches continue to dominate national mental health priorities, they clearly are not sufficient to achieve understanding of the etiology, diagnosis, treatment, and prevention of mental disorders that differ with gender, age, ethnic minority group, marital roles, parental roles, and economic status.

Second, in applying new paradigms, we must identify the processes by which gender-related personal attributes and social roles contribute to risk for various types of mental disorder for diverse groups of women. Gender-related attributes (particularly those related to instrumentality and perceived control), gender and sex role expectations and obligations (particularly with regard to caring, nurturance, and actual access to and control of resources), and gender-related negative life events, all affect risk for psychological disorder. How they vary with ethnic minority group status has yet to be systematically determined. In particular, the interrelationships among gender and sex roles, ethnic minority status, and expectancies of helplessness and hopelessness must be systematically investigated. Research must identify the extent to which psychopathology in women reflects a "cost of subordination" that reflects the normative expectation that women should respond to the needs of others combined with lack of power and resources associated with women's roles and status.

A stress and coping framework that includes biological, psychological, social, and cultural variables related to gender—and that considers the behaviors of women in their social context—promises significant advances for mental health research and theory applicable to women in all their diversity. Transactional models are particularly needed to sort out the interactions among characteristics of the situation and characteristics of the person in creating risk for mental disorder. In developing such models, however, it is important to listen to the women themselves, and to incorporate the meaning of their experiences into the models. It must also be remembered that stress and coping frameworks are not necessarily feminist; devaluation and stereotyping can permeate them as well.

Third, research on diagnosis and treatment must recognize that diagnostic definitions are social constructions reflecting the values and beliefs of those in power to do the constructing. Disorders that have high prevalence for women overlap with each other as well as with women's gender and sex role stereotypes. Research is urgently needed that seeks to identify and prevent forms of misdiagnosis and inappropriate treatment that result from the stereotyping and devaluation of women. The influence of gender and racial stereotyping has been thoroughly documented, but there remains much to learn about the nature and extent of the processes by which such stereotyping becomes translated into misdiagnosis and inappropriate treatment. In particular, it is critical that we find ways to eliminate misdiagnosis resulting from failure to identify a history of physical and sexual abuse.

A final priority that emerges reflects the need to maintain active policy advocacy on behalf of women's mental health research priorities. The paucity of mental health research on diverse populations of women reminds us of the relationship of the larger social context to the nature and form of knowledge that is pursued. Interest in a women's mental health research agenda emerged in the 1970s. It was not until 1984, however, when congressional action designated women as a priority population for the Alcohol, Drug Abuse, and Mental Health Administration, that women's mental health issues became formally part of the federal research agenda. It was public demand for such information, not the innovative leadership of those persons controlling the agencies, that broadened the national perspective.

Will implementation of the women's research agenda become translated into funding for research that goes beyond traditional biomedical
paradigms? Will research that explores psychological, social, and cultural
factors affecting mental health and illness in women of diverse ethnicity
be supported in more than a token fashion? Only time and continued
monitoring will tell. Eternal vigilance and a strong women's movement
appear to be the necessary foundation for achieving alternative visions
and implementing a women's mental health research agenda responsive
to the needs of all women into the twenty-first century.

REFERENCES

Abramson, L. Y., and Andrews, D. E. 1982. Cognitive depression: implications for sex differences in vulnerability to depression. *International Journal of Mental Health* 11:77–94.
Abramson, L. Y., Metalsky, G. I., and Alloy, L. B. 1989. Hopelessness depression: a theory-
based subtype of depression. *Psychological Review* 96:358–72.
Amaro, H., and Russo, N. F. 1987. Hispanic women and mental health: an overview of
contemporary issues in research and practice. *Psychology of Women Quarterly* 11:393–407.
Amaro, H., Zuckerman, B., and Cabral, H. 1989. Drug use among adolescent mothers: pro-
file of risk. *Pediatrics* 84:144–51.
American Psychiatric Association (APA). 1994. *Diagnostic and statistical manual of mental dis-
orders.* 4th ed. revised (DSM-IV). Washington, D.C.: APA.
Aneshensel, C. 1986. Marital and employment role-strain, social support, and depression
among adult women. In *Stress, social support, and women,* ed. S. Hobfoll, pp. 99–114.
Washington, D.C.: Hemisphere.
Aneshensel, C. S., Frerichs, R. R., and Clark, V. A. 1981. Family roles and sex differences in
depression. *Journal of Health and Social Behavior* 22:379–93.
Bassoff, E. S., and Glass, G. V. 1982. The relationship between sex roles and mental health: a
meta-analysis of twenty-six studies. *Counseling Psychologist* 10:105–12.
Belle, D. 1990. Poverty and women's mental health. *American Psychologist* 45:385–89.
Billings, A. G., Cronkite, R. C., and Moos, R. H. 1983. Social-environmental factors in unipo-
lar depression: comparisons of depressed patients and nondepressed controls. *Journal
of Abnormal Psychology* 92(2):119–33.
Brown, C., Bhrolchain, M. N., and Harris, T. O. 1975. Social class and psychiatric disturbance
among women in an urban population. *Sociology* 9:225–54.
Brown, G. W., and Harris, T. 1978. *Social origins of depression: a study of psychiatric disorder in
women.* New York: Free Press.
Browne, A. 1987. *When battered women kill.* New York: Lexington Books.
Browne, A., and Williams, K. R. 1989. Exploring the effect of resource availability and the
likelihood of female perpetrated homicides. *Law and Society Review* 23:75–94.
Bryer, J. B., Nelson, B. A., Miller, J. B., and Krol, P. A. 1987. Childhood sexual and physical
abuse as factors in adult psychiatric illness. *Am J Psychiat* 144:1426–30.
Burnam, M. A., Stein, J. A., Golding, J. M., Siegel, J. M., Sorenson, S. B., Forsythe, A., and
Telles, C. A. 1988. Sexual assault and mental disorders in a community population. *J.
Con and Clin Psychol* 56:843–50.

Carmen, E. (H.), and Rieker, P. P. 1989. A psychosocial model of the victim-to-patient process. *Psychiatric Clinics of North America* 12(2): 431–43.

Carmen E. (H.), Russo, N. F., and Miller, J. B. 1981. Inequality and women's mental health: an overview. *Am J Psychiat* 138, 10:1319–30.

Cleary, P. D., and Mechanic, D. 1983. Sex differences in psychological distress among married people. *Journal of Health and Social Behavior* 24:111–21.

Collins, P. H. 1989. The social construction of Black feminist thought. *Signs: Journal of Women in Culture and Society* 14:745–73.

Comas-Díaz, L.

    1987. Feminist therapy with Mainland Puerto Rican women. *Psychology of Women Quarterly* 11:461–74.

    1991. Feminism and diversity in psychology: the case of women of color. *Psychology of Women Quarterly* 15:597–610.

Cox, J. L., Connor, Y., and Kendell, R. E. 1982. Prospective study of the psychiatric disorders of childbirth. *British Journal of Psychiatry* 140:111–17.

Cronkite, R. C., and Moos, R. H. 1985. The role of predisposing and moderating factors in the stress-illness relationship. *Journal of Health and Social Behavior* 25:372–93.

Deaux, K. 1985. Sex and gender. *Annual Review of Psychology* 36:49–81.

Eichler, A., and Parron, D. L. 1987. *Women's mental health agenda for research.* Rockville, Md.: NIMH.

Fine, M. 1985. Reflections on a feminist psychology of women: paradoxes and prospects. *Psychology of Women* 9:167–83.

Freeman, T. 1951. Pregnancy as a precipitant of mental illness in men. *British Journal of Medical Psychology* 24:49–54.

Fullilove, M. 1988. Ethnic minority women and AIDS. *Multicultural Inquiry and Research on AIDS* 2(2):4–5.

Gater, R. A., Dean, C., and Morris, J. 1989. The contribution of childbearing to the sex difference in first admission rates for affective psychosis. *Psychological Medicine* 19(3):719.

Gelinas, D. J. 1983. The persisting negative effects of incest. *Psychiatry* 46:312–32.

Gelles, R. 1975. Violence and pregnancy: a note on the extent of the problem and needed services. *Family Coordinator* 24(1):81–86.

Golding, J. M. 1990. Division of household labor, strain, and depressive symptoms among Mexican Americans and non-Hispanic Whites. *Psychology of Women Quarterly* 14:103–17.

Goodman, L. A., Koss, M. P., and Russo, N. F.

    1993a. Violence against women: physical and mental health effects. Part 1: Research findings. *Applied and Preventive Psychology: Current Scientific Perspectives* 2:79–89.

    1993b. Violence against women: physical and mental health effects. Part 2: Conceptualizing post-traumatic stress. *Applied and Preventive Psychology: Current Scientific Perspectives* 2(3):123–30.

Green, B. L., and Russo, N. F. 1993. Work and family roles: selected issues. In *Psychology of women: a handbook of issues and theories,* ed. F. L. Denmark and M. A. Paludi, pp. 685–720. Westport, Conn.: Greenwood Press.

Greene, B. 1990. Sturdy bridges: the role of African-American mothers in the socialization of African-American children. *Women and Therapy* 9:205–25.

Hamilton, E. W., and Abramson, L. Y. 1983. Cognitive patterns and major depressive disorder: a longitudinal study in a hospital setting. Journal of Abnormal Psychology 92(2):173–84.

Hamilton, J. 1984. Psychobiology in context: reproductive-related events in men's and women's lives (review of *Motherhood and mental illness*). *Contemporary Psychiatry* 3(1):12–16.

Hamilton, J. A., Jensvold, M., Rothblum, E., and Cole, E., eds. 1994. *Psychopharmacology from a feminist perspective.* Binghamton, N.Y.: Haworth Press.

Hamilton, J. A., Parry, B. L., and Blumenthal, S. J. 1988. The menstrual cycle in context. I: Affective syndromes associated with reproductive hormonal changes. *Journal of Clinical Psychiatry* 49:474–80.

Harlow, C. W. 1991. *Female victims of violent crime.* NCJ-126826. Washington, D.C.: U.S. Department of Justice.

Hobfall, S., ed.

1986a. *Stress, social support, and women.* Washington, D.C.: Hemisphere.

1986b. The limitations of social support in the stress process. In *Social support: theory, research, and applications,* ed. G. Sarason and B. R. Sarason, pp. 391–414. The Hague: Martinus Nijhof.

Hobfall, S. E., and Leiberman, J. R. 1987. Personality and social resources in immediate and continued stress resistance among women. *Journal of Personality and Social Psychology* 52:18–26.

Hobfall, S. E., and London, P. 1986. The relationship of self-concept and social support to emotional distress among women during war. *Journal of Social and Clinical Psychology* 4:189–203.

Hobfall, S. E., and Walfisch, S. 1984. Coping with a threat to life: a longitudinal study of self-concept, social support, and psychological distress. *American Journal of Community Psychology* 12:87–100.

Horwitz, A. V., and White, H. R. 1987. Gender role orientations and styles of pathology among adolescents. *Journal of Health and Social Behavior* 28:158–70.

Kandel, D. B., and Davies, M. 1982. Epidemiology of depressive mood in adolescents. *Arch Gen Psychiat* 39:1205–12.

Kaplan, G., Roberts, R., Camacho, T., and Coyne, J. 1987. Psychosocial predictors of depression: prospective evidence from the human population laboratory studies. *American Journal of Epidemiology* 125:206–20.

Kessler, R. C., and McLeod, J. D. 1984. Sex differences in vulnerability to undesirable life events. *American Sociological Review* 49:620–31.

Kessler, R. C., McLeod, J. D., and Wethington, E. 1985. The cost of caring: a perspective on the relationship between sex and psychological distress. In *Social support: theory, research, and applications,* ed. I. G. Sarason and B. R. Sarason, pp. 491–506. The Hague: Martinus Nijhof.

Kessler, R. C., Price, R. H., and Wortman, C. B. 1985. Social factors in psychopathology: stress, social support, and coping processes. *Annual Review of Psychology* 36:531–72.

Koss, M. P. 1990. The women's mental health research agenda: violence against women. *American Psychologist* 45:374–80.

Koss, M. P., Goodman, L. A., Browne, A., Fitzgerald, L., Keita, G. P., and Russo, N. F. 1994. *No safe haven: male violence against women at home, at work, and in the community.* Washington, D. C.: American Psychological Association.

Lazarus, R. S., and Folkman, S. 1984. *Stress, appraisal, and coping.* New York: Springer.

Lewis, D. K. 1977–89. A response to inequality: Black women, racism, and sexism. In *Black women in America: social science perspectives,* ed. M. R. Malson, E. Mudimbe-Boyi, J. F. O'Barr, and M. Wyer, pp. 41–64. Chicago: University of Chicago Press.

Lopez, S. 1989. Patient variable biases in clinical judgment: a conceptual overview and some methodological considerations. *Psychological Bulletin* 106:184–203.

Loring, M., and Powell, B. 1988. Gender, race, and DSM-III: a study of the objectivity of psychiatric diagnostic behavior. *Journal of Health and Social Behavior* 29:1–22.

McAdoo, H. P., and McAdoo, J. L. 1985. *Black children: social, educational, and parental environments.* Beverly Hills, Calif.: Sage Publications.

McBride, A. B. 1990. Mental health effects of women's multiple roles. *American Psychologist* 45(3):381–84.

McGrath, E., Keita, G. P., Strickland, B. R., and Russo, N. F., eds. 1990. *Women and depression: risk factors and treatment issues.* Washington, D. C.: American Psychological Association.

McKibben, L., DeVos, E., and Newberer, E. 1989. Victimization of mothers of abused children: a controlled study. *Pediatrics* 84:531–38.

Manderscheid, R. W., and Sonnenschein, M. A., eds. 1990. *Mental health, United States, 1990.* National Institute of Mental Health. DHHS Pub. No. (ADM)90-1708. Washington, D.C.: U.S. Government Printing Office.

Myers, J. K., Weissman, M. M., Tischler, G. L., et al. 1984. Six-month prevalence of psychiatric disorders in three communities. *Arch Gen Psychiat* 41:959–67.

Neugebauer, D. D., Dohrenwend, B. P., and Dohrenwend, B. S. 1980. The formulation of hypotheses about the true prevalence of functional psychiatric disorders among adults in the United States. In *Mental illness in the United States*, ed. B. P. Dohrenwend, B. S. Dohrenwend, M. S. Gould, B. Link, R. Neugebauer, and R. Wunsch-Hitzig. New York: Praeger.

Newmann, J. P.
   1984. Sex differences in symptoms of depression: clinical disorder or normal distress? *Journal of Health and Social Behavior* 25:136–60.
   1986. Gender, life strains, and depression. *Journal of Health and Social Behavior* 27:161–78.
   1987. Gender differences in vulnerability to depression. *Social Service Review* 61:447–68.

Nolen-Hoeksema, S.
   1987. Sex difference in unipolar depression: evidence and theory. *Psychological Bulletin* 101:259–82.
   1990. *Sex differences in depression.* Stanford, Calif.: Stanford University Press.

O'Connell, A. N., and Russo, N. F., eds. 1991. *Women's heritage in psychology.* New York: Cambridge University Press.

Plass, P. S., and Strauss, M. A. 1987. Intra-family homicide in the United States: incidence, trends, and differences by religion, race, and gender. Paper presented at the Third National Family Violence Research Conference, University of New Hampshire, Durham, N.C.

President's Commission on Mental Health (PCMH). 1978. Report of the Special Population Subpanel on Mental Health of Women. *Task panel report submitted to the President's Commission on Mental Health.* Vol. 3. Washington, D.C.: U.S. Government Printing Office.

Public Health Service Task Force on Women's Health Issues. 1985. *Report on the task force on women's health issues.* Washington, D.C.: U.S. Government Printing Office.

Reid, P., and Comas-Díaz, L. 1990. Gender and ethnicity: perspectives on dual status. *Sex Roles* 22:397–407.

Rieker, P. P., and Carmen, E. (H.). 1986. The victim-to-patient process: the disconfirmation and transformation of abuse. *Am J Orthopsychiat* 56:360–70.

Rieker, P. P., and Carmen, E. (H.), eds. 1984. *The gender gap in psychotherapy: social realities and psychological processes.* New York: Plenum Press.

Riley, D., and Eckenrode, J. 1986. Social ties: subgroup differences in costs and benefits. *Journal of Personality and Social Psychology* 51(4):770–78.

Robins, L. N., Helzer, J. E., Weissman, M. M., Orvaschel, H., Gruenberg, E., Burke, J. D., and Regier, D. A. 1984. Lifetime prevalence of specific psychiatric disorders in three sites. *Arch Gen Psychiat* 41:949–58.

Rosenfield, S. 1982. Sex roles and societal reactions to mental illness: the labeling of "deviant" deviance. *Journal of Health and Social Behavior* 23:18–24.

Russo, N. F.
1984. Women in the mental health delivery system: implications for research and public policy. In *Women and mental health policy*, ed. L. E. Walker, pp. 21–24. Beverly Hills, Calif.: Sage Publications.
1985. *A women's mental health agenda*. Washington, D. C.: American Psychological Association.
1990. Overview: forging priorities for women's mental health. *American Psychologist* 45:368–73.

Russo, N. F., Amaro, H., and Winter, M. 1987. The use of inpatient mental health services by Hispanic women. *Psychology of Women Quarterly* 11(4):427–42.

Russo, N. F., and Green, B. L. 1993. Women and mental health. In *Psychology of women: a handbook of issues and theories*, ed. F. L. Denmark and M. A. Paludi, pp. 379–436. Westport, Conn.: Greenwood Press.

Russo, N. F., and Olmedo, E. L. 1983. Women's utilization of outpatient psychiatric services: some emerging priorities for rehabilitation psychologists. *Rehabilitation Psychology* 28(3):141–55.

Russo, N. F., and Sobel, S. B. 1981. Sex differences in the utilization of mental health facilities. *Professional Psychology* 12(1):7–19.

Russo, N. F., and Zierk, K. L. 1992. Abortion, childbearing, and women's well-being. *Professional Psychology: Research and Practice* 23:269–80.

Saluter, A. 1989. Singleness in America. In *Studies in marriage and the family*. U.S. Bureau of the Census. (Current population reports, series P-23, no. 162). Washington, D.C.: U.S. Government Printing Office.

Sarason, I. G., Johnson, J. H., and Siegel, J. M. 1978. Assessing the impact of life changes: development of the life experience survey. *Journal of Consulting and Clinical Psychology* 46:932–46.

Segura, D. A. 1989. Chicana and Mexican immigrant women at work: the impact of class, race, and gender on occupational mobility. *Gender and Society* 3(1):37–52.

Selik, R. M., Castro, K. G., and Pappaioanou, M. 1988. *Distribution of AIDS cases, by racial/ethnic group and exposure category. United States, June 1, 1981–July 4, 1988. MMWR CDC Surveillance Summary*. July, pp. 1–10.

Snodgrass, S. E. 1985. Women's intuition: the effect of subordinate role on interpersonal sensitivity. *Journal of Personality and Social Psychology* 49(1): 146–55.

Sobel, S. B., and Russo, N. F. 1981a. Equality, public policy, and professional psychology. *Professional Psychology* 12:180–89.

Sobel, S. B., and Russo, N. F., eds. 1981b. *Sex roles, equality, and mental health*. Washington, D.C.: American Psychological Association. (Special issue of *Professional Psychology* 22 [Whole no. 1]).

Spence, J., Helmreich, R., and Stapp, J. 1974. The personal attributes questionnaire: a measure of sex-role stereotypes and masculinity-femininity. *JSAS Catalog of Selected Documents in Psychology* 4, 43–44 (MSNo. 617).

Stacey, W., and Shupe, A. 1983. *The family secret*. Boston: Beacon Press.

Stack, C. 1974. *All our kin: strategies for survival in a Black community*. New York: Harper and Row.

Staples, R. 1987. Social structure in Black female life. *Journal of Black Studies* 17:267–86.

Stark, E., Flitcraft, A., Zuckerman, D., Grey, A., Robison, J., and Frazier, W. 1981. Wife abuse in the medical setting: an introduction for health personnel. *Domestic Violence Monograph Series, No. 7*. Rockville, Md.: National Clearinghouse on Domestic Violence.

Thoits, P. A.

1984. Explaining distributions of psychological vulnerability: lack of social support in the face of life stress. *Social Forces* 63:463–81.

1986. Multiple identities: examining gender and martial status differences in distress. *American Sociological Review* 51:259–72.

1987a. Gender and marital status differences in control and distress: common stress versus unique stress explanations. *Journal of Health and Social Behavior* 28:7–22.

1987b. Position paper. In *Women's mental health agenda for research*, ed. A. Eichler and D. L. Parron, pp. 80–102. Rockville, Md.: NIMH.

1987c. Negotiating roles. In *Spouse-parent worker: on gender and multiple roles*, ed. F. J. Crosby, pp. 11–22. New Haven, Yale University Press.

Tolman, R. M., and Bennett, L. W. 1990. A review of quantitative research on men who batter. *Journal of Interpersonal Violence* 5:89–118.

Towne, R. D., and Afterman, J. 1955. Psychosis in males related to parenthood. *Bulletin of the Menninger Clinic* 19(1):19–26.

Travis, C. B. 1988. *Women and health psychology: mental health issues*. Hillsdale, N.J.: Lawrence Erlbaum.

Turner, R. J., and Avison, W. R. 1989. Gender and depression: assessing exposure and vulnerability to life events in a chronically strained population. *Journal of Nervous and Mental Disease* 177:443–55.

U.S. Bureau of the Census. 1989. *Household and family characteristics: March 88*. (Current populations reports, series P-20, no. 162.) Washington, D.C.: U.S. Government Printing Office.

van der Kolk, B. A. 1988. The trauma spectrum: the interaction of biological and social events in the genesis of the trauma response. *Journal of Traumatic Stress* 1:273–90.

Waisberg, J., and Page, S. 1988. Gender role nonconformity and perception of mental illness. *Women and Health* 14:3–16.

Weissman, M. 1987. Advances in psychiatric epidemiology: rates and risks for major depression. *American Journal of Public Health* 77:445–51.

Weissman, M., Leaf, F., and Bruce, M. 1987. Single parent women? a community study. *Social Psychiatry* 22:29–36.

Whiffen, V. E. 1988. Vulnerability to postpartum depression: a prospective multivariate study. *Journal of Abnormal Psychology* 97:467–74.

Whitely, B. E., Jr. 1985. Sex role orientation and psychological well-being: two meta-analyses. *Sex Roles* 12:207–25.

Wolf, B. 1987. *Low-income mothers at risk: the psychological effects of poverty-related stress*. Unpublished doctoral dissertation. Harvard Graduate School of Education, Cambridge, Mass.

Wortman, C., and Brehm, J. W. 1975. Responses to uncontrollable outcomes: an integration of reactance theory and the learned helplessness model. In *Advances in experimental social psychology*, ed. L. Berkowitz. Vol. 8. Orlando, Fla.: Academic Press.

Wyatt, G. 1985. The sexual abuse of Afro-American and White-American women in childhood. *Child Abuse and Neglect* 9:507–19.

Zill, N. 1978. *Divorce, marital happiness and the mental health of children: findings from the OCD national survey of children*. Unpublished report.

Zinn, M. B. 1990. Family, feminism, and race in America. *Gender and Society* 4:68–82.

A Brief History of the Center for Minority Group Mental Health Programs at the National Institute of Mental Health

T HE Center for Minority Group Mental Health Programs (CMGMHP, or the Center) was established as part of the National Institute of Mental Health (NIMH) in November 1970, and it ceased formal operations in 1985. During that fifteen-year period, it was the nucleus of NIMH research, manpower development and training, and technical assistance activities judged to bear on the mental health status and improvement of the quality of life of minority group people in the United States—American Indians, Alaskan Natives, Asian Americans and Pacific Islanders, Blacks, and Hispanics.

Conceived in the late 1960s, the Center was established in an atmosphere of urgent need, forceful demands, and high expectations. It matured during the most programmatically and politically tumultuous period in the now nearly half-century-long history of the NIMH. Indeed, by the time of the Center's official demise, the NIMH itself had been dramatically reshaped from what it was fifteen years before, and the Institute's evolving mission and reconfiguration figured prominently in the Center's dismantling.

In 1985, the Center's research and clinical training grants were mainstreamed into existing NIMH divisions, and a new Minority Research Resources Branch was created for developing minority scientists and for further expanding the nation's capacity for research on minority-relevant mental health issues. A subsequent reorganization eliminated that unit as well; reponsibility for oversight of its function was assigned to a new statutorily mandated office, that of the NIMH Associate Director for Minority Concerns.[1] Still, the legacy of the CMGMHP is a rich, ongoing one: today, programs and, more importantly, the vision set by the NIMH Center for Minority Group Mental Health Programs continue to contribute to the scientific strength of the nation and, inseparably, to yield benefits to minority group members.

This chapter offers an account of the politics and policies of minority mental health programs at the NIMH over a crucial, fifteen-year span, addressing issues involved in the Center's establishment and major directions in the areas of research, training, and services development. We shall revisit the key issues identified in our original chapter in *Racism and Mental Health* and shall retrospectively evaluate our initial perspective. While emphasizing the Center's programs, we necessarily discuss the evolution of the Center's "home," the NIMH itself. Also, for purposes of closure, we shall review briefly the status of minority-focused programs at the NIMH in the years since the Center ceased operations.

One prefatory note: In the previous edition of this volume, Brown and Ochberg concluded their chapter on the development of a minority mental health program at NIMH with a promise: this much is clear: in the next edition of this book, the chapter on minority centers will more likely be written by the staff of the Center for Minority Group Mental Health Programs than by two White administrators." In fact, the Center now is history and one of us (BSB) is writing again. Now a *former* federal program administrator, I am more appreciative than I could have imagined twenty years ago of the dedication and contributions of countless individuals—an original "Rainbow Coalition"—who have made this account possible: James Ralph, Juan Ramos, Jim Pittman, Marian Primas, Bill Denham, Claude Thomas, Rhetaugh Dumas, Jim Goodman, Dick Shapiro, Frieda Cheung, and numerous others at the NIMH both past and present; and others outside the NIMH, from Arthur Fleming to Elliot Richardson to the late Justice Thurgood Marshall.

NIMH: The Early Years

The NIMH today is the largest research and research-training facility in the world devoted to the study of mental disorders and to the exploration of social, behavioral, and neurobiological mechanisms relevant to mental illness and health. Authorized in 1946, the Institute was one of the initial four components of the National Institutes of Health (NIH). Until the very recent past, however, NIMH's mission was defined more broadly than those of other NIH programs; in addition to the research mandate it shared with all NIH units, NIMH also was authorized to train mental health clinical—as well as research—personnel, and to assist states and communities in developing improved mental health service systems.

Throughout its early years, when little empirical data existed about mental illness or health, NIMH encouraged a liberal interpretation of its research mandate. It accurately perceived early on the breadth of factors, from biological to psychological to social, that impinged on mental illness and health, and it maintained a diverse research portfolio. Public perceptions of the relevance of NIMH research and its programs broadly were enhanced in the mid 1960s by two events.

One was the enactment of the Community Mental Health Centers (CMHC) Act, President Kennedy's "bold new approach" to mental health care service delivery that promised to exhibit, in communities throughout the nation, tangible evidence of the federal government's commitment to the mental health needs of all Americans. One outcome of the community mental health centers legislation was that the CMHC program—and, by implication, NIMH and the mental health field—was to act as a lightning rod for a range of previously inchoate issues, extending from citizen involvement and consumer participation in the design and delivery of health care to more critical appraisals of the knowledge base underlying mental health services, including their relevance to minority and other "special need" and/or disenfranchised groups. Not only did the CMHC program mark a novel role for the federal government in the health care arena, but it also dictated that the mental health field would be linked closely to key social, as well as health care–related, issues of the day. In the mental health field, the Civil Rights Act of 1966, for example, translated into heightened attention to civil rights advocacy for persons with mental illness. This attention spawned the Mental Health Law Project, now the Judge David L. Bazelon Center for Mental Health Law; over the years, its activities have been of direct, continuing relevance to the minority community.[2]

The second influential event was President Lyndon Johnson's pledge to refocus the nation's scientific prowess on social ailments such as poverty, crime, urban problems, and drug and alcohol abuse. The response of then NIMH director Stanley Yolles to this "Great Society" call for the application of research relevant to pressing social problems included the creation, within NIMH, of several problem-focused "centers." Contending that traditional vertical lines of research and training grant programs reporting to an Associate Director for Extramural Programs was insufficiently responsive to targeted needs, Yolles proposed the use of such "centers," to ensure that basic and applied research, training, demonstrations, technical assistance and consultation, information dissemination, and related activities would be devoted to critical program targets in an intensified, coordinated way.

The Centers that NIMH established were of two types. (1) *Comprehensive*, or operating, centers had their own budgets and were responsible for stimulating, reviewing, and funding activities in a given area (such as metropolitan problems, crime and delinquency, suicide). (2) *Coordinating* centers did not possess actual funding authorities; rather, their staff acted as expert advocates within NIMH for particular issues (such as child and family mental health).

The promise of the CMHC program, together with the high-profile position taken by NIMH with respect to social problems, underscored NIMH's unique mission within the NIH. This mission afforded NIMH a degree of public and political visibility and presence unlike that claimed by other NIH research institutes, and it offered Americans a sense of proprietorship of the Institute that was unlike that experienced by the other research units of NIH. The unique role and identity of NIMH led to its separation from NIH in 1968,[3] a bureaucratic status that would hold until NIMH itself was programmatically dissected in 1992, its research and research-training components returning to the NIH, and its service and other activities re-created as a new Center for Mental Health Services within the Substance Abuse and Mental Health Services Administration, the successor agency to ADAMHA.

The organizational precedent and framework provided by NIMH's special problem centers presented the Institute with an opportunity to respond directly to escalating minority mental health concerns. If this opportunity was not exploited immediately by the NIMH leadership, neither was it ignored by the cadre of Black psychiatric leadership in the 1960s.

Key Issues in Developing the NIMH Minority Program

Not surprisingly, the social ferment that drove much of the Great Society's agenda was felt keenly in the mental health field. Civil rights legislation, the enactment of Medicare and Medicaid, and (in mental health) the CMHC movement all represented real gains, but they also generated hopes, many of which remained unmet as the nation entered the era of cities in flames, campus disturbances, the poor people's march, and other fundamental societal awakenings. Opportunities and frustrations that emerged during this period encouraged focused efforts by minority groups—and others—to attack and amend inequities in organized structures at all levels of society. In 1968, the Kerner Commission Report identified racism as a primary cause of violence in the nation. The following year, the Joint Commission on Mental Health of Children, Inc., endorsed a widespread conviction that racism was America's number one public health problem.

As recounted by Pierce, the destructive influence of racism had long been glaringly evident to the scattering of minority mental health professionals in the country. The turmoil of the 1960s steeled the resolve of leaders in the minority community to combat the issue systematically. Their perseverance resulted in the formation of the Black Caucus of the American Psychiatric Association, which immediately used its voice to characterize the NIMH as a "racist bureaucracy," faulting it, along with other federal agencies, for failing to include more Blacks in decision-making roles and failing to accelerate equal employment opportunities.

One of the authors (BSB) was NIMH deputy director, under Yolles, at the time of this pronouncement and was assigned to head a Yolles-appointed work group to review and respond to the charge of the Black psychiatrists. Brown already had been introduced to the politics of race in the mental health field. One of his earliest tasks at NIMH had been to recruit a new superintendent for Saint Elizabeths Hospital, in Washington, D.C., which was then (and remained until the late 1980s) an NIMH unit. With the choice of two excellent candidates—one a Black psychiatrist, and one a White psychiatrist—Brown selected the former, and immediately found himself the object of an EEO complaint and lawsuit filed by the rejected White candidate. Undaunted by that experience, Brown and the work group proceeded to develop an ambitious NIMH response aimed at correcting problems identified by the Black psychiatrists. That effort led to a commitment on the part of NIMH to establish an identifiable organizational unit to foster the development of mental health programs for minority groups and to step up efforts to recruit minority personnel for NIMH.

The work group effort overlapped with the presidential campaign of 1968 and concluded just as the wholesale political firings of Johnson administration appointees and other senior federal officials began. Among the first to go in the restaffing of the Department of Health, Education, and Welfare (HEW), was NIMH director Yolles. Appointed by the new administration to head NIMH, Brown would receive, and be called to act upon, the report of the minority concerns work group he had headed.

The NIMH's commitment to creating a new program devoted to minority mental health concerns ran counter to the position of the incoming Nixon administration regarding new national categorical programs. In a sharp reversal of the Great Society's emphasis on federally directed, activist approaches to domestic needs, the new administration placed high priority on grant consolidation, revenue sharing, and regionalization of federal programs—"gospel" to successive administrations, across the life span of the CMGMHP. Nonetheless, NIMH's planning for the administrative creation of the Center proceeded, a decision that was encouraged by the support of the new HEW secretary, Elliot Richardson.[4] In November

1970, the outcome of two years of formal and informal negotiation between NIMH and the minority community as represented by the Black psychiatrists, was an announcement by Secretary Richardson of the establishment of the Center for Minority Group Mental Health Programs, within the Division of Special Mental Health Programs.

Though the Center was a reality, fundamental issues regarding its philosophy and operation were yet to be resolved. These were identified and discussed in depth by Ochberg and Brown and are only summarized here.

Definition of Minority. Though Black psychiatrists had been at the forefront of efforts to bring NIMH to task for its record in minority-relevant staffing and programming, the Black leadership was quick to acknowledge the importance of including in the new initiative other minority groups designated in HEW's 1970 Equal Employment Opportunity program—Spanish Americans, American Indians, and Asian Americans. Because prejudice based on ethnicity and sex were judged to be less destructive than that stemming from racism, White ethnic minorities and White women were excluded from the definition of minority, though women's concerns would be brought under the mandate of the NIMH Associate Director for Special Populations in 1985.

Relationships Among Minority Groups. While open to the inclusion of other than Black minority group members, several of the Black leadership also believed that combining ranks among minority groups would tend to dilute, rather than strengthen, the voice of the new Center. Disagreeing with NIMH staff, the Black psychiatrists argued that as the "majority minority" they should be in charge. Opposition to this claim was voiced first by Spanish American representatives, who expressed concern that their interests risked being superseded. American Indians and Asian Americans were less vocal about the issue, possibly because of the former's traditional channels within the Bureau of Indian Affairs and Indian Health Service, and the latter's disinclination to ally with other American racial minorities in demanding targeted federal intervention programs. NIMH countered that organization along racial lines, with funds allocated on a capitation basis, would lead to quadruplication of bureaucratic processes and deprive the Center of a central voice and its funds of critical mass; this position ultimately prevailed.

"Segregation" of a health Program. The decision to establish the Center notwithstanding, debate persisted about the legality, morality, practicality, and effectiveness of having a separate minority program. One argument against separation was a fear that the much larger research, training, and service divisions of NIMH would divest themselves of all accountability, including budgetary and personnel practices, in favor of

minority concerns. The opposing view was that Center staff would constitute a critical mass that would attract more minority employees for other
Institute components and catalyze its minority-relevant programming.

Maintenance of Professional Standards. Linked to the issue of the Center's autonomous status was the question of standards of quality, both in
staffing and in grant awards criteria applied by the Center. At issue were
contentions that White-administered programs or standards of research,
training, and education generally had never broken the cycle of minority
group degradation, powerlessness, and ignorance, and that White insight
was blind to Black or other minority problems. Others argued that science
knows no color distinctions. The NIMH policy decision at the time the
Center was established was to maintain traditional scientific standards
and methods, and at the same time, to seek innovative means of making
programs more relevant to minorities.

Scope and Focus. Would the CMGMHP be a comprehensive center
wherein chief responsibility for all NIMH minority programs could be in
the hands of minority people? This would allow, it was argued, for the
best overview of minority mental health programs in America, development of the most exhaustive registry of minority mental health personnel,
and stimulation of the greatest amount—and most germane—minority
mental health grants in all areas. Or, would relatively inexperienced
people operating a comprehensive program have only a token impact on
nationwide problems? Should the support of research, or training as a
precursor to research and minority-relevant services, be the primary
focus? Favoring research was (1) its prestige within NIMH; (2) the fact
that curricula for training programs and basic concepts for developing
service programs require research-based information; and (3) the fact that
research grants tended to be funded for shorter periods than training
grants and would thus permit a more constant flow of new and uncom-
mitted funds. Training, on the other hand, had proponents both inside
and outside the minority communities, who argued that minority role
models in the mental health professions and high quality minority men-
tors in research would influence the quality and, thus, the relevance of
research.

Style and Emphasis. A lively debate addressed questions of "paraprofessional" versus "professional" training in both the clinical and research spheres and, following that, of a CMGMHP emphasis on "innovative" research as opposed to traditional biomedical and behavioral
mental disorders research. If the Center were to train a new breed of mental health worker lacking all of the specialized education of the core mental health professions, would the result be an expansion of needed services for minority populations, or simply a disparity between "White"

professional mental health programs and "minority" paraprofessional programs? Similarly, would a traditional focus on research into the etiology and treatment of mental disorders in minority populations direct attention away from studies of White racism or the impacts of racism on physical and mental health?

These, then, were what NIMH staff and its consultants and advisors from the various minority and other groups viewed as the critical "developmental" questions concerning the directions and ultimate success or failure of the CMGMHP. That the issues were raised speaks well of the gritty determination of all parties to address the hard questions concerning the function of the bureaucratic entity that would be responsible for dealing with racism and mental health. That many questions were not answered directly or immediately speaks tellingly of their complexity. Later, against the backdrop of the program as it actually evolved, we will look back at these questions and attempt to appraise if and how well they were resolved by the Center during the years of its existence.

In April 1971, less than five months after the creation of the Center had been announced, these and other issues suggesting both the promise and the pitfalls of the new NIMH Center for Minority Group Mental Health Programs were presented to James Ralph, M.D., an outstanding young Black psychiatrist newly recruited by NIMH to build and manage the program. As suggested above, the Center's mission was broad, comprising the following tasks:

- To stimulate and support research to elucidate the deleterious effects of racism on White populations and to identify and facilitate institutional and organizational changes to eliminate racism;[5]
- to support innovative training programs and fellowships;
- to devise methodologies to measure the manifestations of, and progress in combatting, institutional racism;
- to collaborate with non-NIMH entities in furthering CMGMHP objectives;
- to disseminate information by means of conferences, committees, and publications.

The Early Years of CMGMHP

The immediate need was to spread word of the new center to the target populations—groups which, at that time, were likely to be outside primary communications channels of the mental health field. In a two-year span from 1971 to 1973, the Center convened approximately five national conferences and an additional ten regional workshops targeted to minority populations. Designed both to identify the mental health needs and interests of various minority groups and to begin generating grant applications, these sessions proved to generate much heat as well as light; yet out of them evolved a comprehensive minority group agenda that recommended each group's primary needs and priorities for mental health research and research training, and clinical personnel development. First, predictably, was a national conference for Black professionals, convened at Meharry Medical College, in Nashville, Tennessee. Given the by-then-extensive groundwork laid by the early years of confrontation—then negotiation and collaboration—between the Black community and NIMH, that first session was task oriented and productive. It was not, however, a bellwether for those to follow.

At the second conference, on the topic of Hispanic mental health, suspicion and hostility toward the NIMH proved more treacherous. Held at the University of Chicago, the plenary session concluded with NIMH director Brown sitting in the center of a large room, flanked by senior NIMH staff, fielding questions—and challenges—as to the nature of NIMH-funded research, training, and service programs to be made available to the "Spanish-speaking, Spanish-surnamed" population. Despite the hostility expressed, the ultimate yield of the conference was positive: formation of the Coalition of Spanish-Speaking Mental Health Organizations (COSSMHO), an entity that, under the leadership of Rudy Sanchez, would evolve over the 1970s and 1980s into an effective educational body and formidable lobbying force for Hispanic mental health interests.

The National Conference on Indian Mental Health—convened at Deganawidah-Quetzalcoatl Universidad, in Davis, California, in late 1971—was noteworthy less for high drama and confrontation than for a somber realization of the immensity of the task before the new center. The springboard for the session, as noted by Brown, was the long national legacy of societal neglect of American Indian populations, punctuated by overt racism and bigotry. Brown conceded in his keynote address, "add [to indicators of Native American health and social status] the long list of special mental problems in the mental health area—the high rate and peculiarities of the alcohol problem among Indians, or the high suicide rate among Indian youth, for example—and you have the topic for a very gloomy conference" (Brown, pers. files).

The challenge, Brown said, would be to focus not on the deprivations and stresses faced by the Indian population, but rather on adaptive behaviors. "There is considerable merit in focusing our attention on some of the strengths and positive mental health features that exist in Indian tribal structures," he urged. Urging conference attendees to participate in the follow-up regional workshops already being planned by Center staff, Brown noted that overdue efforts were already under way. In response to the president's directive in July 1970 for special funding for Indians' health needs, NIMH had reprogrammed $750,000 to augment programs to treat and prevent alcohol abuse among Indian groups; a similar earmarking of funds would occur in 1972, Brown said. Continuing attention to Indian problems would be enhanced by the appointment of American Indian professionals to the CMGMHP's initial review group (IRG), the advisory body responsible for advising the Center and the larger NIMH on Indian-relevant concerns and for evaluating funding applications to the Center. The first Native American appointed to the IRG, Brown announced, was Dr. Carolyn L. Attneave, who at the time was field director of the Public Service Careers Program in the Massachusetts Department of Mental Health.

The risks—and, eventually, benefits—of the novel cross-cultural outreach undertaken by the CMGMHP perhaps were most dramatically underscored in the Center's initial interactions with the Asian American population, which began auspiciously, but then, at the 1972 annual meeting of the National Association of Social Workers, Center director Ralph failed to mention any initiatives for the Asian–Pacific Islander population. When questioned, he responded to the effect that Asians, the "model minority" whose educational attainment and income typically outstripped those of other minority groups, had no special needs. He then embellished his remarks with complimentary comments about the success of Japanese products in the United States marketplace. His well-intentioned talk quickly generated more than a hundred letters of protest from Asian American social workers to the NIMH director, as well as a flurry of congressional inquiries regarding the omission of Asian American concerns from the CMGMHP agenda.[6] Given the capacity of the focused attention of an incensed congressman to capture the attention of federal program heads, Brown immediately dispatched Okura, then executive assistant to the director, to meet with representatives of the Asian American social workers and assure them that their concerns would be addressed at the first national Asian American mental health conference in 1972.

Funds allocated for that conference, which met in San Francisco, permitted the invitation of eighty-seven participants representative of the ethnic, gender, and geographic distribution of Asian American mental health professionals. Upon announcement of the conference, however, NIMH was besieged with requests to participate; on opening day, more than seven hundred Asian American mental health workers registered. Ten scheduled workshops were expanded to twenty, and pre-arranged hotel facilities were buttressed by a hastily negotiated arrangement for meeting space with a neighboring church. Although the "model minority" group proved to be angry, vocal, and disorderly, two specific courses of action emerged: (1) to establish a national coalition to promote the mental health, social, and human development aspirations of the Asian and Pacific Island peoples, and (2) to conduct commuity-based research of the needs—and unmet needs—of this population.[7]

Minority-Targeted Research

Having been presented with an array of urgent, controversial, and unanswerable questions when he assumed his post, CMGMHP director Ralph opted to design as broad and flexible a program as funds and policies would permit. In deciding upon the strategy, he and his staff took the same route chosen by the first NIMH director, Robert Felix, some twenty-five years earlier, in building the NIMH. Felix's strategy had been a resounding success. From a program authorized in 1946 but granted no appropriation, the NIMH had burgeoned in its first quarter-century. By 1968, when the Institute moved out of the NIH, it all but dwarfed the other NIH components.

Ralph organized the Center into two sections: Minority Group Mental Health Programs, headed by Mary Harper, Ph.D.; and Racism and Mental Health Programs, headed by Richard Shapiro. Between the two sections, the Center attempted to address both the cause and consequences of racism. Requests for funding applications (RFAs) were developed in numerous areas. Priority was given to the identification and development of models and demonstration programs aimed at reducing the multigenerational dependency of minority group members on public assistance; to improve the quality of mental health services to minority groups; and to study theories and strategies of social change within minority groups. At the same time, other RFAs sought grants to study such issues as preventing exploitation of minorities in human experimentation; examining the mental health implications of institutional racism and desegregation; and establishing graduate-level training programs specifically to facilitate the reduction of racism in mental health service settings.

For immediate start-up, in fiscal year 1970, other NIMH operating divisions transferred a number of existing grant projects to the Center. Included in the shift were seven research grants focusing on Blacks and Hispanics, and three training grants, which included all four racial and ethnic groups. Whereas that initial trickle of transfer projects intensified in successive years, one concern—that the mainline research, services, and training divisions would abdicate their role and responsibility in the minority arena—proved never to be realized (as discussed below in our "retrospective look," at the lifespan of the CMGMHP).

Efforts also were accelerated to provide clinical services training as well as research training opportunities to minority group members. Clinical training models would be pursued along both paraprofessional and professional tracks, thus defusing the concern that minority trainees would be relegated to lower-skill, lower-paying jobs in the mental health field. Paraprofessional training offered an immediate, short-term response, and by 1972 (the second full year of Center operations), a sizeable portion of the NIMH's request of Congress for a CMGMHP budget increase of over a quarter-million dollars would be directed to paraprofessional training. Illustrative of the training efforts were programs in New York City and Detroit to train Black youth (many of whom could not meet prevailing academic standards for entry into graduate schools) for careers in social work in urban center areas. A similar program in social work was designed principally for Native American students at Brigham Young University and the University of Utah. The CMGMHP joined forces with the Indian Health Service to fund a program at the University of Montana, to train Northern Cheyenne Indians as indigenous mental health workers. In Los Angeles, funds were made available to train Chicanos as mental health specialists, capable of providing counseling and referral services to members of their communities.

Urgent and valid as they were, these training initiatives constituted only a first step. As had been true historically, both money and the muscle at NIMH resided with the research programs, and it was to these that the Center turned its attention.

Minority Mental Health Research and Development Centers

Perhaps the key Center-driven initiative in its first years of operation occurred in 1973 when Ralph and Brown encouraged then HEW secretary Casper Weinberger to approve an NIMH/CMGMHP proposal to include a new program of Minority Research and Development centers in an HEW-wide effort designed to target health-related services to minorities. The R&D centers were designed as institutional-based mechanisms to design, conduct, and implement research programs relevant to minority groups; as ongoing, interdisciplinary research "programs," rather than discrete research "projects," the R&D centers would also provide a setting for training minority students as researchers. In fact, each grant would provide support for research associates and assistants; for senior scholars-in-residence; for technical assistance; for information dissemination activities; and for underwriting an advisory board comprising members from academia and the community.

To launch the program, the CMGMHP provided a five-year grant of $200,000 annually to five applicants, each focused on a single minority group, for culture-specific studies. First, in 1973, was the Spanish-Speaking Mental Health R&D Center at the University of California, Los Angeles. The following year, three more were funded: an Asian American R&D Center, at San Diego State College; the Mental Health R&D Center in Black Communities, at Howard University, Washington, D.C.; and the Fanon Mental Health R&D Center, at Charles Drew Postgraduate Medical School, Los Angeles. A fifth R&D Center, for Native American programs, was funded through the National Tribal Chairmen's Association in 1975. The Minority R&D centers proved to be a durable support mechanism. Whereas principal investigators and host institutions have shifted frequently and continuously over the years, the core concepts have survived and continue to thrive well into the 1990s (the current status of the R&D centers is discussed later).

An in-depth review of the R&D program conducted by NIMH in 1985–1986 to assess gains and needed future directions in minority research and research training programs judged the R&D program a success, notwithstanding a conclusion that the R&D centers "have made their major contribution in non-research activities, although these activities were highly pertinent to developing minority research resources in the early years of these Centers." The NIMH evaluators found the research programs to vary considerably from center to center, even though a majority used a common conceptual frame of reference—a stress-coping model—to organize their research. Individual projects within the centers were found to include, for example, an examination of the symptom patterns of depressive disorders and variations in symptomology across age, gender, and SES; a study of factors associated with adolescent pregnancy; an effort, focused on Mexican Americans, to develop measurement instruments to assess life event changes, stress, social support networks, coping responses, and personal resources; a project to translate the Diagnostic Interview Scheduled (DIS) into Vietnamese and Korean; a study of primary care and mental health status in a Chinatown; and a project to identify pertinent mental health or illness indicators of Asian Americans in the 1980 census.

Of concern to the evaluation team, however, was evidence that, with few exceptions, the R&D centers had not been successful in developing large-scale project support—that is, independent, investigator-initiated research applications (RO-1s) that could compete with all others submitted to the NIMH. At the same time, the R&D centers were judged to have provided invaluable assistance in those exceptional instances where grants were approved. The evaluators noted that two successful RO-1 proposals from R&D centers each had benefited from approximately two years of developmental work and pilot studies before being funded; similar support for a prolonged preparatory period likely would not have been found outside the R&D centers program.

Minority Mental Health Research and Clinical Fellowship Program

Another historical landmark in the CMGMHP's history occurred in 1973 when the American Sociological Association, concerned about the underrepresentation of minorities in graduate training and research careers, sparked a new era of clinical and research training for minority populations. While the Center, under Ralph's direction, already had begun building its research program, the request for a targeted training program not only made good sense, but it answered one of the tough questions that had been on his desk upon his arrival at NIMH: Should the Center's focus be research (the urgent need for which was undisputed) or on training (as a foundation for future research)? The answer, clearly, was both. Quickly, inquiries and formal funding applications were received from the other "core" mental health disciplines—psychiatry, initially for clinical training only (American Psychiatric Association); psychology (American Psychological Association); nursing (American Nurses Association); and social work (Council on Social Work Education).

In 1974, NIMH announced its Minority Fellowship Program (MFP), a major new structure designed to increase the number of minorities in the mental health professions; to improve the quality of training available; and to improve the responsiveness of the professions to minority concerns. To launch the effort, the CMGMHP had initially available $5 million to establish graduate fellowships for students in disciplines that fell under the aegis of the professional associations listed above. MFP students could choose their doctoral training institutions, and receive academic support as well as advice and counseling. Program directors of each fellowship program were instrumental in negotiating collaborative arrangements at the students' chosen schools and in monitoring each student's training, ensuring that they participated in research and clinical activities relevant to the given profession. The initiative—particularly the financial aid and honorific aspect of selection as an MFP fellow—had a dramatic effect on the students' academic achievements. An initial, NIMH-internal evaluation of the program conducted in 1977 found the overall retention rate for MFP fellows to be 96.5 percent, pointing to attrition well below that of other students in the same departments.

Although the MFP program set and maintained an enviable record in encouraging minority students to pursue doctoral and postdoctoral training, a major drawback was that, given the orientation of the co-sponsoring professional organizations, research training provided under the program focused nearly exclusively on social and behavioral sciences—and this at a time when much of the attention and funding opportunities of the mental health field were shifting increasingly to the biological sciences, and the rapidly developing discipline of neuroscience. Not until 1988 was this problem rectified, with the introduction of two new MFP research training programs in neuroscience, sponsored by the American Psychological Association and the Society for Neuroscience[8]. In the same year, the American Psychiatric Association, which heretofore had supported only clinical training under the MFP, broadened its support and involvement to include research training for minority medical graduates in psychiatry, a specialty that was leaning increasingly toward the biological model in its research as well as practice patterns.

The President's Commission on Mental Health

Though not an NIMH/CMGMHP program activity, an evaluation of the Center by the Carter administration's President's Commission on Mental Health (PCMH), provided strong endorsement for the Center's thrust as well as specific program activities.[9] In its extensive report, the Research Task Panel of the PCMH stated that:

One of the most promising areas for future research on the relationship between race and mental health is in an area that social scientists have identified only in the last decade, "institutional racism." The concept has generated more discussion than research, but that is in part to be explained by the very organization of the research establishment that resists formulations that would call its own operations into question . . . one could be discriminating, i.e., against a racial minority, without being prejudiced. (This latter formulation was a breakthrough, and set the stage for the concept of "institutional racism" (pp. 1784–85).

The task panel noted that research had by then solidly linked contact with mental health facilities with economic depression, and suggested, from this perspective, that institutional racism helped "to account for high rates of Black unemployment," and went on to link "the high rates of unemployment among Black youth, a rising suicide rate among Black youth, a high crime rate among Black youth, and the institutional practices that exclude or subordinate Black youth" (pp. 1785–86).[10]

The Research Task Panel buttressed its appraisal with specific recommendations, focusing on the need for more facilitated access of minority group members to mainstream mental health research funding channels, and enumerated "compelling . . . needs for minority scientists." Among those recommendations made by the task panel were the access to minority populations that would be afforded to minority scientists and the capacity of minority scientists to generate especially relevant questions and hypotheses about the needs of minority populations. But the panel noted that the impact of legislative and regulatory processes on the 1960s promise of predoctoral support for minority researchers had been "to abort the very takeoff of a needed minority research manpower initiative" (p. 1553). The panel chastised the NIMH for having failed to implement a Minority Access to Research Careers (MARC) program of the sort that allowed NIH institutes to identify, in college, and to recruit and support potential minority researcher candidates.

Though the legislative impact of the PCMH was attenuated by President Carter's defeat in 1980, the commission's report served effectively as a "sourcebook" for a range of policy issues and needs. More immediately pertinent to this account, the PCMH critique of and recommendations for NIMH policies in minority mental health research—and, particularly, research training—underscored the need and set the stage for programs that would extend well beyond the life of the CMGMHP.

Focus on Research Training: MARC and MBRS

Shortcomings noted in the mental health research training sphere by the PCMH Research Panel had been perceived several years earlier to affect all quarters of biomedical science, prompting initiation by the NIH, of two minority-focused research training programs: the Minority Access to Research Careers (MARC) and the Minority Biomedical Research Support (MBRS) programs.

The PCMH was not alone in recognizing the need for a more aggressive tack to correct the shortage of minority research training opportunities in mental health. In 1977, the CMGMHP organized an Institute-wide conference on minority research and research training. In this forum, too, the underrepresentation of minority researchers and graduate students was clear, particularly in the biological and neurological sciences. Existing NIMH research training programs in these disciplines reported difficulty in recruiting qualified minority graduate students and recommended that NIMH provide undergraduate, as well as graduate, support for future scientists. Responding to both of these analyses in 1979, NIMH—in concert with its parent agency, ADAMHA—"bought into" the NIH's MBRS program and duplicated its MARC program.

The MBRS was designed to support faculty research projects in colleges and universities with a substantial minority enrollment, and to strengthen institutional research capabilities through providing funds for purchase of equipment and supplies. It also provided salary support for both undergraduate and graduate students. Unlike the MFP or the

MARC program described below, the MBRS was funded with research, not research training money, given its primary purpose of supporting mental health research by faculty in minority institutions; in a majority of cases, these were Historically Black Colleges and Universities.[11]

The program was administered through the NIH Division of Research Resources (DRR) at NIH, with NIMH staff responsible for program development through site visits and sponsorship of symposia and workshops. Applications generated were reviewed by NIH mechanisms—specifically, the General Research Support Review Committee and the DRR Advisory Council—and applications with fundable priority scores were submitted to the NIMH for approval by its advisory council. Grants selected for payment were funded by NIMH through a reimbursable agreement with NIH.[12]

The NIMH-MARC program, first funded in 1980, provided support to honors undergraduate students, in their junior and senior years, to interest them in pursuing graduate training in mental health–related disciplines. Applications were accepted from facilities in which a majority of students were drawn from one or more minority groups. In addition to academic expenses, the program provided curricula and research experience in the junior and senior years, as well as summer study and research assistant opportunities during the junior-year summer. A second focus of the MARC program involved enhancing the research capabilities of faculty at institutions with substantial minority enrollments. Both pre- and postdoctoral faculty who had arranged for their acceptance into a doctoral or postdoctoral program were eligible.

Collectively, the three programs—the older MFP, the MBRS, and the MARC—had an impressive impact on minority access to and benefit from federally funded research training opportunities, one that was felt within the first few years of their operation. The 1985 NIMH analysis found that, outside these three programs, minorities (who then comprised approximately 20 percent of the U.S. population) constituted 7.1 percent of students in mainstream graduate training programs in mental health–related disciplines. With the programs up and running, minority representation at the graduate level increased to 19 percent in these same disciplines, though their presence in the biological sciences continued to be disproportionately low. Not until the early 1990s, with the introduction of the MFP awards (noted above) focused on neuroscience and psychiatry, did this imbalance begin to be redressed.

Mental Health Services for Minorities

We provide only a cursory review, in this chapter, of issues pertaining to mental health services for minorities during the era of the CMGMHP.

The abbreviated treatment of minority mental health services in this chapter does not minimize the importance of the topic; rather, it reflects the fact that research and clinical personnel needs necessarily preceded and served as a foundation for improved services to minorities. Meeting those initial imperatives demanded the bulk of the Center's energies and resources in its early years.

Indeed, a 1977 status report on mental health services for minorities, produced by the NIMH Division of Mental Health Service Programs, focused on services research, noting that a key shortcoming of research on minority-relevant service delivery issues was that the bulk had been conducted primarily in clinical and social services and/or community agencies, and that it needed to be stimulated in hospitals and large municipal facilities, which tended—then, as now—to treat a relatively larger volume of minority people. The "Status Report" called specifically for more research on (1) culture-specific alternatives for diagnosis, treatment, and service delivery; (2) community/social support systems and coping strategies; (3) lack of fit of existing services and minority group needs; and (4) minority group perceptions of mental health and alternative delivery systems.

Had the direct, categorical mental health service delivery responsibilities of the NIMH has not phased out by virtue of the introduction of block grants during the early years of the "Reagan revolution," and had the Center survived, its role in mental health services most likely would have expanded. As it is, principal responsibility for service delivery concerns in the future will fall under the purview of the Center for Mental Health Services. NIMH does maintain a strong services research program, and throughout the early 1990s, special minority group needs were addressed through the mainline research funding sources.[13] Whereas all research projects funded by NIMH are required to include minority populations, several services research grants being funded in the early 1990s focused exclusively on the use of mental health services by minorities and/or the delivery of care to minorities with mental illnesses. Among the categories of this research were:

- Naturalistic Service Use Studies, to determine the mental health service needs and service use patterns of various minority groups. One grantee has found that 26 percent of Native American adolescents meet criteria for at least one current psychiatric disorder and that friends and relatives are the most common sources of care for mental health problems.
- Treatment Trials, including, for example, a clinical trial of a culturally targeted treatment for Spanish-speaking primary care patients with major depression.

- Service System Evaluations to evaluate how well the service system works for minority populations seeking care.
- Service System Experiments, for example, developing and testing the effectiveness of a program for improving recognition and management of depressive disorders in Indian Health Service primary care clinics.

In addition, the NIMH Office of Programs for the Homeless Mentally Ill, with the Division of Applied and Services Research and the NIMH Associate Director for Special Populations, co-sponsored a two-phase Minority Technical Assistance Program in 1991. Phase 1 was a three-day workshop for minority investigators that was designed to familiarize participants with the review process and included a panel discussion on ethnic and cultural dimensions of service delivery to the homeless mentally ill population. Phase 2 consisted of linking each participant with an established researcher as a mentor, a mock review of participants' draft grant applications, and submission of their revised grant applications in 1992. The program was to serve as a model for encouraging and supporting promising young investigators until they receive their first independent support.

But in beginning to describe activities of the 1990s, we have bypassed the "official" closing point.

Changing with the Times: Phaseout of the CMGMHP

On October 1, 1985, during the tenure of NIMH director Shervert Frazier, M.D., the Center for Minority Group Mental Health Programs was dismantled as part of an extensive NIMH reorganization that was implemented to emphasize the new principal and defining mission of NIMH, research. In Frazier's view, several factors contributed to a need for restructuring—progress in research; changing legislative and administrative mandates that were stripping NIMH of authority for any activity but research; and need for clearer lines of responsibility within NIMH. The rapid growth during NIMH's early lifespan, Frazier said, had resulted in considerable overlap of programs by the early 1980s; combined with the shift of service monies to block grants, and continuing uncertainty about NIMH's role in the support of clinical training, "it seemed an appropriate time for a thorough assessment of the NIMH mission and structure" (p. 1265).

The reorganization abolished three longstanding NIMH headquarters divisions and established a new research-oriented structure in their place. Among those abolished were the Division of Prevention and Special Mental Health Programs (DPSMHP), which had housed the CMGMHP since its inception.

The Center, too, was closed down, and to carry on key programs, a new Minority Research Resources Branch was created in the Division of Biometry and Applied Sciences. Functions of the new minority unit were (1) to plan, support, and conduct programs of research, research training, and resource development in the basic, applied, and clinical sciences, including research and development centers; (2) to review and evaluate research developments in the field; (3) to recommend new program developments; (4) to coordinate with the NIMH intramural program; and (5) to coordinate with the Office of Scientific Information to disseminate research knowledge. The core programs of the Minority Research Resources Branch were the research training component of the Minority Fellowships Program (MFP), the Minority Access to Research Careers (MARC) program, and the Minority Biomedical Research Support (MBRS) program, which NIMH continued to participate in through the NIH; and the minority Research and Development Centers program, consisting of the five university-based centers. As Frazier noted in his report to the field,

With these programs continuing to recruit and train minority researchers—thus expanding our capacity for attention to minority mental health issues—we anticipate an acceleration of the trend toward increased support of minority-relevant research in the mainline research divisions. In 1984 [that is, the last year of CMG-MHP operations], NIMH funded 147 grants in which minority groups were studied; of these, 126 were supported by units other than the Center for Studies of Minority Group Mental Health (p. 1266).

Other than a few congressional inquiries to the NIMH to ascertain that the Institute's few minority senior staff members would not be adversely impacted by the reorganization, the demise of the Center did not appear to precipitate an outcry from the minority community. After fifteen years, the Center closed its doors, and the bulk of its programs continued in other settings. The fifteen-year-long experiment ended on Frazier's upbeat note: "The reorganization of NIMH both reflects the directions and strengths of the field, and charts a course for rational scientific policy-making and resource development over the next several years" (p. 1270).

NIMH Minority Mental Health Programs, 1985–1990s

Since the phaseout of the Center itself, its scientific legacy has continued to grow—in some respects, to flourish—and its programmatic identity has continued to evolve. In 1990, in the wake of Jim Ralph's departure from NIMH, another reorganization phased out the five-year-old Minority Research Resources Branch. As part of this restructuring the successor programs to MARC and MBRS were assigned to the office of the NIMH Associate Director for Special Populations. The Minority Fellowship Program and the Minority Research and Development Centers program were mainstreamed into the contemporary configuration of NIMH extramural research divisions, as RO-1 project grants had been five years previously.

In the early 1990s, MARC was reestablished as the NIMH Career Opportunities for Research Education (CORE) program, while retraining the strategic goals of its predecessor. CORE's Honors Undergraduate program provides support during the junior and senior years of college. Grants are made to institutions with substantial minority enrollments to provide high-level research experiences for promising college students working closely with a faculty sponsor. By 1992, some 80 percent of MARC/CORE graduates had completed or were enrolled in graduate programs in mental health or related fields, such as alcohol or drug abuse, en route to research careers. An additional 6 percent had completed degrees in other disciplines.

In 1991, in recognition of the need to tap talented minority students even earlier during their academic careers, NIMH launched a Minority High School Science Education Program, an initiative unique to AD-AMHA at the time of its introduction. Consisting of supplemental awards to active CORE grants, the program encouraged minority students to select career disciplines related to research on mental and addictive disorders by providing them with hands-on experience working on research projects with faculty and CORE trainees over a two-year period. Students are expected to devote sufficient effort to a given research project and related academic activities to gain insight into the process of scientific discovery. At its advent, the High School Science Education program was administered by CORE programs at the State University of New York/College at Old Westbury, Grambling University, and Howard University.

The Minority Fellowship Program continues to support research training for graduate students in the key disciplines of psychiatry, psychology, sociology, nursing, social work, and neuroscience, with grants funded through the national professional associations in the respective disciplines. MFP directors and selection committees at the associations recruit, select, and closely monitor highly qualified graduate students in accredited doctoral programs throughout the country. In addition to stipend support, personal support and networking opportunities are provided.

NIMH's participation in the NIH-administered Minority Biomedical Research Support (MBRS) program was supplanted in 1990 when AD-AMHA instituted its own Minority Institutions Research Development Program (MIRDP). Like CORE, the MIRDP also adheres to its parent program's objectives: to provide grant support to develop and/or expand, in institutions with a substantial minority enrollment, the capacity for conducting mental health research and to enhance the research capability of faculty to conduct neuroscience, behavioral, biological, and social science research in mental health. Undergraduate and graduate minority students benefit directly from participation in research projects as research assistants and are encouraged to pursue careers in mental health research. By 1992, NIMH had funded eight MIRDP grants, five of them at Historically Black Colleges or Universities.

Also in 1990, in a further attempt to encourage minority scientists to pursue research in the mental health field, NIMH announced a new program of supplemental awards available to established principal investigators with active grants who would use the funds to bring a minority student or faculty member onto a given project. In two years, more than a hundred supplements totaling over $4 million were awarded.

More recently still, the Institute has requested additional funding for 1994 and subsequent years to expand a new program designed to enhance the research infrastructure in schools of medicine at prestigious Black universities: Howard University, in Washington, D.C.; Meharry Medical College, Nashville; Charles R. Drew School of Medicine, Los Angeles; and the Morehouse School of Medicine, Atlanta.

Finally, the initial "research flagship" of the CMGMHP—the Minority R&D centers—continues to survive in the increasingly competitive mainstream research support environment. The five Minority R&D centers active in early 1993, and a sampling of their major research thrusts, are listed below.

Research Center on the Psychobiology of Ethnicity. Researchers at Harbor University of Los Angeles Medical Center are investigating the differential effects of variations of drug dosage among minority patients, examining several genetically influenced biological systems and environmental differences, such as diet, that may be implicated in variations of response among racial and ethnic minority group members. Other lines of research address how different groups perceive psychiatric disorders.

National Center for American Indian and Alaskan Native Mental Health Research. Fewer than seventy doctoral-level investigators around the country were actively engaged in mental health research among American Indians and Alaskan Natives in 1992. More than half of these—four, American Indian themselves—were research associates of the Center, located at the University of Colorado Health Sciences Center. The Center, which offers methodological and cultural technical assistance to investigators interested in the mental health needs of this population, emphasizes methodologic innovations for use with these populations. Emphasis also is given to ensuring that the Indian and Native communities receive reciprocal benefits for participating in research. For example, a contract with the Cherokee Nation of Oklahoma supported the development of intake and treatment progress measures for a tribal adolescent substance abuse treatment program and established the Sequoyah High School biennial survey to determine incidence and prevalence of substance abuse among these Indian and Native adolescents. No invitation to collaborate on research with tribes, villages, or other community-based organizations has been rejected in recent years, a reflection of the cooperative nature of the Center's research undertakings.

Research Center for Black Mental Health. Situated at the University of Michigan, the Center is accumulating needed information on African American mental health by examining in detail the functions of social support, and the relationships between mental disorders such as depression and the seeking of both informal and professional help. In 1992, the Center was working with the State of Michigan to test and understand a misdiagnosis hypothesis—that is, that Black patients who have major depression are more likely to be misdiagnosed as having chronic and undifferentiated schizophrenia—and to test the hypothesis that Black clinicians will make fewer errors in diagnosing Black clients than White clinicians because of fewer social and cultural differences.

National Research Center on Asian American Mental Health. A landmark community epidemiologic study of mental disorders among Chinese Americans conducted out of this NIMH-supported R&D center at the University of California at Los Angeles has estimated the prevalence of selected mental disorders among Chinese Americans and is attempting to identify factors associated with mental health problems in this population. The prospective investigation was slated to obtain seventeen hundred completed household interviews with Chinese Americans living in Los Angeles County, and to follow up with the same respondents one year later. The target population for the study includes Chinese immigrants to the United States and U.S.-born residents of Chinese ancestry.

Hispanic Mental Health Research Program. At Fordham University in New York, this center's work focuses on epidemiologic-clinical studies, with five priority areas of research: emergence of problems, use of services, assessment, effective therapies, and rehabilitation. Another goal is to increase the small pool of scholars trained in Hispanic mental health research.

As all of these ambitious programs have advanced, new public health crises ranging from AIDS to violence have emerged and been recognized as having a disproportionate and devastating impact on the minority community. The disproportionate impact of AIDS on minority groups has been evident since early in the epidemic, even as estimates of rates of HIV-infection and the incidence of full-blown AIDS in the population at large have continued to be adjusted. By 1991, for example, the Centers for Disease Control identified AIDS as the leading cause of death for Black women between the ages of 15 to 44 in two states, New York and New Jersey. In New York City, autopsy results in the early 1990s found rates of HIV positivity of 36–38 percent for Black men from 31 to 50 years old. Minority children, too, are overrepresented among pediatric AIDS cases. Black children, who represent 15 percent of the nation's children, make up 53 percent of all childhood cases of AIDS. Hispanic children, who represent 10 percent of the child population, account for approximately 22 percent of pediatric AIDS cases.

NIMH initiated and has expanded a series of activities to increase the number of minority investigators who serve as principal investigators on HIV-related mental health research. Efforts have included individual technical assistance and a mock review meeting to provide feedback from outside experts on applications to be submitted by early career minority scientists. A handbook on how to develop a successful research application aimed at early career investigators, especially ethnic minority scientists, was prepared and disseminated widely. By 1991, NIMH was supporting fourteen minority investigators using a supplementary research mechanism designed to train minorities in research methodology and design. A special focus of research consisted of efforts to test culture-specific prevention approaches in ethnic and racial minority groups that have been disproportionately represented among U.S. AIDS cases.

An even more recent, still evolving thrust regards initiatives taken by the NIMH, along with other components of the Public Health Service and the health care community broadly, to understand and address violence as a health crisis that disproportionately affects the nation's minority communities.

Retrospective Analysis: Impact of the CMGMHP

In 1972, its first full year of operations, the CMGMHP budget totaled $2.5 million; of that amount, $1.1 million was for research grants. By 1977, the CMGMHP budget had tripled to $7.6 million, $4.7 million of which was for research; minority-focused research supported by other components brought the 1977 total to $7.1 million. Minority-relevant research accounted for 4 percent of all research grants in 1972, and nearly 10 percent in 1977. In 1993, some eight years after the formal dismantling of the CMGMHP, total estimated spending for minority-relevant research and research training activities at NIMH was put at $145 million, 24.8 percent of NIMH's $583 million budget in the first year of the Institute's return to the NIH.[14]

Whereas the numbers suggest an impressive rate of growth, we note that although the NIMH's "current dollar" research budget increased from $129 to $583 million over the period from 1970 through 1993, its "constant dollar" budget just held its ground over the same period, moving from $129 to approximately $134 million. The latter calculation offers a better sense of real changes in research purchasing power by applying a standardized research deflator index to a base year—1970, in this instance. Whereas the rate of the minority-relevant research budget is not quite as remarkable as it first appears, the fact remains that in certain categories—most notably, research training—budget growth for minority programs has outstripped the overall NIMH rate of growth.

Viewed in retrospect, the early debates over various facets of the operation of the CMGMHP were remarkably prescient. Certain of the "developmental" issues discussed above (for example, whether or not to define "minority" so as to include women) proved to portend issues yet to emerge in the health care field. Other concerns, including debates over Center policies and procedures that were seen in 1970 as having an impact on the quality of CMGMHP's portfolio similarly highlight dilemmas with which NIMH and the mental health field broadly have had to deal in more recently.

Questions about the need for the federal research establishment to sharpen its focus on the health and mental health needs of women were answered forcefully in 1992 with the decision of then NIH director Dr. Bernadine Healy to launch a $625 million Women's Health Initiative; involving 150,000 women in a study of the causes of disability and death, the program promises to be the largest single clinical study ever undertaken in the United States. One of us (BSB) accurately foresaw, in the late 1960s, the immense voice, power, and needs of women in the health and mental health spheres; yet the power of women's movement then—unlike that of the nation's minorities—was not sufficiently focused to drive a major federal program. If our decision in 1970 not to include women as a "minority group" was strategically correct, our inability to exploit more effectively subsequent opportunities—such as that offered by the congressionally mandated establishment within NIMH in the mid 1970s of a National Center for the Prevention and Control of Rape—was simply that: an inability to focus the underlying concern in a manner that would translate into sustained political support, public credibility, and programmatic growth.

With respect to the question of relationships among minority groups, NIMH's position that organization of the CMGMHP along racial lines would lead to redundancies in "overhead" while muffling the voice of the Center was correct. But the next step—one favored by these authors—was never taken. In a 1975 speech to the Midwest Regional Conference on Hispanic Mental Health, Brown said, "I am convinced that our CMGMHP has been a good thing; a wise investment. The money has been well spent, for example, in the R&D Centers for research and training; but [I am also convinced] that what the minority community needs is its own legal, legislated structure, a National Institute of Minority Concerns. . . . This way, one will have the law of the land; one will have an authorization level; one will have a critical mass of each of the groups" (Brown pers. files).

In 1975, that proposal was not as far-fetched as it might seem in retrospect; within the previous several years, two of NIMH's original centers—those focused on alcoholism and drug abuse—had evolved into full-fledged institutes that, with NIMH, comprised the ADAMHA. In the years since, numerous HHS secretarial initiatives have focused on specific minority health needs, and an Office on Minority Health was established, but none of these has proved to have the recognition factor or programmatic strength of a federal biomedical and behavioral research institute.

Those well-intentioned concerns over the quality of programs that would be established in a new, autonomous Minority Mental Health Center had no clear answer then—or now. As suggested by the inability of the Minority Research and Development Centers to generate a steady stream of competitive mental health project grant applications even ten years into the program, quality was variable. But this unevenness was never a reflection of the quality of the individuals seeking and pursuing careers in the mental health field. It said much more about the pervasive issue of "institutional racism" that the Center was created to combat. The struggle has been arduous. The CMGMHP was five years in existence before the initiative was taken to extend NIMH-funded science education programs into high schools, and thus level the playing field for many minority students before they encountered "make-or-break" situations and decision points during their undergraduate and graduate academic careers.

Concerning the question of the Center's autonomy, it is interesting that by the 1980s, when pressure began to build among mental health—and, particularly, mental illness—constituencies for an organizational return of NIMH to the NIH, an oft-heard protest was that "separate is not equal" under any circumstances, science included; that by being outside the biomedical science mainstream, mental health science—and thus mental health care and reimbursement issues—were inevitably relegated to second-tier status. Yet when the reunion of NIMH research with NIH was achieved in 1992, provisions were fought for and written into the reorganizing legislation to "protect" the mental health institute's initial review groups, or scientific peer review panels, from being merged with standing NIH review groups.

At the root of the opposition to consolidation was an acknowledgment that funding proposals in the yet maturing, often cross-cutting fields that characterize much mental health research may require more liberal or tailored review criteria than are needed in traditional biomedical science where the disciplinary consensual base for research protocols tend to be broader (if not more rigorous) than for multidisciplinary fields of inquiry into complex social and behaviorial phenomena. A direct parallel can be drawn between these challenges to the mental health field in its entirety, and those with which minority scientists, concerned with minority mental health concerns, have been grappling for well over twenty years.

Early debates over an emphasis on professional as opposed to paraprofessional training for minorities clearly identified a critical issue. Whereas programs to train "new mental health workers" responded quickly and, in many cases, effectively to real needs, a more sustained emphasis on professional training such as that made available through the MFP was the wiser choice. In making it, the mental health field avoided, to a great extent, the less than salutary experience of those involved in the substance abuse treatment fields, in which paraprofessional workers with little appreciation of the role of research in either the development or the evaluation of clinical treatments disadvantaaged those fields, as health care policy considerations have become more data-driven.

Conclusion

By the year 2000, Black Americans, Hispanic Americans, Asian Americans, American Indians, and Alaska Natives collectively will comprise almost one-third of our nation's population. Members of racial and ethnic subgroups will share equally, we now know, in the burden of severe mental illnesses such as schizophrenia, manic depressive illness, major depression, or other severe conditions, as these are distributed among the population at large. As the mental health field focuses more directly on conditions such as these, it is reassuring to know that the CMGMHP set a foundation for minority-relevant research, training, and services that are fully capable of independent growth in the future to ensure and enhance the responsiveness of the mental health service delivery system to diverse populations.

Beyond the issue of severe mental disorders, there is a lasting value and importance to research and training activities—whatever the organizational funding source—that address differences in language and cultural meaning as these affect the experience of mental illness and health and that direct our attention to the strengths as well as the needs many minority individuals bring to treatment. Here, too, the Center is proving to have had a most significant impact, which has extended well beyond the brief fifteen years of its existence.

What was lost with the demise of the Center (a loss linked to the overall reorientation of NIMH to its current, more sharply delimited focus on mental disorders) was an extraordinary institutional locus for combating racism in society, and for viewing mental health for all Americans not exclusively through the lens of pathology, but also of hopeful possibility.

NOTES

1. The Mental Health Systems Act (P.L. 96-398), the principal legislation to come out of the Carter administration's President's Commission on Mental Health, established the position of Associate Director for Minority Concerns. This was one of the few provisions of the Systems Act that was not superseded by the Omnibus Budget Reconciliation Act of 1981 (P.L. 97-35), the early centerpiece of the Reagan administration's "new federalism," under which block grants to the states replaced categorical grants, including those for mental health services. In 1984, the Alcohol, Drug Abuse, and Mental Health Amendments (P.L. 98-509) re-created the NIMH position as Associate Director for Special Populations and included women as a priority population.

2. The mental health advocacy movement historically has had substantial impact on the quality of mental health services over the years, particularly services available to the minority community. Throughout the late 1960s and 1970s, patients in public institutions and service systems most frequently were the plaintiffs in class action suits seeking improved standards and quality of care. Minority group individuals with mental illness typically were overrepresented in these facilities, and thus tended to be among the principal beneficiaries—and precipitants—of progressive change.

3. NIMH experienced several brief placements within the U.S. Public Health Service—for example, as an independent agency equal in bureaucratic status to the NIH, and as a component of the short-lived Health Services and Mental Health Administration—before serving, in 1973, as the kernel from which the new Alcohol, Drug Abuse, and Mental Health Administration (ADAMHA) was formed. In ADAMHA, it was joined by the National Institute on Drug Abuse and the National Institute of Alcohol Abuse and Alcoholism, both of which had originated in the late 1960s as NIMH centers.

4. By 1972, political opportunists in the Nixon White House had realized that NIMH's minority program, though discordant with the administration's overall policy thrusts, also represented a means of reaching out to a population that tended to be highly suspect of, if not hostile toward, the White House leadership. Thus, albeit for cynical political reasons, the fledgling program received funding that made feasible initiation of the Minority Research and Development Centers, discussed subsequently.

5. Throughout much of its early history, "research" was defined by NIMH to include

demonstration programs; thus, "facilitating change" was categorized as a valid research activity. In more recent years, and particularly with the transfer of NIMH to the National Institutes of Health, a stricter definition of research increasingly has precluded the support of demonstration projects that straddle the line between pure, controlled research and service demonstration/intervention activities. The latter are under the purview of the Center for Mental Health Services.

6. A leader among his colleagues on Capitol Hill, Senator Daniel Inouye has been both vigilant and effective in his advocacy of Asian American mental health concerns, especially in the context of moving forward minority mental health programs at the NIMH.

7. Soon after the stormy session, the Pacific Asian Coalition (PAC) was chartered, comprising representatives of Chinese, East Indian, Filipino, Guamanian, Hawaiian, Japanese, Korean, Samoan, Thai, and other Asian ethnic groups. It remains a powerful force within the mental health community today, valued as much for its effectiveness in bridging the interests and contributions of discrete, widely dispersed Asian–Pacific Islander groups as for its service as a link to the NIMH and other mainstream mental health organizations.

8. By 1991, the NIMH MFPs in neuroscience graduated a total of nine doctoral students, more than double the minority doctoral output of U.S. neuroscience programs in 1989.

9. The "President's" Commission was really the brainchild and successful product of First Lady Rosalyn Carter. In the year of Hillary Rodham Clinton's hands-on direction of the national health care reform debate (with informed leadership of mental health care–related issues assumed by psychologist and vice-president's wife, Tipper Gore), media pundits as well as those directly involved in mental health policy and programs have pointed to Rosalyn Carter's role in the PCMH as a standard-setter for the involvement of White House spouses in substantive policy formulation processes.

10. This strong statement and its implicit call for more research and whatever possible application of research to U.S. social policies was made by the overall Research Task Panel. Stronger statements—and condemnations of existing practices—were issued by each minority group contributing to the Task Panel on Minority Mental Health, also issued under the imprimatur of the PCMH.

11. Executive Order 12320, signed by President Reagan in September 1981, established the goal of significantly increasing the participation of Historically Black Colleges and Universities in federally sponsored programs. By fiscal year 1983, ADAMHA was expending nearly $2 million in furtherance of this presidential directive.

12. By the mid 1980s, this arrangement came to be viewed as problematic by NIMH. Applications from HBCUs and other institutions often were submitted as a "package" of proposals, out of which discrete projects were peeled off and referred to the appropriate NIH or ADAMHA institute. Because NIMH-funded research projects came out of the larger NIH application, the visibility of NIMH research support was diminished, to the extent that, occasionally, neither students nor faculty knew that they were receiving NIMH funding. The issue was less one of bureaucratic chauvinism, than a concern that, when applying for additional, non-MBRS funds, investigators who had received NIMH-MBRS funds would not be aware of or pursue career opportunities in the mental health field.

13. Services research remains a key element of NIMH's research portfolio; a congressional directive specifies that, beginning in fiscal year 1994, 15 percent of NIMH's research funds be dedicated to services research.

14. A complete 1993 accounting of minority mental health funding that is a direct legacy of the CMGMHP also would include $843,000 for the clinical training portion of the MFP program, now administered by the new Center for Mental Health Services. The CMHS also budgeted $18 million for "minority-related" service demonstration programs in 1993.

REFERENCES

Brown, B. S., and Goldstein, H. 1978. The lightning rod of human service delivery. In *Contro-versy in psychiatry*, ed. J. P. Brady and H. K. H. Brodie, pp. 1041–54. Philadelphia: W. B. Saunders.

Frazier, S. H. 1985. Director's report: the reorganization of NIMH. *Hospital and Community Psychiatry* 36(12):1265–70.

Joint Commission on Mental Health of Children. 1969. *Crisis in child mental health: challenge for the 1970s.* Washington, D.C.: Joint Commission on Mental Health of Children.

Lutterman, K. G., Bivens, L., Griggs, J., Jenkins, J., Lash, L., Mitnick, L., Parron, D., Pawlow-ski, A., Primas, M., Ragland, S., Ralph, R., Roberts, R., Schneider, S., and Smith, J. P. 1986. *Minority mental health: research training and research centers.* Report of the Task Force on Minority Research Training. Rockville, Md.: NIMH (published for administrative circulation to the National Advisory Mental Health Council, September 15).

National Advisory Commission on Civil Disorders (Kerner Commission). *Report to the presi-dent.* 1968. Washington, D.C.: U.S. Government Printing Office.

Ochberg, F. M., and Brown, B. S. 1973. Key issues in developing a national minority mental health program at NIMH. In *Racism and mental health*, ed. C. V. Willie, B. M. Kramer, and B. S. Brown. Pittsburgh: University of Pittsburgh Press.

Pierce, Chester, M. D., 1973. The formation of the Black Psychiatrists of America. In *Racism and mental health*, ed. C. V. Willie, B. M. Kramer, and B. S. Brown. Pittsburgh: University of Pittsburgh Press.

President's Commission on Mental Health. 1978. *Report to the president.* Vol. 4, *Report of the Research Task Panel*, pp. R-126–30, R-265–69. Washington, D.C.: U.S. Government Print-ing Office.

NOTES ON CONTRIBUTORS

ELLEN L. BASSUK is Associate Professor of Psychiatry at Harvard Medical School in Boston, Massachusetts. She is co-founder and president of the Better Homes Fund.

EVALINA W. BESTMAN is Research Associate Professor at the University of Miami School of Medicine and Executive Director of New Horizons Community Mental Health Center in Miami, Florida.

ELAINE R. BROOKS, formerly with the Department of Psychiatry at the University of California at San Diego, is currently working with the Mental Health Association of San Diego County to advocate locally for comprehensive services for mental illness and substance abuse prevention and treatment in national health care reform.

BERTRAM S. BROWN is former director of the National Institute of Mental Health.

ELAINE (HILBERMAN) CARMEN is Professor of Psychiatry at Boston University School of Medicine. Formerly the Medical Director of the Dr. Solomon Carter Fuller Mental Health Center in Boston, Massachusetts, she is now Medical Director of the Brockton Multi-Services Center.

JAMES P. COMER is Maurice Falk Professor of Child Psychiatry and Director of the Yale Child Study Center School Development Program. He is Associate Dean at Yale University School of Medicine, New Haven, Connecticut.

RUBY M. GOURDINE is Director of Field Instruction and Assistant Professor at the Howard University School of Social Work in Washington, D.C.

JEAN A. HAMILTON is Professor of Psychology in Social and Health Sciences and in the Women's Studies Program at Duke University in Durham, North Carolina.

M. KAY JANKOWSKI is a Ph.D. candidate in clinical psychology at the University of Vermont in Burlington and a former research assistant at the Dana-Farber Cancer Institute in Boston, Massachusetts.

BERNARD KRAMER is Professor of Psychology, Emeritus, at the University of Massachusetts at Boston, Massachusetts.

JOYCE A. LADNER is Acting President and Professor of Social Work at Howard University in Washington, D.C.

429

HARRIET P. LEFLEY is Professor of Psychiatry and Behavioral Science at the University of Miami School of Medicine and former Director of Research and Evaluation at New Horizons Community Health Center in Miami, Florida.

K. PATRICK OKURA is President of Okura Mental Health Leadership Foundation, Inc., in Bethesda, Maryland, and former Assistant Director for International Mental Health at the National Institute of Mental Health.

NOLAN E. PENN is Professor of Psychiatry and head of the Social Psychiatry Research Unit at the School of Medicine at the University of California at San Diego, California.

CHESTER PIERCE is Professor of Education and Psychiatry in the Faculty of Medicine, the Graduate School of Education and the Faculty of Public Health at Harvard University in Boston and Cambridge, Massachusetts.

PATRICIA PERRI RIEKER is Associate Professor of Psychiatry (Sociology) at Harvard Medical School and Director of Psychosocial Research, Division of Cancer Epidemiology and Control, at the Dana-Farber Cancer Institute in Boston, Massachusetts.

NANCY FELIPE RUSSO is Professor of Psychology and Women's Studies at Arizona State University, Tempe, Arizona.

JAYMINN SULIR SANFORD is Assistant Professor of Education and coordinator of the Five-Year Teacher Preparation Program in the College of Education at Temple University in Philadelphia, Pennsylvania.

JOHN MARSHALL TOWNSEND is Associate Professor of Anthropology in the Maxwell School at Syracuse University, Syracuse, New York, and Adjunct Associate Professor, College of Medicine, State University of New York Health Science Center, Syracuse.

CASTELLANO B. TURNER is Professor and Director of the Clinical Psychology Program at the University of Massachusetts at Boston, Massachusetts.

CONSTANCE WILLARD WILLIAMS is Associate Professor affiliated with the Family and Children's Policy Center of the Florence Heller Graduate School for Advanced Studies in Social Welfare at Brandeis University in Waltham, Massachusetts.

CHARLES VERT WILLIE is Professor of Education and Urban Studies at the Graduate School of Education at Harvard University in Cambridge, Massachusetts.

MARIA E. ZUNIGA is Professor of Social Work at San Diego State University and a member of the Board of Directors of San Diego County's Chicano Federation. She serves as a state and national consultant in the provision of culturally competent services to underserved populations.

INDEX

abortion, 199
abused women, 380–82; chronic mental illness among, 217–34; homeless, 242
Adams, G. L., 319
addiction medicine, 60
adolescents, 61–62; African-American, 151–69; childbearing by, 199–213; in criminal justice system, 79–80, 83; in gangs, 85–90; homeless, 249–50
Adoption Assistance and Child Welfare Act (1991), 184
adoptions, transracial, 171–95; agency requirements and, 175–77; data on, 177–79; future directions in, 180–93; mental health issues and, 185–87; organizational positions on, 179–84; review of literature on, 174–75; studies of, 187–80
Adult Children of Alcoholics (ACOA), 64, 65
African Americans, 5, 94, 139–40, 358, 397, 411, 419, 423; adolescent, 151–69; adoption into White families of, see adoptions, transracial; on college campuses, 253, 257, 268–71; culturally sensitive treatment for, 359–65; diagnosis of, 9, 21, 134; direct services to, 10, 11; early childbearing among, 201–10, 212; epidemiological data on, 353–56; frustration aggression among, 264–66; gang violence and, 85, 86, 88–90; gender differences in mental disorder in, 374, 375; HIV infection in, 223, 232, 420; among homeless, 6; impact of stereotypes on treatment of, 4, 11, 12; imprisonment of, 6, 72, 78, 93, 104, 105, 107, 108; incidence of mental illness among, 8–9; in institutions, 14–15; in mental health professions, 4, 18, 22, 400, 401, 403, 405, 407,

408; in military, 67; poverty among, 382; as research subjects, 16–17; self-help movement and, 64–67; violence against, 260–61, 263; vocational rehabilitation for, 68; women, 33–36, 45, 217, 239, 244
Aid to Families with Dependent Children (AFDC), 202, 204, 208, 212, 237, 239, 240
AIDS, 217, 218, 222–23, 232–34, 379–80, 382, 419–20. *See also* HIV infection
Alanon, 65
Alaska Natives, 356, 358, 397, 418–19, 423
Alcohol, Drug Abuse, and Mental Health Administration (ADAMHA), 390, 400, 412, 417, 422
Alcoholics Anonymous (AA), 64, 65
Allen, W. R., 253
Altstein, H., 174
American Council on Education, 254
American Medical Association, 220
American Nurses Association, 410
American Psychiatric Association, 136, 137, 230, 401, 410, 411; *Practice Guidelines for the Treatment of Major Depression*, 299; *Women and Depression* task force report, 320–21
American Psychological Association, 20, 261, 410, 411
American Public Welfare Association (APWA), 177
American Sociological Association, 410
amitriptyline, 331
Anderson, Elijah, 206, 207
antidepressants, 298–301, 303–26, 329–31, 334–40
Arizona, University of, 256
Asian-Americans, 94, 358, 397, 402, 406–07, 409, 419, 423; adoption of, 174–75; chronic mental illness among, 217; on